Ayurveda, Nation and Society

New Perspectives in South Asian History

The New Perspectives in South Asian History series publishes monographs and other writings on early modern, modern and contemporary history. The volumes in the series cover new ground across a broad spectrum of subjects such as cultural, environmental, medical, military and political history, and the histories of 'marginalised' groups. It includes fresh perspectives on more familiar fields as well as interdisciplinary and original work from all parts of South Asia. It welcomes historical contributions from sociology, anthropology and cultural studies.

Series Editors

SANJOY BHATTACHARYA *Head of School of History and Professor of Medical and Global Health Histories, University of Leeds, UK.*

NIELS BRIMNES *Associate Professor in History and South Asian Studies, Department of Culture and Society, Aarhus University, Denmark*

NITIN SINHA *Senior Research Fellow, Centre for Modern Oriental Studies (ZMO), Berlin*

Editorial Advisory Committee

Cristiana Bastos *Professor, Institute of Social Sciences, University of Lisbon, Portugal*

Rajib Dasgupta *Professor and Chairperson, Centre of Social Medicine and Community Health, Jawaharlal Nehru University, India*

Gordon Johnson *University of Cambridge, UK*

Amarjit Kaur *Emeritus Professor of Economic History, University of New England, Australia*

Gyanesh Kudaisya *Associate Professor, South Asian Studies Programme, National University of Singapore*

Erez Manela *Professor, Department of History, Harvard University, USA*

Ayurveda, Nation and Society

United Provinces, c. 1890–1950

SAURAV KUMAR RAI

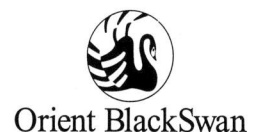

Orient BlackSwan

All rights reserved. No part of this book may be modified, reproduced or utilised in any form, or by any means, electronic or mechanical, including photocopying, recording or by any information storage and retrieval system, in any form of binding or cover other than in which it is published, without permission in writing from the publisher.

AYURVEDA, NATION AND SOCIETY: UNITED PROVINCES, C. 1890–1950

ORIENT BLACKSWAN PRIVATE LIMITED

Registered Office
3-6-752 Himayatnagar, Hyderabad 500 029, Telangana, India
e-mail: centraloffice@orientblackswan.com

Other Offices
Bengaluru, Chennai, Guwahati, Hyderabad, Kolkata,
Mumbai, New Delhi, Noida, Patna

© Orient Blackswan Pvt. Ltd 2024
First Published by Orient Blackswan Pvt. Ltd 2024

Series cover and book design
© Orient Blackswan Pvt. Ltd. 2011

ISBN 978-93-5442-851-7

Typeset in Minion Pro 10/13 by
Jojy Philip, New Delhi 110 015

Printed in India at
Avantika Printers Private Limited, New Delhi 110020

Published by
Orient Blackswan Private Limited
3-6-752 Himayatnagar, Hyderabad 500 029, Telangana, India
e-mail: info@orientblackswan.com

039242

For my mentor and guide
Dr Biswamoy Pati

Contents

List of Tables, Figures and Appendices	ix
Map of the United Provinces	xii
Acknowledgements	xiii
Publishers' Acknowledgements	xvii
Glossary	xix
Preface	xxiii
Introduction	1
1. Ayurveda as 'Indigenous' Medicine: Historical Backdrop and Complexities	23
2. Indian National Congress and the Late Colonial Ayurvedic Movement	59
3. Creating an Ayurvedic Discourse: Print, Organisation and Mobilisation	83
4. Healing the Society: Social Culture of the Late Colonial Ayurvedic Discourse	106
5. Ayurveda in the Market: Economic Underpinnings of the Late Colonial Ayurvedic Movement	149
6. Ayurveda at the Crossroads of Independence: *c.* 1946–50	190

Conclusion 221
Appendices 227
Bibliography 242
Index 257

Tables, Figures and Appendices

TABLES

5.1	Ayurvedic Pharmacies in the Late Nineteenth and Early Twentieth Century India	164
5.2	Popular Ayurvedic Pharmacies of the United Provinces in the First Half of the Twentieth Century	165

FIGURES

1.1	Certificate of *Vaidraj* issued by The Old Indian Medical College (a bogus medical institution)	37
1.2	Registration form for vaids and hakims (under the United Provinces Indian Medicine Act, 1939)	40
1.3	Ayurvedic flag and anthem	45
2.1	Estimated annual expenditure on the basis of proposals received from various District Boards	70
4.1	Effect of Food: Pandit ji (patron) alarmed by the unexpected behaviour of his cook (servant), who after scratching his ring is putting his fingers in the milk he has brought for Pandit ji.	108

4.2	*Stridharma Sikshak*: One of the advertisements at the back of her book by Yashoda Devi.	119
4.3	Then and now: Caricatured comparison between students belonging to *gurukul* and a modern educational institution	128
5.1	Book list at the beginning of an Ayurvedic text; Ganga Granthagar, Lucknow	154
5.2	An illustration of advance booking of forthcoming text by Yashoda Devi.	155
5.3	*Anupam Sahitya*: For common householders and vaids	157
5.4	An advertisement by Yashoda Devi's Devi Pustakalaya, Allahabad	158
5.5	Testing times: An advertisement cautioning people against the substandard Ayurvedic drugs available in the market	163
5.6	Are you ill: An advertisement by Dhanvantari Aushadhalaya, Aligarh, offering free postal assistance to those facing health related problems	167
5.7(a)	An advertisement by Dhanvantari Aushadhalaya (Aligarh) for the sale of agency	168
5.7(b)	Another advertisement by Dhanvantari Aushadhalaya (Aligarh) for the sale of agency	168
5.8	Manhar Tel: An advertisement by Mahashakti Aushadhalaya (Benares) containing testimonials of prominent personalities, including Premchand	173
5.9	An advertisement of Ayurvedic injection by G.A. Mishra Ayurvedic Pharmacy, Jhansi	176
5.10(a)	Some of the advertisements of panacea (*Mahashakti Churna* and *Mahashakti Vati*) by Mahashakti Aushadhalaya, Benares	177

5.10(b) *Makardhwaj Vati*: A panacea made by the Dhanvantari Aushadhalaya, Aligarh — 178

5.11(a) *Mahashakti Modak*: An advertisement of an aphrodisiac — 179

5.11(b) *Kamdīpak Tila*: An advertisement of an aphrodisiac — 180

5.12 Advertisement of *Stri Chikitsak* (a monthly magazine published by Yashoda Devi) — 182

APPENDICES

1. Rules related to the Admission of Patients to the European Civil Hospital, Allahabad (June 1920) — 227

2. Principal Features of Scheme for Establishing Subsidised Dispensaries of 'Indigenous' Medicine in the United Provinces, 1938 — 228

3. District-wise List of 'Genuine' Ayurvedic and Unani Pharmacies Drawn by the Board of Indian Medicine, United Provinces — 230

4. Suggestions Made by Mool Chand Rastogi Trust Aushadhalaya — 233

5. List of Ayurvedic Journals being Published from Different Parts of the United Provinces — 234

6. Syllabus of the Paper on Swasthavratta — 236

7. Lord Dhanvantari — 239

8. Vaid Guru Prasad Tripathi — 240

Map of the United Provinces

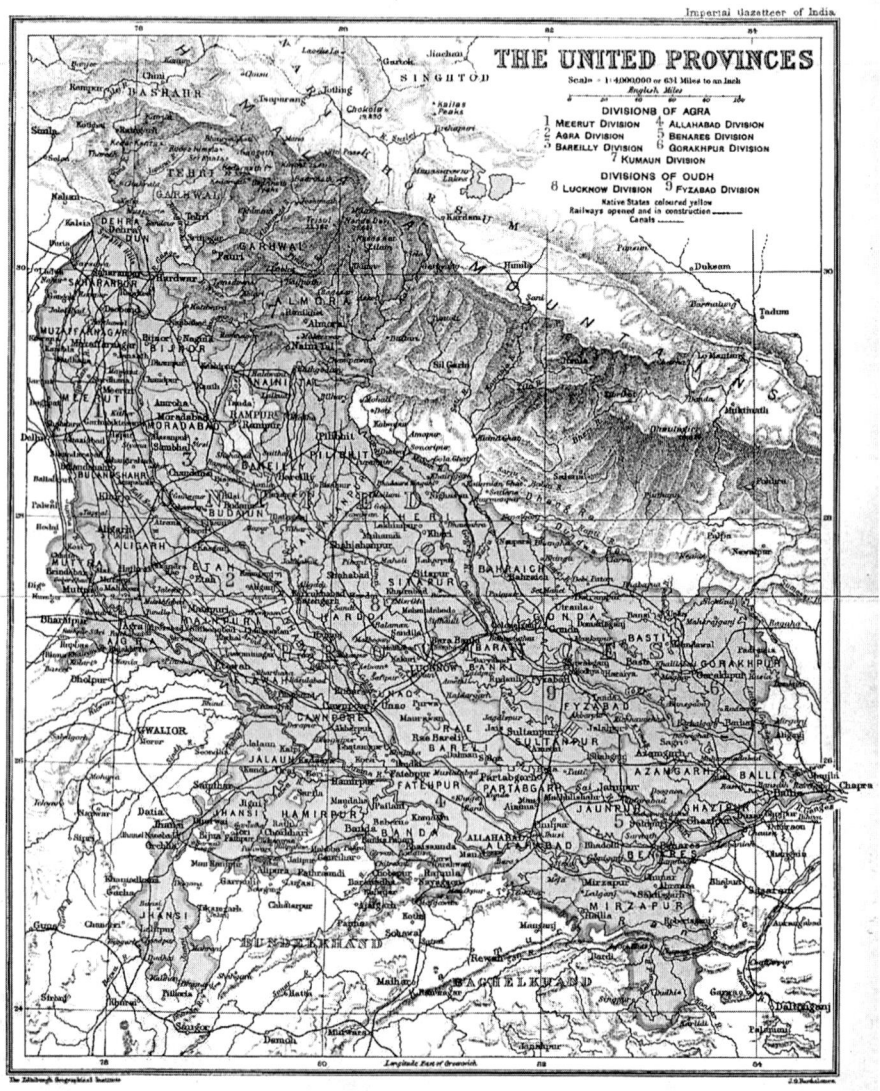

Source: The Imperial Gazetteer of India, Vol. 24, new edition, published under the authority of His Majesty's Secretary of State for India in Council. Oxford: Clarendon Press, 1907–09, opposite p. 250.

Acknowledgements

This monograph grew out of the unwavering support of my mentor and research guide, the late Dr Biswamoy Pati, at each and every stage of my research work. He always responded so promptly and enthusiastically to all my queries and confusion that I was overwhelmed. His faith in me as a research scholar was always a major source of inspiration for me, which kept me moving with my research even in hard times. Above all, his expertise in the social history of health and medicine made things easier for me, naturally. Without his guidance, this work would not have taken its present shape and depth. Unfortunately, he is no more to see this monograph of mine in published form, 'the fruit of my labour', as he would have quirkily called it.

I am also grateful to Dr Pati for inviting Dr Madhuri Sharma to deliver a lecture at one of the weekly seminars at the Department of History, University of Delhi, way back in 2012. Dr Sharma spoke on her then newly published book *Indigenous and Western Medicine in Colonial India* (New Delhi: Foundation Books, 2012) and shared with us her research experiences. This was the first time I seriously started thinking of working on the social history of health and medicine. The correspondence with Dr Sharma which followed afterwards helped me a lot in shaping my research topic. A brief interaction with her at the Nehru Memorial Museum and Library was really useful for me in locating my possible primary sources which were scattered in different repositories of Uttar Pradesh (erstwhile United Provinces). I owe my thanks to her.

I express my heartfelt thanks to Professor Amar Farooqui for suggesting the present title of the book, which exquisitely captures the theme I wish to explore in the following pages. Subsequent interactions with him also helped me a lot in shaping my ideas. I am also grateful to Professor Charu Gupta for giving my vague research topic a focused direction. Her book *Sexuality, Obscenity, Community* (New Delhi: Permanent Black, 2001) and her article on Yashoda Devi were, in a way, mines of information for me regarding the vernacular materials available on this topic. The occasional inputs by Dr Yasser Arafath on my draft are equally significant in sharpening my arguments. I am fortunate to have such teachers at the Department of History, University of Delhi.

I am deeply indebted to Professor S. Irfan Habib for giving me some useful insights related to interaction between Ayurveda and Unani systems of healing in medieval times. Brief interaction with him at the National University of Educational Planning and Administration was productive in many ways. I owe my sincere thanks to Professor Mohan Rao (Centre of Social Medicine and Community Health, Jawaharlal Nehru University), Professor Raj Sekhar Basu (Department of History, Calcutta University) and Professor Sujata Mukherjee (Department of History, Rabindra Bharati University) as well. Their comments on my thesis, the precursor of the present monograph, were really insightful.

I express my deepest sense of gratitude to Vaid Guru Prasad Tripathi of Rae Bareli and Ahsan Husain of Lucknow who spared their time for personal interviews. To me, they were live windows to peep into the world of the early twentieth century when the Ayurvedic revivalist movement was going on. I was really thrilled to interview them.

I owe my sincere thanks to the staff of the Partha Sarthi Gupta Library and Central Reference Library (University of Delhi) for providing many of the secondary sources related to my work. The Nehru Memorial Museum and Library and the All India Ayurvedic Congress Library (both in New Delhi) also provided various kinds of primary and secondary sources concerning my topic. In this regard, I am particularly thankful to Mr Awadhesh Kumar Shrivastava for introducing me to the hitherto unexplored repository located at the campus of the All India Ayurvedic Congress. It proved vital for my research providing a plethora of late colonial Ayurvedic tracts and journals, including various issues of the *Vaidya Sammelan Patrika*.

I am deeply indebted to the staff at the National Archives of India (New Delhi), the Uttar Pradesh State Archives (Lucknow) and the Regional

Archives (Allahabad) for furnishing various archival files which created the skeleton of my present work. I am particularly thankful to Shri Amitabh Pandey and Dr Meera Singh of the Uttar Pradesh State Archives and Ghulam Sarwar and Rakesh Kumar Verma of the Regional Archives (Allahabad) for their cordial support during my visits to these places. Here I would like to especially thank Jaskaran *ji* of the Uttar Pradesh State Archives for his great dedication towards research scholars. He was always there to help me whenever I needed any file.

I also acknowledge the due cooperation of the staff at the Nagari Pracharini Sabha Library, Carmichael Library and Central Library, Banaras Hindu University (Varanasi); and Hindi Sahitya Sammelan Library, Hindustani Academy Library and Bharti Bhawan Library (Allahabad), who gave all possible help in the course of my research work. Particularly the support of Shri S. N. Mishra at Nagari Pracharini Sabha Library, Smt. Sadhana Chaturvedi at Hindi Sahitya Sammelan Library and Shri Gopalji Pandey at Hindustani Academy Library deserves special mention here.

I also take this opportunity to acknowledge my debt to all my teachers who taught me as an undergraduate and postgraduate student at the University of Delhi. I owe my sincere thanks to Professor Shahid Amin, Professor Vinay Lal, Professor Basudev Chatterjee, Professor Anshu Malhotra, Dr Jagdish N. Sinha, Ms Namrata Singh, Ms Rashmi Seth, Ms Gayatri Bhagwat Sahu and Dr Sidheshwar Prasad Shukla for shaping my consciousness and ideas as a history student.

It has been a long and arduous journey. I am fortunate to have numerous supportive friends both within and outside academia without whom I would not have the energy and zeal to pursue this work. I gracefully acknowledge the support of two of my friends, Piyush and Ajay, who proved to be wonderful hosts during my research trips to Varanasi and Allahabad, respectively. Their presence at these two places respectively made my multiple research trips a pleasurable experience. I am also indebted to my office colleagues at the Nehru Memorial Museum and Library and the Gandhi Smriti and Darshan Samiti for their cooperation. I am grateful to Arun for helping me out with the quality of photographs used in this monograph.

I convey my endless thanks to the series editors for considering my manuscript worthy enough to be included in the prestigious

'New Perspectives in South Asian History' series by Orient BlackSwan. It is really enthralling to see my manuscript among the works of seasoned scholars who embellish this series. I owe a debt of gratitude to the anonymous reviewers of this work whose precise comments allowed me to enrich this monograph further. I also extend special thanks to Veenu Luthria and the entire team at Orient BlackSwan for their interest, patience and support throughout the production of this monograph.

Earlier versions of some of the chapters have been published in the journals *Indian Economic and Social History Review* (October–December 2019), *Summerhill: IIAS Review* (Winter 2019), *History and Sociology of South Asia* (January 2016) and the Occasional Paper series of the Nehru Memorial Museum and Library (2020). I thank the editors and publishers of these journals for allowing me to include the revised versions of these articles in this book.

I take this occasion to pay tribute to my mother, the late Mrs Neeta Rai. Without her love and affection I could never even think of coming this far in my academic life. She played a crucial role in this work as well without even realising that ever. I so wish she could hold this book in her hands.

Words are insufficient to express my gratitude to Shikha. I owe a debt to her which is beyond words. Together, we have faced so many ups and downs in a short span of partnership that it becomes unimaginable to many. This book, I am sure, is one of the reasons to celebrate our collective journey through life. The 'arrival' of our daughter Anaya will remain an important personal 'event' for me in the journey of this book. She keeps reminding me that there is a world outside books and office work.

Finally, for any errors of fact, style or argument, which might have crept into this book, the responsibility is entirely mine.

Publishers' Acknowledgements

The publishers would like to thank Sage Publications for their kind permission to reuse the following works by the author in the present volume.

Parts of Chapters 3 and 4 of the present volume have been published earlier as 'Gendering Late Colonial Ayurvedic Discourse: United Provinces, c. 1890-1937'. *History and Sociology of South Asia*, 10, no. 1, 2016; and as 'Invoking "Hindu" Ayurveda: Communalisation of the Late Colonial Ayurvedic Discourse'. *The Indian Economic and Social History Review*, 56, no. 3, 2019.

The publishers would also like to thank the Indian Institute of Advanced Study (IIAS), Shimla for their kind permission to reproduce with revisions the following article by the author.

Parts of Chapters 1 and 4 of the present volume were first published as 'Brahmanizing Ayurveda: Caste and Class Dimensions of Late Colonial Ayurvedic Movement in Upper India'. *Summerhill: IIAS Review,* 25, no. 2, 2019.

Glossary

angrezi dawai	allopathic medicines
antur ghar	a dark unventilated small room/hut, generally built outside the main quarters, for pregnant women; also called *Sutika griha*
*aushadhalaya*s	Ayurvedic dispensaries
bachcha	male child
bachchi	female child
balak	male child
Bhagat	folk healers engaged in the treatment of snakebite
Brahmacharya	celibacy; also the first stage in the *asrama* system (refers to stages of life) of Hinduism
burhi vidhwa	elderly widows practising household remedies
Chamar	an 'untouchable' caste in pre-modern India, which traditionally handled dead animals; officially designated as Scheduled Caste (or Dalit) in independent India
*Chuhrri*s	a downtrodden caste from Punjab
Daad	dermatophytosis or ringworm
dai	midwife
*dawakhana*s	Unani dispensaries
dhai	wet mother
dhiwar	fisherman
dhobi	washerman

garbhavyapta	diseases specific to the uterus
Gṛihastha	householder; also the second stage in the *asrama* system of Hinduism
grihastha shiksha	education related to domestic affairs
groh	group
gurukul	a traditional school in India with students living near their teacher/mentor
Hadis or Doms	an 'untouchable' caste in pre-modern India, which traditionally dealt with sweeping as well as disposal and cremation of dead bodies; officially designated as Scheduled Caste (or Dalit) in independent India
hakim	A Unani practitioner
ilm	knowledge
kahar	water or palanquin bearers
kalima	Muslim sacred utterance
kapha	the watery element
kobiraj	the occupational title of an Ayurveda practitioner in Bengal
kochwan	coachman
ksheer-sagar	celestial ocean, according to a legend, which was churned by the gods and the demons to acquire nectar *(amrit)*
ladka	male child
ladki	female child
mahanth	the chief priest of a temple or the head of a monastery
mali	gardener
mofussil	non-urban districts
mulk	nation
nadi-parikshan	pulse examination
nai	barber
namardi	impotency
nautch girls	dancing girls

niyog	a conjugal practice in which a childless widow may have sexual intercourse with her husband's younger brother in order to beget a child
pir	a Muslim spiritual guide
pitta	the fiery element
prameha	a syndrome described in the Ayurvedic texts that includes clinical conditions involved in obesity, prediabetes, diabetes mellitus, and metabolic syndrome
purdah	veil
qaum	community
samrajya	territory/empire
santan	progeny
santan palan	nurturing of progeny
Sanyasa	renunciation; also the fourth and last stage in the *asrama* system of Hinduism
shishu	infant
shuddh	pure
suchi-patra	detailed catalogue
sutras	verses
swapnadosh	night-fall or wet dreams
swaraj	self-rule
tridosha	the concept of the three humors (watery, fiery and airy)
upnivesh	colony
vaid	an Ayurvedic practitioner
vanaprastha	forest dwelling; also the third stage in the *asrama* system of Hinduism
vata	the airy elements
virya	semen
viryarakshanopayah	ways to preserve semen
Vishuddhata	ultra-purity
vyabhicharini	sexually corrupt
yonivyapta	diseases specific to the genital area

PREFACE

It was in April 2014 that I met Vaid Guru Prasad Tripathi for the first time during one of my sojourns to Lucknow, the present-day capital of the north Indian state of Uttar Pradesh. An hour-long animated interaction with him precipitated and personified the world of 'new' *vaid*s in which I had already been treading for the past few years through archival gateways. Interestingly, Vaid Guru Prasad Tripathi had chosen a temple located in Charbagh area of Lucknow as the site of his temporary clinic. Upon enquiring how his weekly visit to this place started, he replied that the erstwhile *mahanth*[1] of that temple was his brother-in-law. It was upon his request that Vaid Tripathi started coming there in 'broader public interest'. Hailing originally from Raebareli, a small township situated around 80 km south of Lucknow, Vaid Tripathi was well into the tenth decade of his age (that is, a nonagenarian) when I met him. He used to treat the patients primarily at various places in Raebareli for most part of the week and used to come to Lucknow every Thursday in the afternoon where he remained till late in the evening.

Incidentally, Vaid Tripathi had received the degree of 'Ayurveda Acharya' from the Ayurvedic College, Banaras Hindu University, in 1947. Standing at the crossroads of 'colonial' and 'post-colonial', my interaction with him allowed me to grasp the worldview of an Ayurvedic practitioner trained in the first half of the twentieth century and someone who witnessed closely the developments which followed independence. In many ways he remains a living example of many of the conclusions drawn by me in this book from the archival files/vernacular tracts. His perception on 'How old is Ayurveda?';[2] 'What were the reasons behind the decline of Ayurveda by the nineteenth century?';[3] 'What are the differences, if any, between Ayurveda and Unani?';[4] 'What changes pharmaceuticalisation of Ayurvedic drugs have brought in the area of Ayurvedic treatment?'[5] and on various other issues helped me substantially to stride into the world of the late colonial Ayurvedic practitioners. It was a fascinating account of memory and simultaneous articulation of how Ayurveda and related perceptions were shaped through the late colonial medical revivalist movement. In many ways, the persona of Vaid Tripathi remains with me as a symbol of 'new' vaids and their fractured world which the Ayurvedic revivalism produced and was, in turn, curated by during the course of late nineteenth and early twentieth century.

It is interesting to note that against the growing dominance, or more so hegemony, of the Western medicine in colonial India, an entire movement had come up to revive 'indigenous' healing systems including Ayurveda in the late nineteenth and early twentieth century. However, such medical revivalism was not just limited to the issues of health and medicine; rather, proponents and practitioners of 'indigenous' healing systems readily interacted and intervened in the making of a 'nation' and various aspects of the society. Thus, if one closely examines the 'indigenous' medical discourse(s), it exhibits tremendous socio-political content as well as intent. The present work examines this late colonial phenomenon of whittling down Ayurveda into a 'Hindu' healing system along with its inherent caste-, class- and gender-oriented biases by focusing on the complex intersectional agendas that were shaping the practice and politics of Ayurvedic medicine in north India.

Simultaneously, this study contradicts the conventional division between 'Arts' and 'Science' which often blurs the social content of the 'scientific' discourses. The advocates of 'science' mostly portray their discipline as firmly grounded in 'rationality' and 'objectivity'. Consequently, the 'scientific' discourses are believed to be free from 'subjective' social prejudices/biases. However, the present analyses of the late nineteenth and early twentieth century Ayurvedic discourse emanating from the United Provinces (present-day Uttar Pradesh) challenges this conventional outlook towards the 'scientific' discourses. In fact, as argued by the post-structuralist/post-modernist writers, modernist traditions tried to arrange knowledge around certain major binaries such as science vs literature/magic, fact vs fiction, civilisation vs madness, truth vs imagination, new time vs antiquity/dark age, and so on.⁶ In all these binaries, the second term always occupies a substandard or inferior position. Thus, in 'modern' times, 'true' knowledge became synonymous with 'science' and 'science' became synonymous with the 'objective' and 'proven' facts, free of social subjectivity. However, in reality, the 'scientific' discourses could never shed their social content completely. That is why Immanuel Wallerstein, while discussing the prospects of social science in the twenty first century, argues for the epistemological reunification of the so-called 'two cultures',⁷ that of the sciences and the humanities, in order to understand the real texture of the 'scientific' discourses.⁸ This book makes an attempt in this direction in the specific case of the late colonial Ayurvedic discourse to bring out its real texture.

Here it is important to delineate certain things at the very outset. First is regarding the usages of the term 'indigenous' during the course of the present narrative. In the Indian context, one has to be very careful while using this term as it is very hard to differentiate between 'indigenous' and 'foreign' in Indian society. Most of the supposedly 'indigenous' characteristics of Indian society and culture were actually bestowed by the people who were not the original inhabitants of India, including the Aryans. Moreover, colonial India witnessed the efforts both by the colonisers as well as the colonised to settle this issue of Indian 'indigeneity'. However, eventually they ended up making this category more messy, debatable and more contentious than ever. This work nowhere claims to resolve this contentious category; instead, it explores the complexities associated with what is called 'indigenous' with special reference to medicine. That is why quotation marks have often been used while referring to the term 'indigenous'. Even where it is not put in this way, one needs to bear in mind the complexity of this category in the Indian context.

In a similar vein, even 'Western' medicine was never a homogenous entity in terms of its origins and practices. It changed significantly in due course of history, exhibiting regional variations as well. That is why, more recently, scholars have started using the term 'biomedicine' instead of 'Western' medicine to differentiate between modern system of healing and the traditional healing practices throughout the world. However, having acknowledged the diverse roots of the so-called 'Western' medicine, I have preferred using this term in the case of present work largely because the

Ayurvedic practitioners of the period under discussion used this binary opposition of 'indigenous' vs 'Western' to shape their revivalist nationalist discourse. For them, any healing practice pertaining to Europe fell under the broader umbrella of 'Western' medicine irrespective of its extant multiplicity and, hence, was subjected to nationalist resistance.

Second, the term 'Ayurvedic discourse' in this work has been used in its broadest sense. It includes the texts written not only by the full-time Ayurvedic practitioners but also by those who were invoking Ayurveda and other ancient Indian healing texts to derive legitimacy for their ideas. In fact, the early twentieth century United Provinces witnessed a plethora of non-specialist Ayurvedic writings and health tracts for didactic purposes. The present work incorporates these writings as well while analysing the late nineteenth and early twentieth century Ayurvedic discourse. I have also preferred to use the term 'Ayurvedic discourse' instead of 'Ayurvedic discourses' largely because I am focussing only on those Ayurvedic texts which exhibited some socio-political concerns. It is not to deny that there were Ayurvedic texts which exclusively discussed the diseases and their remedies, and nowhere manifested any such socio-political concerns.[9]

Third, there is no denying the fact that there were various regional Ayurvedic discourses, each of which had its own specificities respectively. Nevertheless, this book focuses entirely on the Ayurvedic discourse emerging out of north India, particularly the United Provinces. Thus, it nowhere claims that the kind of socio-political manifestations and predilections exhibited by the Ayurvedic discourse as delineated had any universal applicability. One should not carelessly generalise the findings of the present work in case of various other Ayurvedic discourses emerging out of different regions in the subcontinent.

Lastly, so far as the time period chosen for the purpose of the present analysis is concerned, it roughly falls between 1890 and 1950. This is largely because it was from the 1890s onwards that the proponents/practitioners of 'indigenous' medicine started coming in a big way against the colonial linkages/motives of Western medical science. In fact, the anti-plague movement of the 1890s politicised the entire health discourse. Health issues and the choice of healing system(s) subsequently became an important socio-political issue to be discussed publicly from various platforms. This manifested in the remarkable proliferation of Ayurvedic tracts/journals and organisational activities among the vaids in the early twentieth century. Moreover, the book goes up to *c.* 1950. The basic idea is to look at the fate of the Ayurvedic revivalist movement and the ensuing change and continuity in the attitude towards 'indigenous' medicine in the years immediately following independence. Here the book stops at the *Report and Recommendations of the United Provinces Ayurvedic and Unani Systems Reorganisation Committee* (1949) and the ensuing discussions/decisions over its various recommendations in the official circle which showed the glimpses of the future role of 'indigenous' healing systems in the health administration of the province.

I hope the ever-growing global fascination towards Ayurveda and its 'ancientness' becomes more sensitive towards its late colonial transformations. This study is not at all aimed to strip Ayurveda as a system of healing of its medicinal value, but to look at the history behind its present form and its positioning in various socio-political and economic manoeuvrings of colonial era which gave it a typical texture worth noticing. In essence, this study looks at the wider socio-political and economic history of the late nineteenth and early twentieth century India through the prism of medical revivalism.

NOTES

1. Refers to the chief priest of a temple or the head of a monastery.
2. Replying promptly to this question, he said, 'It is eternal' (Interview by the author with Vaid Guru Prasad Tripathi, Lucknow, India, 17 April 2014).
3. Answering this, Vaid Tripathi began by saying that India lost its independence way back in AD 712 (he was so precise about the year, which is amazing as this was the year when Muhammad Bin Qasim invaded India). However, according to Vaid Tripathi, despite the 'Muslim' rulers promoting Unani, Ayurveda survived. This was largely because, in his perception, there was 'no real difference' between Ayurveda and Unani. For him, it is just the difference of language which makes the two systems appear distinct; otherwise both the systems have similar medical prescriptions and to an extent similar pharmacopoeia as well. Tripathi further argued that it was the establishment of colonial rule in India which inflicted a serious blow to Ayurveda as the English instilled among the Indians a 'sense of inferiority' in every respect, whether language, culture or knowledge system, including Ayurveda (Tripathi, interview).

4. As already mentioned, Vaid Guru Prasad Tripathi perceives 'no real difference' between the two systems of healing except that of language. Interestingly, among the various Ayurvedic medicines which he gave to treat my cough, there was Hamdard's *Joshina* as well. It should be noted that Hamdard India is the pharmaceutical company renowned for producing Unani medicine (Tripathi, interview).
5. Vaid Guru Prasad Tripathi believes that one should take Ayurvedic medicines only after consulting a qualified vaid. He stresses upon the vaid–patient relationship and laments that these days there are very few vaids who give time to create a strong vaid–patient relationship, which is an integral part of Ayurvedic treatment. He believes that in order to gain monetary profit, these pharmacies have done more harm to Ayurveda rather than promoting it (Tripathi, interview).
6. For some exemplary works in this regard, see Michel Foucault, *Madness and Civilisation: A History of Insanity in the Age of Reason* (London: Tavistock, 1961); Michel Foucault, *The Archaeology of Knowledge* (London: Tavistock, 1969); Hayden White, *Metahistory: The Historical Imagination in Nineteenth Century Europe* (Baltimore: Johns Hopkins University Press, 1973); Jean Francois Lyotard, *The Postmodern Condition: A Report on Knowledge*, trans. Geoffrey Bennington and Brian Massumi (Minneapolis: University of Minnesota Press, 1984); Reinhart Koselleck, *The Practice of Conceptual History* (California: Stanford University Press, 2002).
7. This phrase of 'two cultures' was famously coined and expanded by C. P. Snow in his first part of the Rede Lecture in 1959 and earlier in his article published in the *New Statesman* in 1956. According to Snow, the intellectual life of the whole of Western society was split into two polar cultures—the sciences and the humanities—creating dangerous schism between the two. For details, see C. P. Snow, *The Two Cultures and Scientific Revolution* (New York: Cambridge University Press, 1959).
8. Immanuel Wallerstein, 'The Heritage of Sociology: The Promise of Social Sciences', *Current Sociology* 47, no. 1, 1999, 1–37.
9. It should also be noted that I am using the term 'discourse' in its formal dictionary meaning, that is, a long and serious treatment or discussion of a subject/theme in speech or writing. See *Oxford Advanced Learner's Dictionary*, 6th edn (Oxford: Oxford University Press, 2000).

INTRODUCTION

The Indian subcontinent has traditionally been an abode of an extensive range of healing systems and practices, some of which date hundreds of years back in history. However, 'ancientness' of a healing practice nowhere connotes 'changelessness' despite claims of being 'timeless'. This study unravels changes and associated manifestations and politics, particularly during colonial period, of one such proclaimed 'timeless' healing system called Ayurveda. The late nineteenth and early twentieth century witnessed the rise and growth of 'medical nationalism' in India. Consequently, 'Indianisation' was sought after both in the medical profession as well as in the choice of healing system. So far as the Indianisation of medical profession was concerned, the issue of Indianisation of the Indian Medical Service (IMS) figured in every session of the Indian National Congress between 1893 and 1907.[1] Also, there was constant demand to open more superior positions for 'native' medical graduates who were not part of the IMS.[2] These demands for greater Indianisation of the IMS and superior medical profession continued to grow despite tremendous opposition of various European officials of the IMS throughout the early twentieth century.[3]

Besides Indianisation of the medical profession, simultaneous attempts were made to write off Western medicine completely, thereby replacing it with 'indigenous' healing practices. It was in this context that Ayurveda was posed by its practitioners and publicists as the worthiest 'indigenous' system of healing and a 'true' claimant of 'national healing system' of India. This soon precipitated in an Ayurvedic revivalist movement which altered Ayurveda fundamentally, thereby shaping 'modern' form of a so-called 'timeless' healing tradition. Incidentally, the socio-economic context in which this entire politics of Ayurvedic revivalism unfolded bore huge imprints on the final outcome. This study ventures to capture these overlaps and intersectional musings of modern transformation of Ayurveda, politics of a nation and overarching trends of contemporaneous society and economy.

Further, as the study emphasises, resistance against Western medicine was not essentially and exclusively a result of the nationalist or *swadeshi* zeal. Rather, several other factors played crucial role in fuelling the entire politics of medical resistance and revivalism in colonial India. For instance, fear of losing caste, especially in the case of Brahmins, was one of the driving factors behind their resistance against Western medicine. Similarly, religious concerns played an important role behind opposition to vaccination as it was supposed to attract the wrath of Goddess Sitala. Furthermore, in the case of anti-plague movement of the late nineteenth century, patriarchal concerns were at the centre of the entire discourse. Even pecuniary concerns came into play on some occasions. For instance, in Singhabhum area, certain zamindars opposed the free-of-cost vaccination drive to check smallpox largely because earlier they used to take 25 per cent of the fees as cess from private inoculators.[4] In other words, discourse over medicine and choice of healing system was nowhere a singular discourse simply over medicine or the healing system, rather several other discourses around caste, religion, patriarchy, etc., merged with it. This study chronicles these interwoven threads of varied discourses through extensive analysis of Ayurvedic revivalist movement and associated discourse that particularly emanated from the United Provinces.

Here it is interesting to note that healing practices throughout the world underwent significant epistemological and structural transformations with the onset of modernity. In this regard, Michel Foucault in his pioneering work *The Birth of the Clinic* delineates two significant developments in the field of (Western) medicine in the nineteenth century. First was the broader epistemological shift marked by the development of the idea of 'medical gaze'[5] and second was the shift in the utility of medicine marked by 'a spontaneous and deeply rooted convergence between the requirements of political ideology and those of medical technology'.[6] These two developments, according to Foucault, made modern medicine an important tool of governance/power regimes. Historians like David

Arnold have tried to replicate this model in the colonial setting by looking at the relationship between Western medicine and its involvement in colonial expansion/consolidation.[7] What is missing in such analyses is the study of parallel development even in the case of 'indigenous' systems of healing. By the late nineteenth and early twentieth century, 'indigenous' systems of healing like Ayurveda became equally fraught with such socio-political overtones and indulged in pathological classification of the subject population in binary terms.

In other words, likewise Western medicine, the late colonial Ayurvedic and associated health discourse was not an isolated discourse on 'science' and medicine; instead it was simultaneously a socio-political discourse. Tropes of medical revivalism, social issues and political concerns got readily intertwined in it, thereby transcending the set medical boundaries. That is why, the Ayurvedic discourse of the period under discussion was not only about plague, malaria or any other disease; rather, it was also about *purdah*, *brahmacharya*, language, caste, class, community, nation, colonialism, etc. This work unravels these distinctive non-Ayurvedic engagements of the Ayurvedic revivalist discourse.

COMPREHENDING MEDICAL REVIVALISM: TOWARDS SOCIO-POLITICAL HISTORY OF LATE COLONIAL AYURVEDIC DISCOURSE

Three broad schools of historiography can be discerned so far as the efforts to comprehend medical revivalism in India are concerned. The first school views the 'indigenous' response to Western medicine in binary terms of 'resistance' or 'acceptance'.[8] Scholars belonging to this school have basically shown how 'indigenous' medical systems initially lost their ground owing to the greater importance attached to the Western healing practices by the colonial rule. However, they argue that with the emergence of cultural and political nationalism in the late nineteenth and early twentieth century, the traditional healing practices benefitted from the revival of public support for 'indigenous' cultures. According to them, this kind of nationalist support politicised the entire issue of medicine and paved the way for revivalism of 'indigenous' systems of medicine as Western medicine came to be seen as a 'political weapon' at the disposal of the colonialists. Logical though their arguments are, this kind of historiography failed to look at the multiplicity and complexity of nationalist interaction and encounter with Western medicine. Nationalist resistance and revivalism nowhere denied the possibility of 'interaction' and even 'selective adoption' even in the case of 'purists', and it was nowhere merely a question of complete 'resistance' or complete 'acceptance' of Western system of medicine.

For the first time, it was Charles Leslie who, way back in the 1970s, in his various articles talked about this 'interaction' and 'selective adoption' or, to use his own words, 'the ambiguities of medical revivalism in India'.[9] Leslie drew very clear distinction between 'classical' Ayurvedic and Unani medical practices and 'traditional–cultural' system of Ayurveda and Unani that came into vogue in the late nineteenth and early twentieth century.

After Leslie, over the next three decades, historiography remained silent on the issue of nationalist discourse on medicine and efforts towards the revival of 'indigenous' systems of medicine. Although the 1990s witnessed a tremendous rise in the writings on medical history in India, they basically concentrated on the progress of Western medicine in India and the manner in which it came to establish its hegemony over 'indigenous' systems of medicine.[10] In other words, they largely focused on 'imperialism of medicine'.

Nonetheless, the first decade of the twenty-first century witnessed the flood of writings which clearly brought forth the complexity of nationalist medical revivalism. Significant among them are the works of Seema Alavi, Neshat Quaiser, Claudia Liebeskind (all of whom have concentrated on Unani Tibb, mainly in the United Provinces), and Kavita Sivaramakrishnan, Uma Ganesan, Madhuri Sharma and Projit Bihari Mukharji (who have basically dealt with Ayurveda).[11] They have shown how the colonial context led to the evolution of 'new' vaids and *hakims* who differed remarkably from the hakims and vaids of earlier centuries. In fact, in their revivalist zeal, these 'new' vaids and hakims fundamentally reshaped and redefined 'indigenous' systems of healing in order to compete with the Western system of medicine by incorporating novel traits such as standardisation, professionalisation and institutionalisation. Such refashioning of 'indigenous' systems of healing like Ayurveda as a 'codified', 'literate' 'classical' tradition, separated it from miscellaneous assorted, vernacular traditions of healing practices it was indebted to so far.[12]

Neshat Quaiser, in this regard, goes on to identify four different categories of the Unani practitioners in terms of their response to Western medicine—modernists, purists, synthesists and reformists.[13] In a similar vein, Projit Bihari Mukharji in his recent work goes beyond the institutional changes that were crucial in shaping of 'modern' Ayurveda. He looks at the therapeutic changes within Ayurveda as initiated by modern technologies which brought it closer to the global medical episteme. Here Mukharji particularly focuses on the day-to-day, mundane, small technologies, the introduction of which fundamentally altered the approach of an Ayurvedic practitioner (*kobiraj* in the context of Bengal) towards his patient and the pertaining disease. Pocket watches to check the pulse, thermometers to check the temperature, stethoscopes to hear the patient breath, microscopes through which germs and blood cells could be seen, injections of endocrinal extracts to rejuvenate the patients and even glass phials (rather than carpet bags full of crushed herbs) in which medicines were stored are some of the mundane small technologies which Mukharji has taken up to show the therapeutic changes in Ayurveda in the late nineteenth and early twentieth century. According to Mukharji, these everyday small technologies were 'motors' or 'catalysts' of therapeutic change in modern Ayurveda through their constant presence. Thus, he emphatically argues that strings of broadly Ayurvedic and broadly 'Western' scientific knowledge were pulled together and 'braided' around the technological objects in the late nineteenth and early twentieth century, thereby leading to the emergence of 'modern' Ayurveda which was considerably different from its predecessor.[14]

Now, the third kind of historiography, which is still underdeveloped and glimpses of which can be found in the writings of Biswamoy Pati, Charu Gupta, Kavita Sivaramakrishnan, Rachel Berger, Madhuri Sharma and David Hardiman, transgresses the defined boundaries of medicine in order to write the broader social history of health and medicine.[15] They have shown how the reshaping and redefining of 'indigenous' systems of medicine was not the result only of medical resistance or revivalism; rather several other driving forces were involved in it. They have viewed the medical ideas and clinical interaction in a broader socio-historical context. In their writings, discourse over medicine was not an isolated discourse, rather it merged with several other discourses over caste, class, community, religion, gender, etc.

The present work combines the second and third school of historiography on medical revivalism in order to write about the socio-political concerns of Ayurveda and the associated health discourse emanating from the United Provinces. This work particularly aims at enriching the third school of historiography, that is, the social history of health and medicine by looking at the caste-, class-, community- and gender-oriented reflections of the late nineteenth and early twentieth century Ayurvedic discourse. An analysis of the Ayurvedic print and drug market to look at the commercialisation of the health discourse and healing practices is also an important area of concern of the present study.

Actually, if we carefully examine most of the erstwhile historiography on medical revivalism, we can clearly see that they have either looked at the entire efforts to revive 'indigenous' healing systems as a unilinear political project to counter colonial hegemony or they have looked at it strictly from the medical point of view and tried to hint at the novelties which the 'indigenous' healing practices came to acquire in their course of revival. My effort is to illuminate the social dimensions of medical revivalism in India. I explore how the Ayurvedic discourse of the time got intertwined with facets of caste, class, gender and community-based notions and ambitions. Furthermore, while examining the political dimensions of medical revivalism, the idea is to complicate it by going beyond the unilinear interpretation of medical revivalism as mere reflection of anti-colonial nationalist struggle. In many ways, the present work (especially Chapter 6) complicates the prevalent binary categories of colonialism and nationalism; or colonialism and post-colonialism. The late nineteenth and early twentieth century India had been witnessing many other political processes and not merely anti-colonial nationalism; whether it was the politics of caste, community, gender, and so forth—all of which had equal bearing on the Ayurvedic revivalist movement.

HISTORICISING THE 'ETERNAL' HEALING SYSTEM: AYURVEDA, MYTH AND REALITY

Before moving ahead, let us take a slight detour and briefly discuss the origin myth of Ayurveda as it constituted a significant part of the late colonial Ayurvedic discourse. Simultaneously, it helps in understanding the source of many of the exaggerated claims and arguments made by the proponents of Ayurveda during the late nineteenth and early twentieth century, which in many ways linger on till today.

Juxtaposition of essential and useful knowledge with prevailing belief system and religious faiths was an integral part of pre-modern knowledge system. The Indian subcontinent was not an exception to this phenomenon. One can find healing practices integrally linked with religious myths and magical charms and spells in the ancient Indian healing system(s). Exemplary to this is the origin myth of 'Ayurveda'—the 'Sanskritic' healing system. Ayurveda is believed to be one of the *Upaveda*s or the auxiliary Vedas traditionally associated with the *Atharvaveda*. It is noticeable that the earliest recorded mention of medicines in the Indian subcontinent is to be found in the *Atharvaveda* itself.[16] However, no trace of 'Ayurveda' as a canonical text can be found by the same name even in its mutilated form. The earliest traceable Indian treatises carrying Ayurvedic concepts are *Charaka* and *Sushruta Samhita*s. While *Charaka Samhita* deals with medicinal remedies, *Sushruta Samhita* primarily expounds surgical treatments.

The Myth

Delineating the origin of Ayurveda, *Charaka Samhita* states that '[W]hen diseases appeared as impediments to penances, fasts, study, continence, vows and life of the embodied creatures, then the great sages of righteous deeds, having compassion for all living beings before them, assembled together on the auspicious side of Himavat [the Himalayas].'[17] Considering freedom from diseases as the 'excellent root of religion, wealth, pleasure and salvation'[18] these Vedic sages commissioned sage Bharadvaja to invoke Lord Indra, the chief deity, to receive the sacred 'Ayurveda' or the 'Science of Life'. According to *Charaka Samhita*, Indra had acquired this sacred knowledge of healing through the Ashvins (the heavenly healers) who, in turn, had received it from Prajapati, who was the son of Lord Brahma—the creator of universe and the originator of the entire Vedic knowledge including Ayurveda.[19] Nevertheless, as described by *Charaka Samhita*, having learnt it in its entirety, sage Bharadvaja acquired through Ayurveda unlimited disease-free life and passed on this 'Science of Life' to other great sages as well.[20] Afterwards, sage Atreya Punarvasu, who was part of the great assemblage of sages and had received the auspicious Science of Life from Bharadvaja, out of his compassion for all creatures, passed it to his six disciples—Agnivesha, Bhela, Jatukarna, Parashara, Harita and Kharapani.[21] Invested with the responsibility of spreading the Science of Life for the well-being of all creatures, each of these six disciples of sage Punarvasu compiled their own treatises (with Agnivesha being the first one) containing the sacred knowledge of healing.[22] Although there was no difference in teaching, and the great sages valued all of them equally, the health treatise of sage Agnivesha gained popularity in due course of time. After some time, Agnivesha's treatise was edited and corrected by Charaka and bears his name as *Charaka Samhita*, the earliest traceable canonical text on Ayurveda.

Alternatively, *Sushruta Samhita*, the text dealing with surgical healing, offers a slightly different story regarding the origin of Ayurveda. *Sushruta Samhita* states that it was through Lord Dhanvantari that the Science of Life or Ayurveda was passed on to human beings. According to the prevailing legends, Lord Dhanvantari first appeared as a consequence of the mythical churning of the celestial ocean *ksheer-sagar* and warded off death, disease and decay from the deities by offering them nectar of life.[23] Afterwards, Lord Dhanvantari appeared on the earth as Divodasa, the king of Kashi (present day Varanasi). According to *Sushruta Samhita*, moved by human suffering, the assemblage of great sages (which included Aupdhenava, Vaitarna, Aurabhra, Paushkalavat, Karvirya, Gopur Rakshit, Sushruta, etc.) approached Divodasa to seek the divine Science of Life.[24] Divodasa agreed with them and delivered Ayurveda which was subsequently recorded by Sushruta word-by-word.

Although presenting two different versions of the origin of Ayurveda, what is common in both the stories is the 'divine origin' of Ayurveda. Keeping in mind that ancient societies throughout the world often resorted to admixture of belief systems, religious faiths and useful knowledge, the theory of the divine origin of Ayurveda does not appear strange. The problem arises when the contemporary Ayurvedic practitioners keep following the same line of argument blindly. Interestingly, most of the Ayurvedic practitioners of India even in the twenty-first century believe in the theory of the divine origin of Ayurveda.[25] This sort of 'perpetual hallucination'[26] in which knowledge gets stuck with belief system is a significant hurdle in the scientific appraisal of Ayurveda.

It is interesting to note that faced with the challenge of growing influence of Western medicine in India, the Ayurvedic practitioners of the late nineteenth and early twentieth century strived hard to claim 'scientific status' for the Ayurvedic healing system. This was largely because one of the major charges levelled against 'indigenous' systems of healing by the colonial officials was that such healing systems were grossly 'unscientific' and often dwindled to the extent of quackery. That is why in their revivalist quest, the 'new' vaids of the late nineteenth and early twentieth century dramatically reshaped and redefined the Ayurvedic system of healing to incorporate the traits on the basis of which Western medicine was claiming its superiority (such as scientificity, standardisation, professionalisation and institutionalisation).[27]

At the same time, there was no dearth of the Ayurvedic practitioners who flagged the 'divine origin' of Ayurveda and tried to confer this particular healing system with a sacred aura. An interesting example in this regard was the celebration of 'Dhanvantari Divas' which was promoted in particular by the leaders of the All India Vaidya Sammelan in order to forge a corporate social identity amongst the Ayurvedic practitioners. Dhanvantari, who was now deemed as the incarnation of Lord Vishnu, emerged as 'a common professional deity'. Consequently, as argued by Kavita Sivaramakrishnan, by the 1930s, 'even smaller towns and cities in North India reported the celebration of Dhanvantari festivities, all commonly timed and with an effort at similar forms of worship'.[28] Further, as discussed by Madhuri Sharma, the All India Vaidya Sammelan effectively assimilated the modern ideas of democracy, liberty and parliamentarianism with the worship of Dhanvantari. The following statement of Pandit Jagannath Shukla at the seventeenth session of the All India Vaidya Sammelan exemplifies the aforesaid attempt:

> We want to see our Vaidya Sammelan so strong and well organised that it becomes the government of vaidyas...god Dhanvantari as our king and Ayurveda world our state, acceptance of authenticity and credibility of Ayurveda over other medical systems as our investment, Vaidya Sammelan as our parliament and provincial sammelan as our provincial government.[29]

Thus, one can see the contrasting efforts by the late nineteenth and early twentieth century Ayurvedic practitioners to simultaneously deify as well as rationalise the Ayurvedic system of healing—a trend which continues till this date.[30]

The Reality

As is the case with many other ancient Indian texts, to assign any definite time frame for Ayurveda is a difficult task. The situation gets more complicated in the absence of any such text by the same name, howsoever mutilated. Nevertheless, if we take Ayurveda as one of the Upavedas or auxiliary Veda of *Atharvaveda*, then in no case can the history of Ayurveda be stretched beyond 1000 BC; as historians by and large agree that *Atharvaveda* is a constituent of the later Vedic corpus, that is, texts belonging to the time frame c. 1000–600 BC.[31]

Similar difficulties pertain even in the case of *Charaka Samhita* and *Sushruta Samhita*—the earliest available texts on Ayurvedic healing. The life and times of Charaka and Sushruta are not known with certainty. According to one assumption, Charaka lived before Panini, the grammarian, who in turn is said to have lived in the fifth century BC.[32] This sort of opinion is based on the fact that Panini mentions the name of Charaka in some of the *sutras* (verses) written by him. However, it is not clear from these sutras whether Panini is using the term Charaka as the name of an individual or to denote the followers of a branch of Vedas as there are scholars who believe that the term Charaka basically refers to a group of mendicant healers and not to any individual. According to them, a branch of *Atharvaveda* named *Vaidyacharana* is related to medicine and Charaka may be a group of physicians who had faith in it and 'who roamed from place to place offering medical services to the people'.[33]

Some other scholars have identified Charaka of *Charaka Samhita* with Patanjali.[34] Again, this postulation is based on the myth that both Patanjali and Charaka were viewed as the incarnations of Sesha (the divine serpent), and hence the amalgamation of the two identities takes place. Moreover, confusion prevails even on Patanjali. One cannot say with certainty that the name Patanjali, which comes in connection with three things—commentary on *Charaka Samhita*, a grammarian, and propounder of *Yoga Sutra*—is associated with the same person in all the three cases.

At the same time, the French Orientalist Sylvan Levi identified Charaka with the court physician of the Kushana ruler Kanishka who reigned in the second century AD.[35] Levi reached this conclusion on the basis of finding the name Charaka in the Chinese translation of the Buddhist *Tripitaka*. Incidentally, Jawaharlal Nehru in his magnum opus *The Discovery of India* also forwarded the same opinion by considering Charaka as the 'royal court physician of Kanishka'.[36] However, there are doubts on the Kushana linkages of Charaka. First, there is no way to ascertain that Charaka mentioned in the Buddhist texts is the same Charaka of *Charaka Samhita*, as the Buddhist texts nowhere refer to his work. Second, if Charaka was the court physician of Kanishka, *Charaka Samhita* must have borne the name of the ruler upon whose patronage Charaka was dependent. However, *Charaka Samhita* does not offer any such clue. Lastly, and strangely enough, despite the fact that Buddhist influence dominated Kanishka's court, *Charaka Samhita* does not give any such impression of Buddhism.

Similar doubts prevail regarding the life and times of Sushruta as well. One may consider Sushruta as living sometime around the sixth century BC as the *Shatpatha Brahmana* (a text belonging to the same period) carries an enumeration of bones which shows an amazing similarity with the account in *Sushruta Samhita*. However, an alternative view is that Sushruta lived after Charaka and it is nothing but mere speculation to trace him in the sixth century BC.

Interestingly, the Chronology Committee[37] of the National Institute of Sciences of India in a general meeting held on 6 November 1950 adopted the following chronology for the ancient Indian texts:[38]

Age of *Rigveda*:	2000–1500 BC
Age of *Samhitas* and *Brahmanas*:	1500–800 BC
Age of old *Upanishads*:	900–500 BC
Dharmasutras:	600–200 BC
Subha Sutras:	500 BC and later

Mahabharata, Manusmriti and *Ramayana*:	200 BC–AD 200
Charaka:	AD 100
Charaka Samhita:	Kernel of AD 100, but enlarged in later time
Sushruta Samhita:	AD 200–500

While making the above recommendations, the Committee observed:

> The Committee felt that it is very difficult to ascertain the dates of Indian literary works of the Pre-Christian Era. But after discussing the different views, the Committee recommend that the Chronological Table given in Appendix 1 [re-produced here] may be taken as working hypothesis for this Symposium. The list is based on the *History of Indian Literature* by Winternitz except, where otherwise stated.[39]

Subsequently, *The Gazetteer of India* also dated *Charaka Samhita* back to the first century AD and *Sushruta Samhita* to the fourth century AD. *The Gazetteer of India* further stated that 'the period of rational medicine starts about 800 BC and from that time until about AD 1000 is the golden age of Indian medicine'.[40]

Surprisingly, on the issue of the origin of Ayurveda, the mid–twentieth century political leaders and government institutions/publications (mentioned earlier) appear more scientific as compared to that of the twenty-first century India. The AYUSH Department, which came into existence in November 2003,[41] under the auspices of the Ministry of Health and Family Welfare, interestingly offered the following answer in response to the question, 'What is the origin of Ayurveda?'

> Ayurveda, the ancient most health care system *originated with the origin of universe. With the inception of human life on earth Ayurveda started being applied*. The antique Vedic texts have scattered references of Ayurvedic remedies and allied aspects of medicine and health. *Atharva Veda* mainly deals with extensive Ayurvedic information. That is why Ayurveda is said to be the offshoot of *Atharva Veda*.[42]

Here, tracing the origin of Ayurveda with the origin of universe and the inception of human life on earth is completely nonsensical and unscientific. The fact that such kind of an opinion is being promulgated by a government ministry is more disappointing.

In fact, moving beyond the debate surrounding the life and times of Charaka and Sushruta, it is worth discussing that 'Ayurveda' to what extent is 'Vedic'. In this regard, Debiprasad Chattopadhyaya for the first time brought out strong conceptual and epistemological differences between Vedic notions and Ayurvedic medicine. According to Chattopadhyaya, much of traditional Indian medicine reaches us 'in the form of a strange amalgam of science and its opposite—or, to be more specific, of natural science and regimented religion'.[43] For example, as delineated by Chattopadhyaya, *Charaka Samhita*, while arguing in favour of consumption of beef and alcohol, also expresses great religious reverence for the cow and considers alcoholism as a morbid condition. Explaining this contradiction, Chattopadhyaya argues that since pragmatic medical necessities often required use of tabooed materials, Ayurvedic remedies often came in the garb of religiosity 'to evade the censorship of the lawmakers who insist on abject surrender to the fundamentals of regimented religion'.[44] However, despite these intrinsic contradictions, Chattopadhyaya nowhere considers Ayurveda as outside the fold of Vedic canon. He simply argues in favour of critically approaching the existing medical corpus and unravelling the 'real medical core of Ayurveda'.[45] In fact, in the writing of Chattopadhyaya, the Ayurvedic practitioners appear as 'undercover' scientific rational beings fighting against the hegemonic irrational and un-scientific 'counter-ideology'.

Moving a step ahead, Kenneth G. Zysk delineates the non-brahmanical Buddhist origin of Ayurveda.[46] According to Zysk, although Ayurvedic literature uses Vedic imagery and mythology to evoke a sense of continuity with the past and to draw legitimacy in a society dominated by brahmanical norms, the roots of Ayurveda are firmly grounded in the medical knowledge of wandering ascetics, most probably of Buddhist monks. Zysk corroborates this by his fascinating comparisons between the medical 'case histories' as delineated in the *Tripitaka*s and the diagnoses and therapies described in the Ayurvedic texts. By doing so, Zysk fills an important lacuna of the Sanskrit medical texts, that is, absence of 'case studies'. Even Galen, the Roman physician to whom the Western and Arabic systems of medicine owe their origin, while propounding his medical ideas talks about individuals suffering from various diseases and his involvement with them. However, Sanskrit texts keep propounding medical notions and therapies in abstract without bringing individual case studies and experiences onto the scene, which seems impractical from the viewpoint of a pragmatic healing system. However, Zysk has shown that Ayurvedic theories were heavily based on case studies and subsequently followed the course of action in each case as delineated in the Pali texts.

Furthermore, historians have expressed opinions that *Atharvaveda*, one of the four Vedas and with which Ayurveda is traditionally associated, itself contains such charms and spells which seem to throw light on the beliefs and practices of the non-Aryans.[47] In that case, Ayurveda also appears to be a 'non-Aryan knowledge system' incorporated, developed and brahmanised by the Vedic Aryans at a later stage. While in this case one can push the origin of Ayurveda even beyond the Vedic age, to the Indus Valley Civilisation, any attempt to do so essentially disconnects Ayurveda from its Aryan/Vedic heritage and argues strongly in favour of Ayurveda being a 'stolen system' from the *adivasi*s (tribes) of the country whose contributions were never duly acknowledged by any of the (brahmanical) Ayurvedic texts.[48]

In light of the aforementioned debates, one can plausibly argue that Ayurveda is a system of healing carrying within its fold multiple influences. These influences are often so strong that to locate 'the core of Ayurveda' and its 'origin point' is extremely difficult. It is a system of healing which developed over centuries and incorporated the medical knowledge of various groups, castes, class and communities that was brahmanised, ritualised and sanskritised in due course of time to maintain the power equations of the hierarchical society. In fact, unlike the communalisation of healing practices, which took place in the late nineteenth and early twentieth century (especially in the 1920s and the 1930s), that ripped apart Ayurveda and Unani along communal lines, there is evidence which attests to the healthy interaction between the two systems of healing in the medieval age. Hakim Bahwa Khan, who was in the court of Sikandar Lodhi (1489–1517), while writing a treatise of Unani medicine, advised hakims to learn from Ayurveda because of changed milieu,[49] without any perceived threat of losing identity. In a similar vein, Hakim Yusuf Bin Muhammad, a physician during Babur's reign, composed medical treatises integrating the Ayurvedic and Unani systems of medicine. He brought together relevant material, pertaining to hygiene, diagnosis and treatment of diseases, from both the systems of healing, highlighting their significant aspects.[50] In other words, the perceived threats related to the identity of a particular healing system started appearing primarily in the late colonial period with the politicisation of knowledge systems and healing.

CHAPTERISATION

Chapter 1 begins with a discussion on the historical backdrop against which the issue of 'indigenous' medicine gained prominence along with the complexities of responses invoked by it. At the same time, the first chapter also looks at the cynical tendencies active amongst the claimants of 'indigenous' medicine, and how these tendencies created internal fissures, not just between the vaids and the hakims but also within their own groups. Simultaneously, this chapter also explores themes like 'nationalising Ayurveda' and response of the colonial government towards the medical revivalist movement. In short, in order to prepare the background for the subsequent discussion, this chapter establishes the fact that the late colonial revival/reconstruction of Ayurveda as 'indigenous' and 'national' medicine was not merely a medical phenomenon but a gross socio-political process as well.

Chapter 2 explores the official nationalist response by the Indian National Congress and its leaders to 'indigenous' medicine. Here the opinions of three nationalist leaders who were associated with the Indian National Congress—Hakim Ajmal Khan, Mahatma Gandhi and Govind Ballabh Pant—have been discussed in detail. While Hakim Ajmal Khan was himself a practitioner-cum-activist of 'indigenous' medicine, Mahatma Gandhi and Govind Ballabh Pant were key political figures both at the national and regional levels, holding tremendous influence, who often talked about the issue of 'indigenous' medicine, particularly Ayurveda. Simultaneously, this chapter also explores the nitty-gritty of various decisions taken by the provincial ministry of the United Provinces, headed by the Indian National Congress that came into power in 1937, which favoured the practitioners and pharmacies related to 'indigenous' medicine over Western system of healing. The chapter shows how populist decisions on this front brought forth further challenges, often deepening the internal fissures among the practitioners of 'indigenous' medicine.

The third chapter delineates the emergence and consolidation of the Ayurvedic discourse and movement in the public sphere in the specific context of the late colonial United Provinces. In this regard, this chapter particularly focuses on three crucial factors—print, organisation and mobilisation—as the key to the creation of the upper-caste/-class Ayurvedic discourse. Here, the publication of several Ayurvedic journals and tracts, establishment of the All India Vaidya Sammelan and the United Provinces Vaidya Sammelan, institutionalisation of *Dhanvantari Mahotsava*, etc., have been discussed in detail in order to grasp the pursuit of creating an Ayurvedic discourse and movement having universalising tendencies. It has been shown that through print, organisation and mobilisation, attempts were made to 'standardise', 'institutionalise' and 'sanitise' the entire Ayurvedic discourse to make it appear as a monolithic discourse.

Chapter 4, based on the extensive reading of the late nineteenth and early twentieth century Ayurvedic tracts and journals emanating out of the United Provinces, looks at the caste, class, community and gender-oriented concerns of Ayurveda and the associated health discourse. As argued earlier, the late nineteenth and early twentieth century health discourse was not just about healing of the 'body'; rather it aimed for broader social goals. Incidentally, the kind of social culture which the late colonial Ayurvedic discourse manifested was highly casteist, communal, and gender- and class-biased. In order to catch these social reflections of the late nineteenth and early twentieth century Ayurvedic discourse, in this chapter, I have particularly focussed on two specific issues—brahmacharya and midwifery—which appeared repeatedly in the Ayurvedic discourse during the period under consideration.

The fifth chapter explores how the market and its dynamics played a significant role in shaping the late colonial Ayurvedic movement, the related discourse and its social content. The unique feature of this chapter is the discussion on the Ayurvedic print market which has been a neglected area of research. This chapter also highlights the salient features of the Ayurvedic drug market with special focus on the advertisements for Ayurvedic drugs, which provides rich insights to understand how the visual culture and print media were tapped by the Ayurvedic practitioners and pharmaceutical companies to carve out a niche for themselves in the medical market.

The last chapter captures the fate and place of Ayurveda at the crossroads of independence with particular reference to the United Provinces. Here, I have examined in detail three landmark reports: *Report of the Health Survey and Development Committee*, 1946; *Report of the Committee on Indigenous Systems of Medicine*, 1948; and *Report and Recommendations of the United Provinces Ayurvedic and Unani Systems Reorganisation Committee*, 1949. Simultaneously, this chapter critically explores various other steps/deliberations/decisions taken by the government of the United Provinces for the promotion of 'indigenous' medicine/Ayurveda in the years immediately following independence.

Finally, the Conclusion summarises the main themes examined in this monograph.

NOTES

1. It should be noted that although the doors of the Indian Medical Service (IMS) were thrown open to Indians since the introduction of competitive examinations for recruitment (that is, from January 1855 onwards), by 1905 only 5 per cent of the IMS men were of Indian origin. For details, see Roger Jeffery, 'Recognising India's Doctors: The Institutionalisation of Medical Dependency, 1918–39', *Modern Asian Studies* 13, no. 2, 1979, 310.
2. The 'native' graduates from various Indian medical colleges used to be employed as sub-assistant surgeons (SASs) who worked under constant supervision of the IMS officials. Their desire for independent charge, even of minor civil surgeoncies, was regarded as too ambitious.
3. For details on this theme, see Saurav Kumar Rai, 'Indianisation of the Indian Medical Service, c. 1890s–1930s', *Proceedings of the Indian History Congress*, 75th session, New Delhi, 2014, 826–32.
4. Biswamoy Pati, *Situating Social History: Orissa (1800-1997)* (New Delhi: Orient Longman, 2001), 20.
5. 'Medical gaze' basically implies medical separation of a patient's body from the patient's person through conversation, observation and physio-chemical examinations by the medical practitioners. In other words, 'medical gaze' leads to biological reductionism of a human body by negating supra-natural identities related to soul and mind. It allows the medical practitioners to classify diseases (and, more so, human beings) based on bodily symptoms.

6. Michel Foucault, *The Birth of the Clinic: An Archaeology of Medical Perception* (New York: Pantheon Books, 1973), 38–39.
7. David Arnold, *Colonising the Body: State Medicine and Epidemic Disease in Nineteenth-Century India* (Berkeley: University of California Press, 1993).
8. See R. C. Majumdar, 'Medicine', in *A Concise History of Science in India*, eds D. M. Bose, S. N. Sen and B. V. Subbarayappa (New Delhi: Indian National Science Academy, 1971), 213–68; Poonam Bala, 'Medical Revivalism and the National Movement in British India', *Ancient Science of Life* 10, no. 1, 1990, 1–5.
9. Charles Leslie, 'The Professionalising Ideology of Medical Revivalism', in *Modernisation of Occupational Cultures in South Asia*, ed. Milton Singer (Durham: Duke University Press, 1973), 691–708; Charles Leslie, 'The Modernisation of Asian Medical Systems', in *Rethinking Modernisation: Anthropological Perspectives*, eds John Poggie and R. Lynch (Westport: Greenwood Press, 1974), 377–94; Charles Leslie, 'The Ambiguities of Medical Revivalism in Modern India', in *Asian Medical Systems: A Comparative Study*, ed. Charles Leslie (Berkeley: University of California Press, 1976), 356–67.
10. Some exemplary works in this regard are: Poonam Bala, *Imperialism and Medicine in Bengal: A Socio-Historical Perspective* (New Delhi: Sage Publications, 1991); Arnold, *Colonising the Body*; Mark Harrison, *Public Health in British India: Anglo-Indian Preventive Medicine, 1859–1914* (Cambridge: Cambridge University Press, 1994); Anil Kumar, *Medicine and the Raj: British Medical Policy, 1835–1911* (New Delhi: Sage Publications, 1998).
11. Seema Alavi, 'Unani Medicine in the Nineteenth Century Public Sphere: Urdu Texts and the Oudh Akhbar', *Indian Economic and Social History Review* 42, no. 1, 2005, 101–29; Neshat Quaiser, 'Politics, Culture and Colonialism: Unani's Debate with Doctory', in *Health, Medicine and Empire: Perspectives on Colonial India*, eds Biswamoy Pati and Mark Harrison (New Delhi: Orient Longman, 2001), 317–55; Claudia Liebeskind, 'Arguing Science: Unani Tibb, Hakims and Biomedicine in India, 1900–50', in *Plural Medicine, Tradition and Modernity, 1800–2000*, ed. Waltraud Ernst (London: Routledge, 2002), 58–75; Kavita Sivaramakrishnan, *Old Potions, New Bottles: Recasting Indigenous Medicine in Colonial Punjab, 1850–1945* (New Delhi: Orient Longman, 2006); Uma Ganesan, 'Medicine and Modernity: The Ayurvedic Revival Movement in India, 1885–1947', *Studies on Asia* 4, 2001, 108–31; Madhuri Sharma, *Indigenous and Western Medicine in Colonial India* (Delhi: Foundation Books, 2012); Projit Bihari Mukharji, *Doctoring Traditions: Ayurveda, Small Technologies and Braided Sciences* (Chicago: University of Chicago Press, 2016).

12. For an interesting insight on this phenomenon of codification and standardisation of Ayurveda in modern India and its impact on popular local practitioners (such as nattuvaidyas) and their ways of knowing with specific reference to Kerala, see K. P. Girija, *Mapping the History of Ayurveda: Culture, Hegemony and the Rhetoric of Diversity* (London and New York: Routledge, 2022).
13. Quaiser, 'Politics, Culture and Colonialism', 320–21.
14. Mukharji, *Doctoring Traditions*.
15. See Biswamoy Pati, 'Siting the Body: Perspectives on Health and Medicine in Colonial Orissa', *Social Scientist* 26, nos 11–12, 1998, 3–26; sections on brahmacharya, midwifery, child-care, women's health and indigenous practices, plague and women's honour, etc., in Charu Gupta, *Sexuality, Obscenity, Community: Women, Muslims, and the Hindu Public in Colonial India* (Delhi: Permanent Black, 2001); Biswamoy Pati and Mark Harrison, eds, *The Social History of Health and Medicine in Colonial India* (London and New York: Routledge, 2009); Sivaramakrishnan, *Old Potions, New Bottles*; Rachel Berger, *Ayurveda Made Modern: Political Histories of Indigenous Medicine in North India, 1900–1955* (Hampshire: Palgrave MacMillan, 2013); Sharma, *Indigenous and Western Medicine*; David Hardiman, 'Indian Medical Indigeneity: From Nationalist Assertion to the Global Market', *Social History* 34, no. 3, 2009, 263–83.
16. R. S. Sharma, *India's Ancient Past* (Delhi: Oxford University Press, 2005), 313.
17. Atridevji Gupt, tr., *Charaka Samhita* (Benares: Bhargava Pustakalaya, 1948), Sutra Sthana, Chapter 1, Verses 6–7.

    ('*Vighnabhoota yada rogah pradurbhootah sharirinam;*
    Tapovasadhyayan brahmacharya vratayusham.
    Tada bhooteshvanukrosham puraskritya maharshayah;
    Sametah punyakarmanah parshve Himvatah shubhe.')

    (Author's translation. All translations that appear throughout this book are the author's translations from the original, unless mentioned otherwise.)
18. Gupt, *Charaka Samhita*, Sutra Sthana, Chapter 1, Verse 15.

    ('*Dharma Artha Kaama Mokshanam aarogyam moolmuttamam.*')
19. Gupt, *Charaka Samhita*, Sutra Sthana, Chapter 1, Verses 4–5.

    ('*Brahmanah hi yatha proktamayurvedam Prajapatih;*
    Jagrah nikhilena Davishvanau tu punastatah.
    Ashvibhyam bhagvanchhakrah pratipede ha kevalam
    Rishiprokto Bharadvajastsmachh kramupagamat.')

20. Gupt, *Charaka Samhita*, Sutra Sthana, Chapter 1, Verses 25–27.
21. Ibid., Sutra Sthana, Chapter 1, Verses 30–31.
22. Ibid., Sutra Sthana, Chapter 1, Verses 32–33.
23. Hari Prasad Shastri, tr., *The Ramayana of Valmiki* (London: Shanti Sadan, 1952), 1: Chapter 41, Verses 18, 19 and 21; Pratap Chandra Roy, tr. *The Mahabharata* (Calcutta: Bharata Press, 1884), 'Adiparva', Chapter 18, Verses 38, 39 and 53.
24. Kaviraj Kunjalal Bhishagratna, tr., *Sushruta Samhita* (Calcutta: Self-published by the author-cum-translator, 1907), Sutra Sthana, Chapter 1, Verses 1–6.
25. This was very well reflected at the Eighth International Congress on Traditional Asian Medicine (ICTAM) held at Sancheong, South Korea (9–13 September 2013) which was attended by the author personally. At this conference, Ayurvedic practitioners from different parts of the Indian subcontinent either kept arguing in favour of the divine origin of Ayurveda or pushed the history of Ayurveda ahistorically, without any concrete evidence, 5,000 years back to the Neolithic age in India.
26. At the ICTAM, when one of the Ayurvedic practitioners from the Kayachikitsa Department, Banaras Hindu University, received some historical insights on Ayurveda from a group of historians from Delhi University (which comprised of late Dr Biswamoy Pati and three of his doctoral students, including myself) and was made aware of the ahistoricity of the theory of divine origin of Ayurveda and the myth of 5,000-years-old history, he came up with a reaction that he had been living in a 'hallucination' till that date. Still, there were many others, including those working with the AYUSH Department (the organisation set up by the Government of India under the Ministry of Health and Family Welfare for the promotion of the non-allopathic healing systems such as Ayurveda, Yoga, Unani, Siddha and Homeopathy), who preferred to live in the 'perpetual hallucination' and were adamant to counter each and every historical fact in a grossly ahistorical manner.
27. For details on this theme, see Leslie, 'The Professionalising Ideology of Medical Revivalism'; Leslie, 'The Modernisation of Asian Medical Systems'; Leslie, 'The Ambiguities of Medical Revivalism'; Paul Brass, 'The Politics of Ayurvedic Education: A Case Study of Revivalism and Modernisation in India', in *Education and Politics in India: Studies in Organisation, Society, and Policy*, eds Susanne Hoeber Rudolph and Lloyd I. Rudolph (Delhi: Oxford University Press, 1972), 342–74; Sivaramakrishnan, *Old Potions, New Bottles*; Sharma, *Indigenous and Western Medicine*.
28. Sivaramakrishnan, *Old Potions, New Bottles*, 117.
29. Quoted in Sharma, *Indigenous and Western Medicine*, 80.

80. Incidentally, this representation of Ayurvedic knowledge as 'divine' and 'a heavenly gift' to humanity was consolidated by the upcoming Ayurvedic pharmaceutical companies of the time as well through advertisements and pamphlets largely to reap pecuniary benefits. For a discussion on such sacralisation of Ayurveda at the hands of pharmaceutical companies, see Maarten Bode, *Taking Traditional Knowledge to the Market: The Modern Image of the Ayurvedic and Unani Industry, 1980–2000* (Hyderabad: Orient Longman, 2008), 176–85.
81. See D. N. Jha, *Early India: A Concise History* (New Delhi: Manohar Publishers, 2004), 45; Sharma, *India's Ancient Past*, 117.
82. Sharma, *India's Ancient Past*, 21; Jha, *Early India*, 65.
83. Paliwal Murlidhar and Byadgi P. S., 'Charaka—The Great Legendary and Visionary of Ayurveda', *International Journal of Research in Ayurveda and Pharmacy* 2, no. 4, 2011, 1012, available at http://www.ijrap.net/admin/php/uploads/541_pdf.pdf (accessed on 9 July 2019).
84. Historians generally assign second century BC as time frame for the life and times of Patanjali and his grammatical work (Jha, *Early India*, 104).
85. Cited in P. V. Sharma, *History of Medicine in India: From Antiquity to 1000 A.D.* (New Delhi: Indian National Science Academy, 1992), 181.
86. Jawaharlal Nehru, *The Discovery of India* (New Delhi: Penguin Books, 2004), 116.
87. Following were the members of the Chronology Committee: Professor R. C. Majumdar (chairman); Dr A. N. Singh, Dr S. L. Hora, Dr P. C. Bagchi, Dr A. S. Altekar, Dr D. S. Kothari (members); Dr N. P. Chakravarti and Dr G. P. Majumdar (present by special invitation). The meeting was held on 6 November 1950 in the library room of the physics department of the University of Delhi. See B. L. Raina, *Health Science in Ancient India* (New Delhi: Commonwealth Publishers, 1990), xiii–xiv.
88. List re-produced in Raina, *Health Science in Ancient India*, xiii–xiv.
89. Quoted in Raina, *Health Science in Ancient India*, footnote no. 5, xiii.
40. *The Gazetteer of India: History and Culture*, Vol. 2, 6th edn (New Delhi: Publications Division, 2003), 208.
41. The Department of Indian Systems of Medicine and Homeopathy (ISM&H), which was created in March 1995, was renamed as the Department of Ayurveda, Yoga and Naturopathy, Unani, Siddha and Homoeopathy (AYUSH) in November 2003. Later on, in November 2014, it was raised to the status of a full-fledged ministry, thus renaming it once again as the Ministry of AYUSH.
42. See the official website of AYUSH, section on 'About the Systems'> 'Ayurveda'> 'FAQ'> 'What is the Origin of Ayurveda', available at http://ayush.gov.in/

About-The-Systems/Ayurveda/faq/what-origin-ayurveda (accessed on 9 July 2019); emphasis added.
43. Debiprasad Chattopadhyaya, 'Case for a Critical Analysis of the *Charaka Samhita*', in *Studies in the History of Science in India*, ed. Debiprasad Chattopadhyaya (New Delhi: Editorial Enterprises, 1982), 1: 209.
44. Chattopadhyaya, 'Case for a Critical Analysis of the *Charaka Samhita*', 209.
45. Ibid., 232.
46. Kenneth G. Zysk, *Ascetism and Healing in Ancient India: Medicine in the Buddhist Monastery* (New York and Oxford: Oxford University Press, 1991).
47. Sharma, *India's Ancient Past*, 116.
48. While recently scholars like Poonam Bala have started arguing the case of the pre-Vedic origins of Indian medical tradition (by tracing it from the Indus Valley Civilisation), unfortunately, the idea of non-Vedic origin/content of Ayurveda has still not been emphasised. Conversely, Poonam Bala, even while tracing many therapeutic drugs and ideas to the Harappan culture, goes on to superimpose Vedic identity on the findings of the Indus Valley Civilisation. For instance, in her opinion, the seal of Pasupati (the famous seal found from Mohenjodaro site of the Indus Valley Civilisation) suggests the existence of Rudra (a prominent deity of later Vedic period) as the 'divine physician'. Thus, even the pre-Vedic/non-Vedic medical findings have been interpreted within the broader (Ayur)Vedic paraphernalia. See Poonam Bala, *Medicine and Medical Policies in India: Social and Historical Perspectives* (Lanham: Lexington Books, 2007), 12.
49. In fact, Hakim Bahwa Khan attempted to synthesise the two systems of healing—Unani and Ayurveda—into one, way back in the fifteenth century, which resulted in his text *Madan-us-shifa-i-Sikander Shahi*. According to Hakim Bahwa Khan, the classical Unani system of healing had developed and put into use in the Arabic milieu, having a different climate and availability of drugs as compared to India. Hence, he suggested putting the Unani system into the Indian milieu in order to make it suitable for this land. For this, he directed hakims to look at the Ayurvedic treatises and learn about the locally available drugs and related treatments. To quote Bahwa Khan, 'Unani medicine was not the best suited system for the people of India where the climate and vegetation were different from those prevailing in Greece and Arabia, and that there is need to have a book prepared in Persian that should contain the best of the Ayurvedic system and its drugs' (cited in O. P. Jaggi, *Medicine in Medieval India* [Delhi: Atma Ram, 1977], 114).
50. Poonam Bala, 'State and Indigenous Medicine in Nineteenth and Twentieth Century Bengal: 1800–1947' (PhD diss., Department of Sociology, University of Edinburgh, 1987), 52–53.

1

Ayurveda as 'Indigenous' Medicine

Historical Backdrop and Complexities

Guided by the nationalist feeling and anti-colonial sentiments, the newly emerging reformist elite of the late nineteenth and early twentieth century India tried 'to fashion a "modern" national culture that is nevertheless not western'.[1] In this regard, the idea of 'indigeneity' acquired tremendous significance in the ongoing public discourse of the time. The reformist elite developed a natural attraction for anything and everything representing India's 'indigenous' culture/system/tradition. However, the category of 'indigenous' was quite complex in the Indian context. In a pluralistic society like India, it was/is very hard to determine which cultural artefact, system or tradition truly represented India's 'indigenous' culture or system or tradition. This situation often led to what one may regard as 'cynicalisation' of the claims to 'indigenous' culture, system or tradition where groups or communities or castes or class with certain vested interests of their own, through a combination of organisation, publicity and politics tried to establish their notions as being worthiest for the claim of 'indigenous', often at the cost of 'other' such competing notions. The issue of 'indigenous' medicine in India was not devoid of such cynical tendencies.

The present chapter begins by exploring the historical backdrop in which the category of 'indigenous' medicine, especially Ayurveda, gained significance in the contemporaneous reformist/revivalist discourse. Subsequently, it delineates the construction of Ayurveda as 'indigenous' self and the complexities of the nationalist, both reformist and/or revivalist, quest to fight back the influence of the 'Western' healing system. It illustrates the typical Indian context in which this idea of 'indigenous' medicine, besides being very complex, was also bound to get trapped into the cynical tendencies of the contemporaneous socio-political environment, which resulted in communal, caste, class and gender-based polarisation of healing practices. In other words, the entire discourse over medicine was complex not only at the level of conflict between 'indigenous' and the 'Western' systems of medicine; rather it also pitted one group of 'indigenous' practitioners against another—a tendency which got sharpened in the early years of the twentieth century. This conflict was not just between the 'Hindu' vaid and the 'Muslim' hakim, but also between vaids and hakims who were divided within their 'own groups' respectively.

THE HISTORICAL BACKDROP

Colonialism and medicine always shared an inextricable link. Maintenance of health in distant/unknown lands was one of the major concerns of the early colonisers. That is why the early naval fleet from Europe had a surgeon on it who was not only responsible for looking after the health of those on the ships during exploratory tours, but was also the first one to report about the flora, fauna and resources of these distant lands.[2] However, with the gradual expansion of colonial rule, medicine and medical practitioners assumed a new role in the consolidation of the empire, so much so that according to some scholars, Western medicine in India became synonymous with 'colonial medicine'.[3] In other words, medicine and the related issues in the nineteenth and twentieth century India cannot be studied by overlooking the colonial context.

Medicine became handy in satisfying both the short-term as well as the long-term needs of colonial rule. The short-term needs included proper maintenance of the health of the European officials in the relatively 'hostile' tropical climate of India. In the initial phase of colonial expansion, these short-term needs were, in fact, the primary focus of colonial health policy. It was important from the military and strategic point of view to safeguard Europeans from falling prey to tropical diseases. In fact, until the end of colonial rule, theoretically, the primary function of the IMS was to ensure the health and hygiene of military troops. The IMS officials used to hold civil posts in districts only when the army did not need them, that is, in times of peace. They were bound to revert to their military duty in times of need. In other words, civil posts for the IMS officials were merely a way to house surplus military medical officers in times of peace.[4]

Nonetheless, medicine was significant for the colonial government not just medically but also culturally in satisfying its long-term needs. It is this cultural dimension of medicine and its complexity in creating colonial hegemony which has attracted the attention of recent historians working on the social history of health and medicine.[5] It has been suggested that medicine was 'acting both as a cultural agency in itself, and as an agency of western expansion'.[6] In such works, Western medicine has been characterised as 'the scientific step child of colonial domination and control'.[7]

In the long term, Western medicine not only undermined 'indigenous' healing practices of India but also thoroughly colonised the 'Indian land' and the 'body'. In colonial medical notions, tropics in general and the 'Indian land' in particular appeared as a storehouse of disease and epidemics. In fact, the colonial division of space was officially justified on the grounds of unhealthy practices of the 'natives' and their unhygienic surroundings. David Arnold, in his pioneering work on plague, has described the ways in which colonial medical authorities strived 'to form and give a seemingly scientific precision to abiding impressions of India as a land of dirt and disease, of lethargy and superstition, of backwardness and barbarity...and to contrast this Orientalised India with the cool headed rationality and science, the purposeful dynamism, and the paternalistic humanitarianism of the West'.[8] However, evidence shows that none of the diseases which the colonial sanitary authorities and Western medical notions attributed specifically with the 'Indian land' was unknown to the Europeans. Conversely, recent studies have revealed that colonial rule and its policies were in many ways responsible for the frequent outbreak of epidemics in colonial India.

As, for example, plague turned into epidemics often because of official negligence. Malaria was very much associated with the colonial migration of labourers and their concentration in unhygienic colonies near mines and factories and in the British plantations. Furthermore, European soldiers were the potent disseminators of venereal diseases, such as syphilis, which was often perceived as *firangi rog* (that is, disease of the foreigners).⁹ It is interesting to note that it was in the colonial period that we begin to hear of frequent outbreaks of epidemics. The effective means of communication which ensured colonial expansion and consolidation often raised the localised diseases to the status of epidemics. In fact, this connection between colonial expansion and spread of disease was not exclusive to colonial India. It was a worldwide phenomenon; for instance, smallpox and measles were brought to Mexico and Peru by Spanish conquistadors in the early sixteenth century.¹⁰ That is why a medical historian goes on to characterise colonialism as 'literally a health hazard'.¹¹

Besides colonising the 'Indian land', the colonial health policy tended to colonise the 'Indian body' as well. This became particularly evident in the case of anti-plague measures adopted by the colonial regime towards the end of the nineteenth century.¹² As one scholar remarks, the anti-plague campaign 'was directed more against the natives than the plague bacillus'.¹³ The Epidemic Diseases Act, which was passed in February 1897 in the wake of the outbreak of plague, gave draconian powers to the colonial government. It empowered the authorities to detain the plague suspects, destroy or demolish infected property and dwellings, prohibit fairs and pilgrimages, and examine the passengers at will. In the United Provinces the authorities came up with a unique arrangement of punching a hole of 4/10ths of an inch in the long side of the tickets of plague suspects at railway stations in the Allahabad and Pratabgarh districts.¹⁴ It was like branding a plague victim and raised so much furore that the secretary to the Government of the North Western Provinces and Oudh (erstwhile name of the United Provinces until 1902) had to seek permission for its discontinuation within a week of its introduction.

Particularly emotive was the issue of the 'check-up' of Indian women at railway stations and public places. It was soon translated by the Hindu and the Muslim elites alike as colonial interference in the 'private sphere' and an attempt to 'dishonour' Indian women. In fact, the Plague Riot of Kanpur in April 1900 was fuelled largely by the rhetoric around the issue of women's 'honour'.¹⁵ This rhetoric brought together various sections of Hindu society to 'safeguard' the 'honour' of Indian women. As Charu Gupta puts it, 'interference with women's bodies was effectively used to give an emotive appeal to anger against plague orders, linked as it was to honour, *purdah*, domestic privacy, public examination, and forcible removal to segregation camps and hospitals'.[16]

The aforesaid issue of the 'check-up' of an Indian woman at public places, including hospitals, especially by a male attendant/surgeon continued to be a volatile issue till very late. As late as in 1943, Premvati Mishra,[17] a freedom fighter from the United Provinces, refused to get herself checked by a male surgeon. She categorically wrote to the then district magistrate of Agra that whether she is sent to a safe place or to the jail, but she would not allow in any case to get herself 'checked' by a male surgeon and would lock herself inside the room if force was used.[18]

In fact, such non-medicinal usages of medical theories/discourse in order to colonise the 'Indian land' and the 'body' were in tandem with the broader shift in the history of medicine from being essentially 'clinical' to 'social'. In one of his lectures delivered at the Institute of Social Medicine (Biomedical Centre, State University of Rio de Janeiro, Brazil) in October 1974, Michel Foucault delineated this broader shift in the history of medicine in the case of eighteenth and nineteenth century Europe.[19] According to Foucault, since the eighteenth century, medicine had continually involved itself in what was 'not its business', that is, in matters other than patients and diseases. This, according to Foucault, was marked by four major shifts as follows:[20]

- Appearance of a medical authority, which was not restricted to the authority of knowledge, or of the erudite person who knew how to refer to the 'right authors'. Medical authority was by and large a social authority that could make decisions concerning a town, a district, an institution or a regulation. It was the manifestation of what the Germans called *Staatsmedizin*—medicine of the State.
- Appearance of a medical field of intervention distinct from diseases: air, water, construction, terrains, sewerage, etc. In the eighteenth century all this became the object of medicine.
- Introduction of a site of collective medicalisation: namely, the hospital. Before the eighteenth century, the hospital was not an institution of medicalisation but of aid to the poor awaiting death.
- Introduction of mechanisms of medical administration: recording of data, collection and comparison of statistics, etc.

Thus, as viewed by Foucault, medicine during this period became a 'social practice instead of an individual one' and was endowed with 'an authoritarian power with normalising functions that went beyond the existence of diseases and the wishes of the patient'.[21] This broader shift in Europe allowed the use of medicine/medical discourse in colonial expansion and consolidation as well. Colonial medical authorities were integrally associated with colonialism which was manifested, in the case of colonial India, primarily through the rank and file of the IMS. The cadre of the IMS in their respective capacities as civil surgeons of districts, professors and resident surgeons at the medical colleges, sanitary commissioners and deputy sanitary commissioners of a province performed the socio-political task of Foucauldian 'medical authority' and engaged throughout in consolidating colonial rule.[22]

The racial discrimination in providing health facilities was also a triggering factor behind medical revivalist/reformist movement. The colonial government was interested in promoting Western medicine only as a 'tool' of colonial expansion, as shown earlier, and was never keen to expand the 'practical utilities' of Western medicine in India. That is why the colonial government remained dispassionate when it came to develop the health infrastructure in India. The colonial government's adherence to Victorian notions of the minimalist state provided an ideological background for this. It went on visualising health services as a 'philanthropic' and 'charitable' act, and nowhere perceived it as one of the fundamental tasks of the government.[23] In this regard, in the context of the United Provinces, a circular was issued by the secretary of the chief commissioner of Oudh to the commissioner of Fyzabad division on 21 September 1865 stating that 'The Governor General in Council is of opinion that dispensaries *wholly* supported by Government, should be allowed only in *exceptional circumstances*.'[24] This stated guideline of the governor-general in council clearly shows that the government did not want itself to get seriously engaged in the extension of health services in India. It was rather argued that 'the people of the place [should] evince a sense of the value of the Institution by erecting, at their own cost, a suitable building, and combining to do what they can from their own resources'.[25]

Throughout the nineteenth and early twentieth century, the government kept on emphasising the aforesaid policy of garnering local support for the proper functioning of the civil hospitals and dispensaries. Although some grants-in-aid were given, they were mostly insufficient to meet the expenditure of the dispensaries and civil hospitals. According to a statement showing the accounts of 118 dispensaries and civil hospitals functioning in the North Western Provinces and Oudh during the calendar year 1892, only 24 civil hospitals and dispensaries were able to manage their own expenses and were not in deficit. In other words, the rest 94 civil hospitals and dispensaries were running at a loss. In the light of this fact, the secretary to Government of North Western Provinces and Oudh wrote a letter on 31 July 1895 to all the chairmen and presidents of district boards of the North Western Provinces and Oudh stating categorically that if these hospitals/dispensaries would fail to make up their funds through the income generated from local sources in order to meet their deficits, then the government would have to take stern action, withdrawing whatever grants-in-aid it had been furnishing to these hospitals/dispensaries.[26] Thus, instead of raising grants-in-aid to make up the deficit of the hospitals/dispensaries meant for the common public, the government threatened to withdraw it altogether if enough local income was not secured.[27]

Nonetheless, despite showing its consistent disinterest in extending medical facilities to Indians, proper treatment even of destitute, sick and poor Europeans in India was high on the agenda of the colonial government's health policy. Incidentally, with the establishment of colonial rule in India, a number of poor idle Europeans came to India either looking for work or some private business in the hope of reaping fortunes. While some of them were steady, many of them were 'miserable drunkards' and were often categorised as 'loafers'. Among such persons, disease was common, especially delerium tremens.[28] In the United Provinces, Allahabad was one such place which attracted many idle Europeans. The number of such destitute sick Europeans was so high at Allahabad that by mid-1860s the Government of India started thinking of establishing a separate civil hospital only for Europeans at Allahabad so as to impart the treatment 'which could match the European standard[s]'. This proposal received generous support of J. Irving, civil surgeon, Allahabad, and was forwarded by the government of the North Western Provinces and Oudh.[29]

Similar embodiment of racial/class discrimination in the treatment facilities available to 'native' and European population of India can be seen in the letter sent by C. L. Cox, deputy inspector general of hospitals, Indian Forces, to the brigade major, Umballa, on 30 October 1870. In the letter, Cox writes:

> [A]lthough in the Umballa Station Hospital there is ample room for the reception of Europeans, still, from the nature of the establishment, solely intended for a native hospital, and consisting only of a native doctor, a compounder, *bheesty* and sweeper, without any means for cooking, or for supplying food to cook, - unprovided with bedding for the cold weather (bare *charpoys* being the only furniture), or with *punkhas* or *tatties* for the hot, - unprovided with ward coolies, or in fact, with any of the *essentials of a European hospital*, - it is *ill-adapted for the treatment of Europeans*, who, if they are admitted at all, ought, I think to be taken to where they receive the *treatment suitable to their class*.[30]

Thus, the same hospitals/dispensaries which were deemed fit for 'native' population became 'ill-adapted' and 'unsuitable' for Europeans.

In a similar vein, in another letter to the brigade major, Umballa, on 7 November 1870, C. L. Cox lamented about the condition of a European patient during one of his visits to the Umballa Station Hospital in following terms:

> He [the European patient at the Umballa Station Hospital] appears to be very respectable and well educated. He states that he is the son of a gentleman (a Deputy Inspector General of Hospitals); that he is a Civil Engineer by profession, and lately held a large contract under Messrs. Braseey, Wythes & Company, at the Sutlej Railway Bridge, but that, owing to a suit in the Divorce Court at Lahore, he fell into pecuniary difficulties. He appears to be dying of lung disease. He was lying on a miserable strong bottomed *charpoy*; his bed clothes were filthy razais [quilts] formerly used by soldiers, but long since condemned sold by them in the bazaar for a few annas, and re-purchased for this man. He had not a chair to sit upon, nor a bed-side table on which to place his food which was partly lying on his dirty bedding, and partly stowed away in a window recess, whilst the food itself (the meat portion being goat's flesh purchased in the bazaar) had been cooked for him by the hospital sweeper—his only attendant. Altogether *his plight was pitiable*, and I confess it was *humiliating and distressing to witness a poor respectably brought up Englishman taken into a government hospital* and fed upon very inferior bazaar meat cooked up by a sweeper, *it was a sight well calculated to justly lower us in the estimation of the natives*, who would naturally consider that to consign our distressed countrymen to degradation like this was the treatment we deemed good enough for them.[31]

C. L. Cox further writes that after coming across such a deplorable view, he at once ordered, at his own expense, a proper cook to be entertained and wholesome food and other necessaries to be procured to that patient.[32] Thus, health and proper treatment even of a destitute poor European/Englishman was a matter of great concern for the colonial government and health officials and manifested racial dimensions. Also, this was the case where race subsumed the class differences among the colonisers in colonial context.

In fact, racial division of space seems to have an impact on public health arrangements as well in colonial India. As argued earlier, with the establishment of colonial rule there was a sudden influx of Europeans in India outside the official circle. To cater to their needs, several government hospitals were set up which were intended 'exclusively for the medical relief of civil European and Anglo-Indian government servants and European and Anglo-Indian paupers';[33] as for instance, the European Civil Hospital at Allahabad, Eden Hospital or the European General Hospital in Calcutta.[34] Besides these exclusive 'health islands', there were also wards in other prominent hospitals reserved for the exclusive treatment of European and Anglo-Indian patients. For example, in the United Provinces, there were exclusive European wards at the Balrampur Hospital, Lucknow; King George's Medical College and Hospital, Lucknow; and Thomason Hospital, Agra. Thus, health infrastructure in colonial India also exhibited racial discrimination in terms of space.

It was in the context of the above-mentioned historical backdrop where Western medicine was used by the colonial government to colonise the 'Indian land' and the 'body' and access to Western medical facilities had racial overtones that the revival of 'indigenous' system(s) of healing gained public attention of the reformist elite. The frequent comparison/criticism of Indian system(s) of healing as 'primitive', 'prehistoric', 'stagnant' and 'non-scientific' methods of treatment, amounting to 'quackery', also disgruntled the reformist elite. For them, revival of a 'truly' Indian 'indigenous' system of healing worthier than Western system became crucial to their very identity. However, the multiple responses that came up on the issue of 'indigenous' medicine in this regard were very complex due to a multitude of factors. The following section examines some of these multifaceted responses related to 'indigenous' medicine.

THE IDEA OF 'INDIGENOUS' MEDICINE AND ITS COMPLEXITIES

The pursuit of the revival of 'indigenous' system(s) of healing in India against the aforesaid backdrop had its own intricacies. There were two fundamental questions which the practitioners and proponents of 'indigenous' medicine had to resolve on an urgent basis:

1. Which system represented the 'indigenous' healing system of India?
2. What sort of practices, knowledge and healers precisely constituted that 'indigenous' healing system?

To begin with the first issue: any question regarding which system truly represented the 'indigenous' healing system of India was a tricky one. India was the abode of various healing systems from Ayurveda to Unani to Siddha to other healing practices which did not fall under any 'system' (non-systemic healing practices). Out of these, in the contemporaneous context, Ayurveda and Unani were the two chief contenders for the aforesaid claim of 'indigeneity'. Nevertheless, for the time being, the proponents and practitioners of different healing systems joined hands to fight back the growing (colonial) influences of Western medicine in India. This collaboration between Ayurveda and Unani at the national level was manifested through the writings and deeds of Hakim Ajmal Khan who was associated both with the Indian National Congress and the All India Muslim League, and was an 'indigenous' medical practitioner himself. It was through his efforts that the first meeting of the All India Ayurvedic and Unani Tibbi Conference was convened in 1910. He also established an Ayurvedic and Unani Tibbia College in Delhi.[35]

As Guy Attewell argues, there were three main objectives of the united front thus created for propagating 'indigenous' medicine, all of which were interconnected: first, to further the institutionalisation of Unani and Ayurveda, in separate or combined schools; second, to encourage the horizontal dissemination of knowledge of 'indigenous' medicine, bringing them out of the hereditary control of traditional vaids and hakims; and third, to provide a forum to lobby and bargain with the government for advancement of 'indigenous' medicine.[36] The All India Ayurvedic and Unani Tibbi Conference of Hakim Ajmal Khan was at the forefront of the aforesaid agenda of collaborative action. While it nowhere challenged the standard colonial dichotomy of 'Muslim–Unani' and 'Hindu–Ayurveda', it emphasised on the unity of *ilm* (that is, knowledge) of 'indigenous' medicine in India. In fact, Hakim Ajmal Khan went on to refer vaids and hakims as constituting one *qaum* (community) or *groh* (group) irrespective of their religious affiliations.[37]

However, the early twentieth century simultaneously witnessed intensified polarisation even in the field of 'indigenous' medicine when vaids and hakims throughout north India openly sided with communal forces. They stressed Ayurveda/Unani for the broader agenda of Hindu/Islamic revivalism and the consolidation of Hindu/Islamic religious, cultural and national identity. Despite efforts of conciliation, 'indigenous' healing practices turned into symbols around which communal polarisation could take place.[38] The All India Vaidya Sammelan, which was very much active in the United Provinces, particularly fanned the process of communalisation of the Ayurvedic discourse. The Vaidya Sammelan often claimed itself to be the sole spokesperson of the 'Hindu' vaid interests and stressed that the concerns and interests of 'Hindu' vaids were different from 'Muslim' hakims. That is why the Sammelan was sceptical of the activities of the All India Ayurvedic and Unani Tibbi Conference which had been emphasising on the collaboration and cooperation of the 'indigenous' practitioners of both kinds. In fact, in the discourse of the Sammelan, Ayurveda figured not only as 'distinct' from other existing healing systems but also as most 'original' and 'indigenous' to the Indian soil owing to its local origin vis-à-vis Unani which was deemed as 'foreign'. Further, the Sammelan emphasised Ayurveda as being 'sacred', derived primarily from Hindu Vedic gods and scriptures, thereby associating it with diverse elements of Hindu mythology and sages. Incidentally, for the Sammelan, Ayurveda and Unani represented not merely systems of medicine but distinct cultures, and hence defence of Ayurveda inherently implied the preservation of a 'glorious' 'Hindu' heritage. In this regard, a separate common front of Hindu vaids was advocated by the Sammelan and its leaders such as Jagannath Prasad Shukla to counter the Muslims and their tactics to humiliate the Hindus for selfish gains.[39] More specifically, a collective identity of Hindu vaids was sought by the Sammelan not just to revive and promote Ayurveda but also to associate with politicised networks in order to nourish an overarching 'Hindu' culture as well as nation.

Similarly, in the changing political climate of the early twentieth century, communitarian concerns dominated the Unani discourse of the province as well. The explicit manifestation of this communitarian tilt of Unani was widening rift and clash of egos between the Delhi family of Hakim Ajmal Khan and the Lucknow family of Abd al Aziz, the two prominent Unani families of the time. The Lucknow hakims formed an exclusive association of their own called Anjuman-i-Tibia, in 1911, advocating an unalloyed professional Unani distinct from Ayurveda. Like the All India Vaidya Sammelan, the Anjuman opposed the conciliatory tactics of Hakim Ajmal Khan's All India Ayurvedic and Unani Conference. It went on to make an appeal to the hakims of the province, particularly those of Lucknow, to boycott the Conference. Soon Anjuman-i-Tibia was renamed as the All India Unani Tibbi Conference, thereby claiming for a wider credibility among the practitioners pledged to work for the advancement of Unani alone. Thus, the interests of qaum (that is, community) received an upperhand over the interest of the *mulk* (that is, nation) in the Unani medical discourse of the communally charged atmosphere of the United Provinces.[40]

Moving towards the second contentious issue, as argued in the very beginning, the conflict was not just between the 'Hindu' vaid and the 'Muslim' hakim, but vaids and hakims were also divided within their 'own groups' respectively. This internal division was largely over the question of the nature of practices, ideas, knowledge and healers that precisely constituted the projected 'indigenous' system of healing.[41] This issue became particularly significant as a lot of dialogue/interaction had been going on between Western medicine and/among 'indigenous' systems of healing during this time, often resulting into flow of medical ideas and healing practices across different 'systems'. Here it should be noted that it was by the late nineteenth and early twentieth century that 'fluent' healing traditions were transformed into respective healing 'systems' connoting internal coherence, continuity, discreteness, completeness and homogeneity. Fixed characteristics were drawn pertaining to a 'system' and traditions were reformatted accordingly into a coherent system. Both Ayurveda as well as Unani underwent this politics of reconfiguration into a systemic frame during the period under discussion.[42]

Nevertheless, as argued by David Arnold, a medical practitioner might see himself as belonging to a particular 'system' of healing while actually employing an eclectic mix of diagnostic and therapeutic devices drawn from 'other' systems.[43] Such braiding of healing systems led to multifaceted responses over the practices, ideas and knowledge constituting a particular 'indigenous' system of healing. One can divide these multifaceted responses into two broad categories. The first category included those who advocated selective adoption from Western medicine to enrich 'indigenous' systems of medicine, but keeping the 'indigenous' identity intact. They acknowledged the progress made by Western medicine over the past few centuries and did not reject it outrightly. The second category was composed of purists who made a call to restore the 'pristine purity' of 'indigenous' systems of medicine. They were not ready to acknowledge the superiority of Western medicine in any respect.

However, there were multiple strands within these categories. For example, within purists there were those who denied the medical aspect of Western medicine, but simultaneously adopted its institutional structure to further the cause of 'indigenous' medicine. This ambiguity of revivalist discourse on medicine was analysed for the first time by Charles Leslie in his series of articles.[44] According to Leslie, even while talking of the revivalism of the classical systems of healing—Ayurveda and Unani—both the pragmatic ideologues (also known as 'progressives', who advocated induction of new knowledge alongside classical learning) and the purists (also known as 'conservatives', who emphasised literal revocation of Ayurvedic and Unani texts) resorted to techniques which were alien to the classical system such as institutionalisation of learning, professionalisation of practice and manufacturing of standardised remedies in pharmaceutical factories, all of which were traits of the 'modern' Western system of medicine. Interestingly, Leslie does not find any such deviations in medical revivalism in India to be strange since, according to him, even in Europe, Renaissance and the ideas of Enlightenment while deriving sanctity from classical learning, never literally revived them and altered classical conceptions significantly.[45]

Incidentally, as K. N. Panikkar points out that caught in a paradox to discard the old and create a new cultural milieu, on the one hand, and to preserve or retrieve the traditional cultural tropes so that the past is not swept off the ground, on the other hand; the proponents of 'indigenous' medicine engaged critically with both Western medicine as well as the classical texts in their quest of revitalising Ayurveda.[46] As a corollary, even in their resistance to Western medicine, there was often a tacit acceptance of the standards set by the colonisers. Hence, there is a need to look beyond the singular frameworks of 'resistance' and 'acceptance', thereby exploring the reorganisation of the entire practice in a modern colonial context. In this regard, the first decade of the twenty-first century witnessed a flood of writings which showed how 'new' vaids and hakims evolved during the late nineteenth and early twentieth century and how they were remarkably different from vaids and hakims of the earlier period.[47] In their revivalist/reformist quest, these 'new' vaids and hakims dramatically reshaped and redefined 'indigenous' systems of healing to incorporate the traits on the basis of which Western medicine was claiming its superiority (such as scientificity, standardisation, professionalisation and institutionalisation). These newly incorporated traits in turn introduced long-lasting changes within Ayurveda and Unani thereby altering some of the basic premises of these healing traditions. All this led to the creation of 'modernised traditions' as reflected through the emergence of 'modern' Ayurveda and Unani. This unique combination of oxymoronic traits was peculiar to colonial set-up manifesting 'the rule of colonial difference' in the sphere of medical modernity.[48]

The modern 'Western' standards and traits were adopted by the 'indigenous' practitioners to such an extent that many 'bogus' medical institutions flourished in the early twentieth century, evading the government's eyes to provide certificates not only to unqualified allopathic practitioners but also to vaids and hakims. The very existence of such 'bogus' institutions for providing certificates in 'indigenous' medicine reveals the importance which the system of institutional training had gained even for the practitioners of 'indigenous' medicine by the early twentieth century.[49] One such 'bogus' medical institution providing certificates in Unani, Ayurveda and Homeopathy was The Old Indian Medical College at Barnala in Patiala state (see Figure 1.1). It was opened by Man Singh (son of Narain Singh Ahluwalia of Barnala, Patiala state). According to official records, he was 'a man of poor knowledge and ability; [who] opened this bogus institute and began to earn his

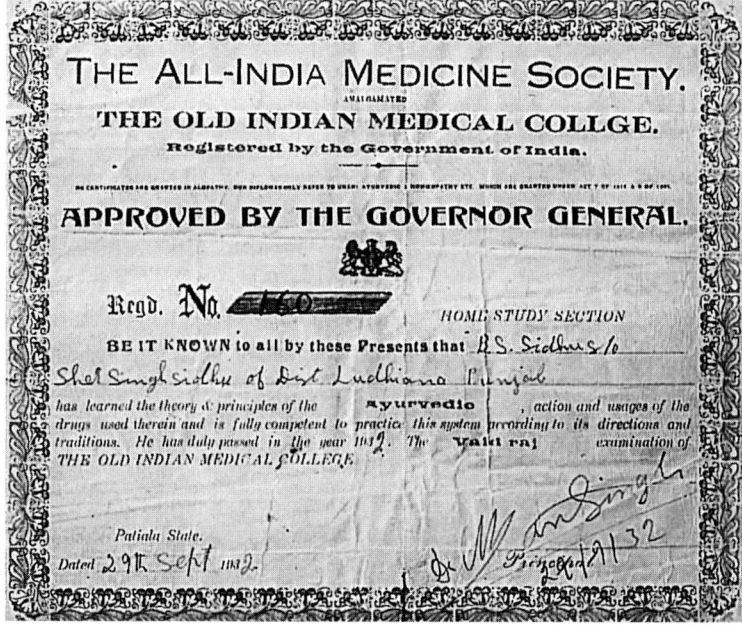

Figure 1.1: Certificate of *Vaidraj* issued by The Old Indian Medical College (a bogus medical institution).[50]

livelihood by false advertisements and selling certificates of this bogus institution'.[51] Throughout the early twentieth century, the Government of India was consistently engaged in restricting the growth of such 'bogus' medical institutions and degrees, both in the field of Western as well as 'indigenous' medicine.[52]

In fact, one of the factors which created internal division amongst the practitioners of 'indigenous' medicine (both vaids as well as hakims) was the kind of training received by them. Earlier vaids and hakims used to learn their skills mostly through the institution of the family or through traditional gurus. *Khandani* (or hereditary) vaids and hakims had more prestige in the society than those who had newly acquired their skills. However, 'new' vaids and hakims of the late nineteenth and early twentieth century started privileging institutional training over traditional individual study under a 'guru'. If we follow this contentious issue carefully, it gives a new insight into the protest of the 'indigenous' practitioners against the medical registration acts which were passed by various provincial governments in the early twentieth century.

Vaids and hakims had been opposing the medical registration acts despite the repeated assurance of the government that such acts were meant only for the practitioners of Western medicine and there was nothing in these acts which could restrict the 'indigenous' practitioners to continue their practice. The very fact that these acts were making a distinction between the 'registered' and the 'unregistered' practitioners or between 'legally/duly qualified' and 'unqualified' practitioners (although only in the case of the practitioners of Western medicine) was unsettling, especially for the newly emerged vaids and hakims of the early twentieth century. This was largely because they believed that their institutional training was at par with the kind of training received by the 'qualified' allopathic practitioners and that there were 'qualified' and 'unqualified' persons even amongst the practitioners of 'indigenous' medicine. However, under the proposed acts while doctors could be 'registered', 'qualified' vaids and hakims could never acquire such a distinction, which the 'new' vaids and hakims found insulting and disrespecting for their status. In other words, they were not against the very idea of 'registration', but they were against its limited scope. Had it been extended to the practitioners of 'indigenous' medicine, then these 'new' vaids and hakims could have possibilities to push themselves ahead of the 'traditional' and 'hereditary' vaids and hakims, owing to the kind of institutional training which they had received.

If we look closely at the debate in the Legislative Council of Bombay which took place in 1911 around the Medical Registration Bill,[53] some hint to this kind of intention of 'new' vaids and hakims can be seen. The government was unwilling to extend the Registration Bill to the practitioners of 'indigenous' medicine, largely because it was argued that the systematic institutional training in their case had still not been evolved. However, some of the members objected to this by stating that there were institutions such as Madrasa-i-Tibbia at Delhi which provided institutional training to hakims and hence the government's argument was not accurate. One can clearly see in this debate the intention of some of the members of the legislative council to get the 'registered' status for the institutionally trained practitioners of 'indigenous' medicine by ignoring the cause of 'hereditary' vaids and hakims.

Incidentally, the All India Vaidya Sammelan and its provincial units such as the United Provinces Vaidya Sammelan, which were dominated by 'new' vaids, actively tried to forward the cause of institutionally trained Ayurvedic practitioners over the 'hereditary' vaids. In fact, even the membership clause of the All India Vaidya Sammelan heavily favoured the institutionally trained vaids. In case of 'hereditary' or non-institutionally trained vaids, only those practitioners engaged in imparting Ayurvedic remedies for more than 10 years could apply for the membership of the All India Vaidya Sammelan, that too on the recommendations of two existing members of the provincial unit and two local notables. In contrast, there was no such clause of experience or recommendation for the institutionally trained vaids in order to take the membership of the Sammelan.[54]

In the United Provinces, these 'new' vaids and hakims eventually succeeded in their above-mentioned pursuit of acquiring 'registered' status when the United Provinces Indian Medicine Act was passed in 1939. Besides resistance of 'new' vaids and hakims, this Act was a product of the post-dyarchic administrative arrangements which had substantially increased the provincial bureaucracy.[55] The Act of 1939 provided for the registration of the practitioners of 'indigenous' medicine as well (see Figure 1.2). The task and authority to supervise this entire process and to maintain a register of 'duly qualified' vaids and hakims was entrusted with the Board of Indian Medicine of the United Provinces. Under this Act, the following persons became entitled to have their names entered in the register of (qualified) vaids and hakims:

- Vaids and hakims who held a degree or certificate of any government Ayurvedic or Unani college or school within the United Provinces or outside it, or a degree in Indian medicine or surgery or midwifery of any university established by law in India.
- Vaids and hakims who had passed the final examinations held by the Board of Indian Medicine, United Provinces, or by any institution affiliated to the Board.

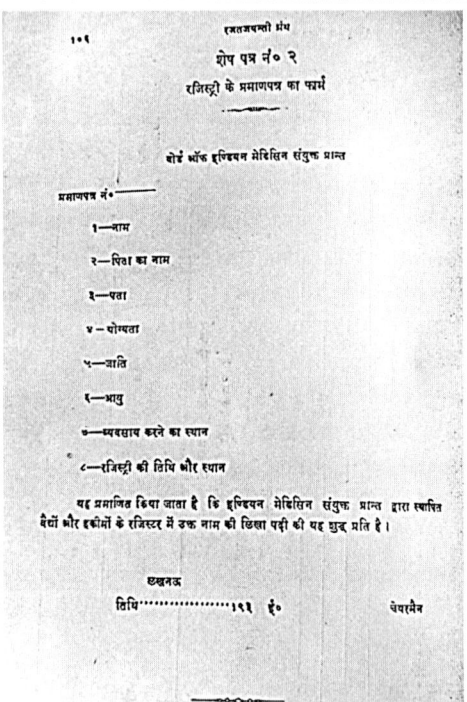

Figure 1.2: Registration form for vaids and hakims (under the United Provinces Indian Medicine Act, 1939).[56]

- Vaids or hakims who had passed an examination from any Ayurvedic or Unani institution in the United Provinces or outside it, recognised by the Board for purposes of registration.
- Vaids or hakims who in the opinion of the Board were of sufficient standing, reputation and ability, and were known for their skill in their profession and who fulfilled the conditions imposed by rules as to the length of their practice.[57]

Now, the first three clauses put the condition of passing some examination or the other to enter the list of registered vaids and hakims. In other words, it was clearly in favour of the institutionally trained 'new' vaids and hakims. The last clause which gave some respite to the 'hereditary' vaids and hakims was actually a tough one. Only after spending several years in the profession a 'traditional' vaid or hakim could gain 'sufficient standing, reputation and ability' as demanded by the Act to get registered; whereas the 'new' vaids and hakims could easily acquire such a reputation immediately after passing the final examinations of their course. Thus, eventually, the institutionally trained vaids and hakims emerged as victors over the 'hereditary' practitioners of 'indigenous' medicine. It also squeezed out many folk healers belonging to the low castes/class whose knowledge had been handed down from generation to generation through the institution of the family.

Similarly, the standardisation of drug manufacturing was another trait of Western medicine which was internalised by the practitioners of 'indigenous' medicine by this time. Earlier vaids and hakims did not merely prescribe the medicines; rather they themselves prepared and gave medicines as well. The skill of determining the quantities in which various elements and herbs were to be mixed to prepare a particular medicine was highly personalised in nature, and vaids and hakims used to decide upon this after looking at the severity of the disease. This skill of making medicine was so personalised in nature that, many a time, the methodology of preparation of a particular medicine disappeared forever after the death of the practitioner.

However, by the late nineteenth and early twentieth century, we see the emergence of some big pharmaceutical companies in different parts of India, standardising the manufacturing of 'indigenous' drugs. For example,

C. K. Sen & Company of Calcutta, established by Chandra Kishore Sen in 1878 and which started large-scale production of 'indigenous' medicines from 1898 onwards; N. N. Sen & Company of Bengal, which was established in 1898; Shakti Aushadhalaya of Dacca, established in 1901; and Arya Vaidyasala of Kottakkal (Kerala), established in 1902 by P. S. Varier. Some of the nationalist leaders like P. C. Ray also pushed for the manufacturing of standardised Ayurvedic remedies. In fact, P. C. Ray himself hawked some of the Ayurvedic products, manufactured by his firm, on the streets of Calcutta.[58] Similarly, Madan Mohan Malviya opened an Ayurvedic pharmacy in Benares after consulting eminent vaids of the city. Interestingly, the establishment of the Ayurvedic pharmacy preceded the establishment of the Ayurvedic College at the Banaras Hindu University (BHU).[59] It shows the importance that the practitioners of 'indigenous' medicine were attaching to the standardisation of manufacturing of 'indigenous' drugs.

Besides these giant pharmaceutical companies manufacturing 'indigenous' drugs, there were numerous small pharmacies in different cities operating at the local level. In fact, the rise and growth of patriotic fervour, particularly following the partition of Bengal in 1905, wherein boycott of foreign goods was adopted as one of the tools of anti-colonial nationalist agitation, gave fillip to Ayurvedic pharmacies as well.[60] The contemporary newspapers often carried the advertisements of these pharmacies and medicines prepared by them and the tall claims that they used to make about their products. Consequently, by the early twentieth century, a kind of medical entrepreneurship came to develop even in the field of 'indigenous' medicine.[61] Actually, vaids and hakims found the standardisation of remedies as one of the factors behind the rapid growth of Western medicine. This was largely because the standardisation of remedies liberated the medical relief from the clutches of a personalised knowledge system. One could buy medicines anywhere by producing the same prescription again and again, and there was no need to visit the practitioner located at some distant place merely to get the renewed dose of medicine. In other words, it was more consumer-friendly. Hence, 'new' vaids and hakims continuously laid emphasis on the standardisation of manufacturing of 'indigenous' drugs and medicines. Besides this, many vaids and hakims saw the opportunity of handsome profit as well in the mass production of 'indigenous' medicine. Hence, we see the mushrooming of Ayurvedic and Unani pharmacies in the early twentieth century, where an established vaid or hakim often owned a pharmacy as well. Such pharmacies often gave postal guidance to the sufferer also and dispatched medicines using the postal services.

Furthermore, the social structure also played an important role in creating fissures within the practitioners of 'indigenous' medicine around the issue related to precise practices/knowledge/healers constituting a particular system of healing. As K. N. Panikkar remarks, '[T]he quest to revitalise indigenous medicine reflected a multi-pronged struggle for cultural hegemony, not only between the coloniser and the colonised, but also between the classes within the colonised society.'[62] In other words, the entire project to recast 'indigenous' medicine which was going on in the late nineteenth and early twentieth century cannot be studied by ignoring the paradigms of both caste and class. While the newly emerging vaids were contesting the dominance of Western medicine, they were also trying to purge the tribal and low-caste healing practices and influences (all of which constituted an important part of folk healing) out of the fold of Ayurveda. This was part and parcel of the creation of an upper-caste/middle-class identity of Ayurveda during this time. Simultaneously, it also manifests the process of urbanisation of Ayurveda as most of these 'new' vaids belonged to the urban landscape.

However, this entire process was not so simple and was marked by its own contradictions and ambiguities. On the one hand, upper-caste/class vaids were condemning the tribal and low-caste methods of treatment which were in vogue particularly in the rural areas, but at the same time they were appropriating some of these methods by Hinduising or Brahmanising them. For example, in Orissa, the treatment of snake bite was largely the domain of low-caste healers.[63] This was largely because while treating snake bites one had to touch the body or even the feet of the patient (who could even be from a low caste), which was 'insulting' for the upper-caste healers. However, over the late nineteenth and early twentieth century, we see Oriya medical texts coming up which not only urged the Brahmins to take up this job, but also provided the treatment of snake bite with a 'ritualised Brahmanical slant'.[64]

Similarly, in the United Provinces, the early twentieth century vernacular medical texts condemned *dai*s (midwives) and *dhai*s (wet mothers) for their alleged 'unclean and polluting' habits and behaviour as they belonged mostly to the low/untouchable castes. That is why one can find a middle-class/upper-caste urge to get rid of these 'lowly' midwives in the name of their professionalisation. In this regard, the reformist elites of the United Provinces openly sided with the governmental drive to professionalise midwifery. Widows of the 'good families' were motivated to take up the profession of midwifery and suggestions were made to always employ wet mothers of one's own caste.⁶⁵ Hence, it was not just the 'hegemony' of Western medicine or the prejudiced efforts of the colonial government that the professionalisation of midwives was called for, rather traditional caste and class concerns were involved in this process as well. Thus, the 'indigenous' practitioners were also divided among themselves along caste, class and community lines in determining the practices, knowledge and healers constituting their respective system of healing that claimed 'indigenous' identity.

NATIONALISING AYURVEDA

Despite the contradictions and complexities, as discussed in the preceding section, attempts were made by the proponents of Ayurveda during the late nineteenth and early twentieth century to pose it as the true claimant of the 'national healing system' of India.⁶⁶ In this discourse, Ayurveda became a true representative of 'time-tested' 'authentic' 'indigenous' healing culture of India. The Ayurvedic practitioners frequently engaged in the political discourses of the time, especially that of the nation-state, so much so that by the mid–twentieth century they came up with an Ayurvedic flag and an Ayurvedic anthem having tremendous similarities with the proposed design of the national flag and a very popular patriotic song, '*Vijayi vishwa tiranga pyara*', respectively (see Figure 1.3). Issues like the 'enslavement' of India (both by the Muslims and the English), drain of wealth, 'emaciation' of the 'Hindu' race and possible remedies frequently appeared in the Ayurvedic tracts/advertisements.

In fact, the upper-caste/middle-class reformist elite of the time felt a desperate urge to invoke and reinterpret the classical Ayurvedic texts and to cast them into the discourse of 'indigenous science' and the 'nation'. This was largely because, as Gyan Prakash puts it, '[T]o be a nation was to be endowed with science, which had become [the] touchstone of rationality.'⁶⁸

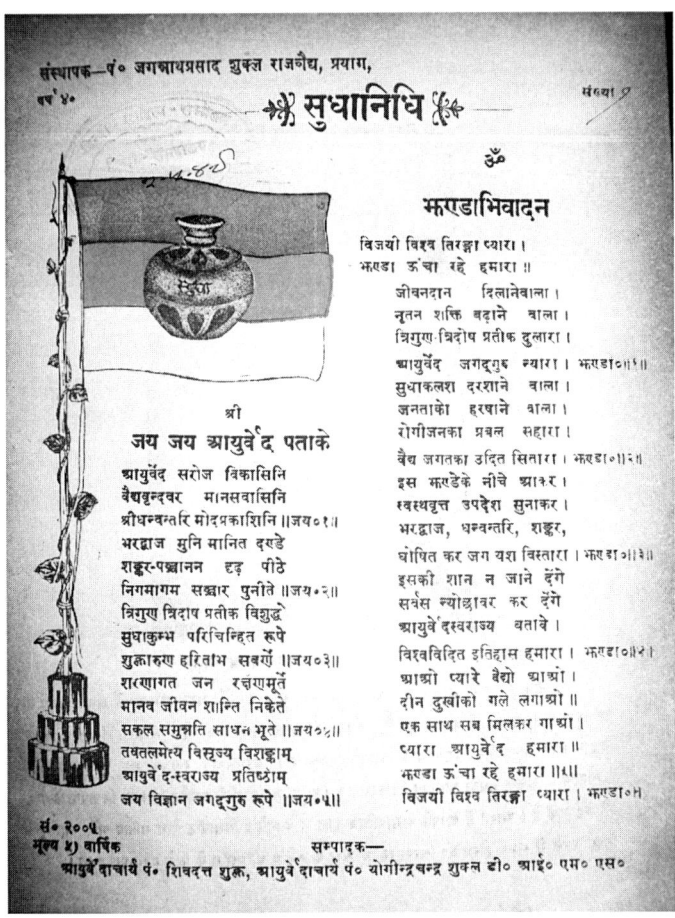

Figure 1.3: Ayurvedic flag and anthem[67]

Hence, the reformist elite lent their full support to the nationalisation of Ayurvedic discourse. Even the Indian princes/chiefs soon joined in this movement to regenerate Ayurveda as 'indigenous' self. The princely states of Jaipur, Alwar, Gwalior, Mysore, Patiala, Baroda, etc., were well-known for their encouragement towards Ayurvedic studies. In fact, one can find many Ayurvedic learning centres being established in these princely states financed by royal donations.[69] Bhagvat Sinhji, the Maharaja of

Gondal, even commissioned a treatise on *Aryan Medical Science* in 1895 which argued in favour of the Aryans being the most enlightened people of their day, pioneering several fields of scientific knowledge, including medicine.[70] Ayurvedic revivalism, thus, became crucial to forge the identity of a 'rising' nation.[71]

However, the emergence of the idea of a 'national' medicine was not an exclusively colonial phenomenon. One can find such ideas floating even in the metropolitan world where pharmacies often invoked national sentiments to increase the sale of their products in the national and international market.[72] Nevertheless, what was 'colonial' about the idea of 'national' medicine in the colonial context was its association with the anti-colonial nationalist struggle against the existing (colonial) regime. Thus, Ayurveda was seen as a remedy to ameliorate the Indian/'Hindu' masses and to restore their vigour and to reinstate their 'lost' independence. In the Ayurvedic discourse of the time, one can see the merging of the discourse over the healthy 'body' and the healthy 'nation'. The stress on brahmacharya (celibacy) by the Ayurvedic practitioners/publicists was part and parcel of the entire project of building a healthy and strong 'nation'. Similar was the logic stated behind the urge for the professionalisation of midwifery by the Ayurvedic practitioners since traditional dais were seen as 'enemies' of the 'health of the nation', as they were blamed for the high infant and maternal mortality of India.

THE COLONIAL GOVERNMENT AND THE 'INDIGENOUS' MEDICAL DISCOURSE

It would be equally interesting to see how the colonial government visualised/reacted to the aforesaid movement/discourse related to 'indigenous' medicine. As argued earlier, medicine was significant both to satisfy the short-term as well as the long-term needs of colonialism. It was precisely against this backdrop that a medical discourse emerged by the late nineteenth century stressing on 'indigenous' medicine. In the early twentieth century, these demands acquired political fervour in the wake of the ongoing nationalist struggle and it became impossible for the colonial government to ignore the demands raised by the practitioners of 'indigenous' medicine and their sympathisers.

However, there were other pragmatic reasons owing to which the colonial government could not ignore the voices of vaids and hakims. The progress of Western medicine in India was so slow that it could hardly meet the demands of the Indian masses. As late as 1913, there were only 2,820 civil hospitals and dispensaries, treating a little over 515,000 in-patients and over 30 million out-patients; 851 state special and railway hospitals treating a little over 98,000 in-patients and 2,331,000 out-patients; and 697 private non-aided institutions treating over 57,000 in-patients and 4,828,000 out-patients. In other words, there were about 4,400 hospitals and dispensaries all over British India, treating about 38 million patients, for a vast population of 240 million.[73] It means that around 84 per cent of the population was still resorting to 'indigenous' medicine/folk healing. Further, there were other problems as well associated with Western medicine. It was costlier than 'indigenous' medicine and the fees demanded by the practitioners of Western medicine were quite high compared to what was charged by the local vaids and hakims, who had flexible fee slabs. Besides, newly qualified Indian medical men (in Western medicine) hardly used to go out to the remote *mofussil* districts and the rural areas. Most of them were either concentrated in the presidency cities or the large towns.[74] An interesting literary depiction of this phenomenon can be found in the novel *Maila Anchal* written by Phanishwar Nath 'Renu'. In the novel, when the protagonist of the story *Daktar Babu* (Prashant) decided to go and serve in the countryside, instead of taking a scholarship and going abroad, his colleagues and other people trained in Western medicine (including some of the professors) came up with sarcastic remarks describing him an 'emotional fool' and 'crazy'. In contrast, the Madras Medical Gazette praised him for his exemplary stance. However, his colleagues believed that Prashant would regret later on for his decision. It shows the reluctance of the majority of the Indian men newly trained in Western medicine to serve in the rural areas.[75]

At the same time, as Rachel Berger points out, the expansion of the bureaucracy following the Montagu–Chelmsford reforms of 1919, resulting in the incorporation of a new class of 'native' servants into the provincial administration, who were subject to the same rules that had governed their European counterparts, also forced the colonial government to take into consideration the services of 'indigenous' practitioners. According to Berger, 'the province, newly responsible for its medical responsibilities to both administrators and subjects, could no longer afford the expensive biomedical bureaucratic measures it had used in the past to certify the [ill] health of its bureaucrats'.[76] The provincial government of the United Provinces consequently decided that lower-class officials could consult 'indigenous' practitioners of their 'preferred' healing system in order to get a certificate of ill health. As a corollary, a Board of Indian Medicine of the United provinces was also established in 1921 to resolve the complicated issues involved while resorting to 'indigenous' practitioners for official purposes such as identification of 'qualified' vaids and hakims, determining the basis of their qualification and gauging the extent of their expertise in the given field.[77] This, in turn, initiated a series of regulations and legislations making 'indigenous' medicine one of the targets of governmental reform in the post-dyarchic period in response to changing medical needs of colonial governance.

Thus, in the aforesaid context, the colonial government could hardly dispense off with the practitioners of 'indigenous' medicine altogether. Noticeable in this regard is the statement made by J. C. Fergusson [under secretary to the Government of India, home (medical) department] in reply to G. Bomford's (director general, IMS) suggestion of the employment of vaids and hakims by local bodies to meet the demands of public health:

> When western medicine in India is so much in need of funds, *it seems a waste of money to subsidise systems* which belong to the dark ages. *It may be politic, however, not to refuse the small degree of recognition* suggested and as Director General recommends these proposals, we may accept them.[78]

This statement clearly brings out the dilemma of the colonial government. The aspirations of the government and the pragmatic necessity of the health administration were pulling its health policies in two different directions. Despite having exclusive faith in allopathy, the government often had to defend itself on the question of encouragement made to 'indigenous' systems which had been serving more than 80 per cent of the population.

That is why, in turbulent political conditions of the early twentieth century, the colonial government never openly came out against the 'indigenous' systems of medicine. In fact, on certain occasions, it showed its concern and sympathy towards these systems and gave verbal assurances to the sympathisers of 'indigenous' medicine to encourage these systems; however, ultimately it followed the policy of negligence silently. The lobby of IMS officials was also at work behind the official negligence of 'indigenous' systems of medicine. The Indian members of provincial assemblies could do little in this regard due to the lack of funding. This entire situation has been well summarised, particularly in the context of the United Provinces, in the following report of a newspaper dated 5 September 1935:

To-Day
Neglected System

> So far as official patronage is concerned, the indigenous systems of medicine have made little headway in the United Provinces, judging from the report of Sir Wazir Hussain, Chairman of the Board of Indian Medicine of the United Provinces in his latest report. In itself utterly inadequate, the amount of Rs. 50,000 originally placed at the disposal of the Board for distribution among Ayurvedic and Unani dispensaries, has been gradually cut down to Rs. 35,000. While some of the institutions have been lucky enough to get a pittance of Rs. 60 each many others have had their claims overlooked. And thus in a country whose people very largely depend on the home systems of medical treatment. Under the Montford political scheme public health and medicine are transferred subjects but have gained little by ministerial patronage. If there is to be retrenchment, the axe falls on them first. Want of money is the handy pre-text but the real reason is the want of sympathy of the vested interests represented by the IMS which virtually rules the department, on which would spend and maintain one allopathic dispensary rather than ten Unani dispensaries, though all of them put together might cost the same amount.[79]
>
> (*National Call*, 5 September 1935, Delhi)

Even earlier, in 1924, when the government of the United Provinces was considering the options at its disposal to extend medical facilities to rural mass, it thoroughly negated the much feasible option of the opening of a large number of Ayurvedic and Unani dispensaries. Rather, it went for the encouragement of private medical practitioners in Western medicine, granting them subsidies and supply of medicines from public funds to settle them in the villages for practice. This was despite the fact that the government itself was sceptical regarding the number of medical practitioners of Western medicine who would be forthcoming to accept this rural assignment. Incidentally, the aforesaid scepticism proved correct when some of the district boards such as Allahabad, Unao and Hardoi expressed their incapability in attracting allopathic medical practitioners on their own and requested the government to make arrangements for this.[80] The allopathic practitioners preferred remaining unemployed/underemployed than going to rural areas. Eventually, it was the Congress government, in 1938, which came up with the scheme of establishing subsidised dispensaries of 'indigenous' medicine throughout the province in order to extend medical relief in rural areas.[81]

CONCLUDING REMARKS

Thus, by the late nineteenth and early twentieth century we see the emergence of Ayurveda as 'indigenous' medicine along with its own complexities. Like Western medicine, it was equally involved in the socio-political landscape of the time and in many ways performed similar functions for the Indian upper-caste/middle-class reformist elite as did Western medicine in the case of the colonial authorities. In other words, early twentieth century revival/reconstruction of Ayurveda was not merely a medical phenomenon; rather it was a gross socio-political process as well. In this regard, it becomes essential to look at the official nationalist response to the late colonial Ayurvedic movement, which would be discussed in detail in the following chapter. What perhaps needs emphasis is that even the official nationalist response to the Ayurvedic movement was never monolithic and exhibited a complex and nuanced picture.

NOTES

1. Partha Chatterjee, *The Nation and Its Fragment: Colonial and Postcolonial Histories* (Princeton: Princeton University Press, 1993), 6.
2. Kumar, *Medicine and the Raj*, 10.
3. The term 'colonial medicine' does not merely refer to Western medicine/medical practices which came to be disseminated through colonial regimes;

rather, as defined by David Arnold, it was 'the operation of colonial power within and through medicine in a colonial setting'. See David Arnold, *The New Cambridge History of India III.5: Science, Technology and Medicine in Colonial India* (Cambridge: Cambridge University Press, 2000), 15.

4. However, as the British Empire in India after the upheavals of 1857 was in the state of perpetual peace (at least militarily), civil posting of the IMS officials was perpetuated for all practical purposes.
5. Some exemplary works in this regard are Bala, *Imperialism and Medicine in Bengal*; Arnold, *Colonising the Body*; Harrison, *Public Health in British India*; Kumar, *Medicine and the Raj*.
6. Roy Macleod, 'Introduction', in *Disease, Medicine and Empire: Perspectives on Western Medicine and the Experience of European Expansion*, eds Roy Macleod and Milton Lewis (London: Routledge, 1988), 1.
7. Lenore Manderson, *Sickness and the State: Health and Illness in Colonial Malaya, 1870–1940* (Cambridge: Cambridge University Press, 1996), 10–14.
8. Arnold, *Colonising the Body*, 292.
9. K. Ballhatchet, *Race, Sex and Class under the Raj* (London: Weidenfeld & Nicholson, 1980).
10. Motolinia, a member of the first group of Franciscans to land in Mexico in 1524, describes the spread of smallpox, which was brought by one of Narvaez's soldiers, in following tragic words: 'As the Indians did not know the remedy for the disease and were very much in the habit of bathing frequently, whether well or ill, and continued to do so even when suffering from smallpox, *they died in heaps, like bedbugs*. Many others died of starvation, because, as they were all taken sick at once, they could not care for each other, nor was there anyone to give them bread or anything else.' Interestingly, Motolinia in his book *Historia* considers such a tragic occurrence a divine intervention to chastise the land of barbarians. Cited in Tzvetan Todorov, *The Conquest of America: The Question of Other* (New York: Harper Perennial, 1992), 136.
11. Donald Denoon, *Public Health in Papua New Guinea: Medical Possibility and Social Constraint, 1884–1984* (Cambridge: Cambridge University Press, 1989), 52.
12. See David Arnold, 'Touching the Body: Perspectives on Indian Plague, 1896–1900', in *Subaltern Studies V*, ed. Ranajit Guha (Delhi: Oxford University Press, 1987), 55–90; Arnold, *Colonising the Body*.
13. Kumar, *Medicine and the Raj*, 197.
14. 'Punch Marking of Railway Tickets Issued at Railway Station in the Allahabad and Pratabgarh Districts', F. No. 109–111, Sanitary Branch, Home Department, April 1900, National Archives of India, New Delhi (hereafter NAI).

15. 'Plague Riot at Cawnpore', F. No. 291–302, Public Branch, Home Department, June 1900, NAI.
16. Gupta, *Sexuality, Obscenity, Community*, 191–92.
17. Premvati Mishra was born in Agra (Firozabad tehsil) in 1915 and was arrested during the Quit India Movement of 1942. Incidentally, she was pregnant when arrested. Hence, she was sent immediately to Sarojini Naidu Hospital of Agra as pregnant women were not kept at the jail. See memoirs of Premvati Mishra in Rekha Trivedi, ed., *Smriti Ke Prishth: Swatantrata Senaniyon ke Sansmaranon par Aadharit* (Lucknow: UP State Archives, Department of Culture, 1998), 26–34.
18. Trivedi, *Smriti Ke Prishth*, 34.
19. Michel Foucault, 'The Crisis of Medicine or the Crisis of Antimedicine?' trans. Edgar C. Knowlton Jr, William J. King and Clare O'Farrell, *Foucault Studies* 1 (December 2004): 5–19, available at https://rauli.cbs.dk/index.php/foucault-studies/article/view/562/607 (accessed on 2 July 2019).
20. Foucault, 'The Crisis of Medicine', 13.
21. Ibid., 13–14.
22. For details on the multifarious functions performed by the cadre of the IMS, see D. G. Crawford, *A History of the Indian Medical Service, 1600-1913* (London: W. Thacker & Co., 1913–14), 2 vols, and Crawford, *Roll of the Indian Medical Service, 1615–1930* (London: W. Thacker & Co., 1930). Additionally, for the racial biases and predilections prevalent in the IMS and the consequent nationalist demand for its Indianisation and subsequent colonial reactions, see Rai, 'Indianisation of the Indian Medical Service'.
23. For details on this theme, see Samiksha Sehrawat, *Colonial Medical Care in North India: Gender, State and Society, c. 1840–1920* (New Delhi: Oxford University Press, 2013). Sehrawat clearly shows that there was an underlying intent of the colonial government to keep the expenditure on medical infrastructure at its lowest. According to Sehrawat, this, in turn, left a colonial legacy of poor medical provision, regional disparities, neglect of rural patients, and over-reliance on the private and voluntary sectors—all issues with contemporary resonance in India.
24. 'Dispensaries and Hospitals', Serial No. 45, Bundle No. 45, 1865, Commissioner's Office Records, Fyzabad, Regional Archives, Allahabad (emphasis added).
25. Ibid.
26. 'Grants-in-aid to Civil Hospitals and Dispensaries in the North Western Provinces and Oudh', F. No. 78, S. No. 14, Box No. 25, 1895, Commissioner's Office, Allahabad (Post-mutiny Records), Regional Archives, Allahabad.

27. In fact, the colonial government always refrained from the massive 'non-colonial' public investments. There was a belief that such investments were 'unfruitful' and 'undesirable' as it could demoralise private initiatives besides adding to the budgetary deficits and national debt. Commenting on this narrow conception of state in terms of financial management on public expenditure, Sabayasachi Bhattacharya argues that the colonial government was under the influence of the principles of Gladstonian finance with some minor adjustments in the case of military expenditure. For details, see Sabyasachi Bhattacharya, *Financial Foundations of the Raj: Ideas and Interests in the Reconstruction of Indian Public Finance 1858–1872* (Hyderabad: Orient Longman, 2005), 41–47. Adding to this, in the specific context of the colonial health expenditure, Mark Harrison argues that the colonial state's investment in expanding medical infrastructure in India was severely restricted by this sort of fiscal conservatism (see Harrison, *Public Health in British India*, 166–67).
28. 'Establishment of a New Civil Hospital at Allahabad for European Patients', F. No. 18, Serial No. 16, Box No. 285, 1868, Commissioner's Office, Allahabad (Post-mutiny Records), Regional Archives, Allahabad. (I owe knowledge of this file to Mr Ghulam Sarwar of the Regional Archives, Allahabad, who brought it to my notice.)
29. Ibid.
30. 'Medical Treatment of Sick Europeans', Serial No. 42, Bundle No. 52, 1870, Commissioner's Office Records, Fyzabad, Regional Archives, Allahabad (emphasis added).
31. Ibid. (emphasis added).
32. Ibid.
33. 'Rules for the Admission of Patients to the European Hospital, Allahabad', F. No. 65, Box No. 31, 1919, Medical Department, Uttar Pradesh State Archives, Lucknow (hereafter UPSA).
34. For rules related to the admission of patients to these European hospitals, see the Appendix 1.
35. For details on Hakim Ajmal Khan, see Chapter 2 of the present work.
36. Guy N. A. Attewell, *Refiguring Unani Tibb: Plural Healing in Late Colonial India* (Hyderabad: Orient Longman, 2007), 152–53.
37. Attewell, *Refiguring Unani Tibb*, 158.
38. It was yet another example of the construction of a communal identity by extracting sacred symbols and spaces out of their context and developing around these symbols/spaces an idiom and a specialised vocabulary so as to express the vision of a 'politically constructed community' and to subsequently mobilise it around these erstwhile sacred symbols/spaces often in opposition

to the 'other' community—a practice which was as such quite pronounced in the late nineteenth and early twentieth century United Provinces. For details on this phenomenon of construction of a community around erstwhile sacred symbols and spaces, especially in the United Provinces, see Sandria B. Freitag, *Collective Action and Community: Public Arenas and the Emergence of Communalism in North India* (Berkeley: University of California Press, 1989).

39. *Sudhanidhi* 2, no. 3 (March 1912–13), 169.
40. For details on national vs. communitarian concerns of late colonial Unani discourse of the United Provinces, see Seema Alavi, *Islam and Healing: Loss and Recovery of an Indo-Muslim Medical Tradition, 1600-1900* (Ranikhet: Permanent Black, 2007), 321-27. However, contrary to the efforts of the All India Vaidya Sammelan and Anjuman-i-Tibia, Kerala exhibited a unique example of Muslim Ayurvedic practitioners. In Malabar, we find distinctive families of hereditary 'Muslim' vaids who had been practising traditional Ayurveda for several generations. For example, the Changampally family settled in Malappuram district. The vaids belonging to this Muslim family were considered to be the masters of *Ashtangahrdayam* and were experts in orthopaedics. Another such family of hereditary 'Muslim' vaids was the Peringattu-thodi family. In the year 1917, vaids of this family also established Peringattu-thodiyil Mammy, Alavi & Company, Vaidyashala for manufacturing Ayurvedic medicines. According to Menon, most of these families probably converted to Islam following the invasion of Malabar by Tipu Sultan in the last decades of the eighteenth century. However, the manner in which these families maintained their hereditary profession and their continued association with the study of Ayurveda and Sanskrit, is indicative of the fact that such pre-modern religious conversions were in many cases highly personal matters. See Indudharan Menon, *Hereditary Physicians of Kerala: Traditional Medicine and Ayurveda in Modern India* (London and New York: Routledge, 2019), 144-45.
41. This was true both for Ayurveda and Unani. However, for the present purpose, the focus is on Ayurveda.
42. For discussion on the transformation of healing traditions into well-organised healing 'systems', see Jean M. Langford, *Fluent Bodies: Ayurvedic Remedies for Postcolonial Imbalance* (Durham: Duke University Press, 2002); Attewell, *Refiguring Unani Tibb*; and Projit Bihari Mukharji, *Nationalising the Body: The Medical Market, Print and Daktari Medicine* (London: Anthem Press, 2009).
43. David Arnold, 'Plurality and Transition: Knowledge Systems in Nineteenth Century India', unpublished paper presented at The Princeton History of

Science Seminar, October 2003, available at http://www.princeton.edu/~hos/Workshop%20I%20papers/Arnold%20History%20of%20Science%20paper.htm (accessed on 23 May 2019).
44. Leslie, 'The Professionalising Ideology of Medical Revivalism'; Leslie, 'The Modernisation of Asian Medical Systems'; Leslie, 'The Ambiguities of Medical Revivalism'.
45. Leslie, 'The Ambiguities of Medical Revivalism', 365–66.
46. K. N. Panikkar, 'Indigenous Medicine and Cultural Hegemony: A Study of the Revitalisation Movement in Keralam,' *Studies in History* 8, no. 2, 1992, 283–308.
47. See Alavi, 'Unani Medicine in the Nineteenth Century'; Quaiser, 'Politics, Culture and Colonialism'; Liebeskind, 'Arguing Science'; Attewell, *Refiguring Unani Tibb*; Sivaramakrishnan, *Old Potions, New Bottles*; Sharma, *Indigenous and Western Medicine*; Berger, *Ayurveda Made Modern*.
48. For discussion over modernity and its impact on medical practices and healing traditions in the colonies, see 'Introduction' of Biswamoy Pati and Mark Harrison, eds., *Society, Medicine and Politics in Colonial India* (London and New York: Routledge, 2018), 1–15.
49. It should be noted that earlier training of vaids and hakims mostly took place through the institution of family.
50. 'Bogus Medical Institution in India', F. No. 52–66, 34-H, Health Branch, Education, Health and Land Department, 1934, National Archives of India (NAI).
51. Ibid.
52. Other examples of such institutions were The Royal College of Homeopathy, Gwalior, and International Medical College, Calcutta. 'Bogus Medical Institution in India', F.No. 52–66, 34-H, Health Branch, Education, Health and Land Department, 1934, NAI.
53. 'Memorial from the All India Ayurvedic and Unani Tibbia Conference against the Medical Registration Act, 1912', F. No. 50/Part B, Medical Branch, Home Department, January, 1914, NAI.
54. *Vaidya Sammelan Patrika* 4, nos 7–9 (July–September 1934), 198–99.
55. For details on post-dyarchic administrative arrangements and emerging need for registration of 'indigenous' medical practitioners, see the section on 'The Colonial Government and the 'Indigenous' Medical Discourse' of the present chapter. The lack of uniform training of 'indigenous' medical practitioners, shifting allegiances and opinions of various factions involved in decision-making, and resistance of district boards dragged this matter of registration of vaids and hakims for almost two decades following the introduction of

dyarchic structure of governance under the Montagu–Chelmsford reforms of 1919. Rachel Berger has particularly delineated this dyarchic moment of Ayurveda in the United Provinces (see Berger, *Ayurveda Made Modern*, 106–27).

56. Kaviraj Pratap Singh, *Nikhil Bharatvarshiya Ayurveda Mahamandal ka Rajat Jayanti Granth* (Benares: Mahashakti Press, 1936), 2: 105.
57. 'Provincial Legislation—United Provinces Indian Medicine Act, 1939', F.No. 46-26, Health Branch, Education, Health and Land Department, 1939, NAI.
58. Anil Kumar, 'The Indian Drug Industry under the Raj, 1860–1920', in *Health, Medicine and Empire: Perspectives on Colonial India*, eds Biswamoy Pati and Mark Harrison (New Delhi: Orient Longman, 2001), 356–85.
59. Sharma, *Indigenous and Western Medicine*, 115.
60. Sujata Mukherjee, 'Ayurvedic Medicine in Colonial Bengal: Challenge and Response', in *India's Indigenous Medical Systems: A Cross-Disciplinary Approach*, eds Syed Ejaz Hussain and Mohit Saha (New Delhi: Primus, 2015), 108.
61. For details on medical entrepreneurship, see Sharma, *Indigenous and Western Medicine*, 105–46.
62. K. N. Panikkar, *Culture, Hegemony, Ideology: Intellectuals and Social Consciousness in Colonial India* (New Delhi: Tulika, 1995), 175.
63. Similar was the case with the United Provinces where treatment of snake bite was generally carried out by low-caste healers known as *bhagat*.
64. Pati, *Situating Social History*, 18.
65. Ayodhya Prasad Bhargava, *Santati Shastra* (Benares City, 1923), 252–54.
66. However, one should always note that even the Indian practitioners of Western medicine were trying hard to 'nationalise' or to make their healing practices less alien in multiple ways. In other words, one should not overemphasise the distinction between 'alienness' of Western medicine and 'indigeneity' of Ayurevda, as has been discussed in the previous section as well. For an interesting narrative of how the Indian practitioners of Western medicine were nationalising their profession, see Mukharji, *Nationalising the Body*.
67. *Sudhanidhi* 40, no. 7 (1 April 1949).
68. Gyan Prakash, *Another Reason: Science and Imagination of Modern India* (New Jersey: Princeton University Press, 1999), 5.
69. Girindranath Mukherjee, *History of Indian Medicine, Vol. 3* (New Delhi: Munshiram Manoharlal Publications Pvt. Ltd., 2003), 2.
70. Hardiman, 'Indian Medical Indigeneity', 270. However, communal overtones can be seen in this treatise as it argues that 'Hindu' medicine, that is, Ayurveda,

reached its greatest glory at the time of the Ramayana and Mahabharata, but had declined with the coming of the 'Muslim' rule and the patronage extended by it to Unani Tibb.

71. However, an interesting anecdote here is of the National Medical Store, Lucknow, which complicates the idea of 'national' medicine. This is the store established by Dr Zafar Husain in the Chowk area of Lucknow in the early twentieth century. This medical store sold (and still sells) exclusively allopathic medicines (*angrezi dawai*). After Dr Zafar Husain, the ownership of the store was passed on to his son Dr Nasir Husain. The fact that both Zafar Husain and Nasir Husain were doctors themselves makes this entire story interesting. Being medical practitioners themselves, both of them must be aware of the politics of 'national' medicine, especially keeping in mind the politics of health and healing in the United Provinces. Still the Husain family not only managed to run a shop by the name of 'National Medical Store' in the first half of the twentieth century, but also laid such a strong foundation that it survives till today, which is in itself remarkable. We have little idea how much opposition they might have faced from vaids and hakims of the province over the name of the medical store claiming itself to be 'national' but selling exclusively allopathic medicines. (Details about the store are based on an interview by the author with Ahsan Husain, Lucknow, India, 14 April 2014). Ahsan Husain belongs to the fourth generation of the Husain family and is the present owner of the National Medical Store. Interestingly, unlike his grandfather and great-grandfather, Ahsan Husain does not hold any professional degree in medical treatment and humorously considers himself as just an 'employee of the shop'.) Here once again the work of Projit Bihari Mukharji (*Nationalising the Body*) is significant as it explains the futility of dichotomous explanation of 'national' vs 'alien/colonial' healing system while discussing Ayurveda and Western medicine.

72. Sharma, *Indigenous and Western Medicine*, 147–48. See the advertisement of Beecham Pills where the advertiser used the picture of Union Jack (national flag of the United Kingdom) along with a phrase 'The National Flag and the National Medicine'.

73. 'Extract from the Proceedings of the Indian Legislative Council Assembled under the Provisions of the Government of India Act, 1915; Resolution Re-Placing the Ancient and Indigenous Systems of Medicine on a Scientific Basis', F.No. 38-50/Part A, Medical Branch, Home Department, July 1916, NAI.

74. 'General Note by the Director-General, Indian Medical Service, on Medical Development for India Generally', F. No. 9-31/Part A, Medical Branch, Home Department, April 1913, NAI.

75. Phanishwar Nath 'Renu', *Maila Anchal* (New Delhi: Rajkamal Paperbacks, 2013), 56.
76. Berger, *Ayurveda Made Modern*, 107.
77. Apparently, the Board of Indian Medicine turned into the apex advisory body to the United Provinces' medical department on issues pertaining to 'indigenous' medicine. It consisted of prominent but lower-level Indian Civil Service members and reputed vaids and hakims of the province. Incidentally, as Rachel Berger argues, the colonial insistence on balancing the numbers of vaids and hakims constituting the Board drew sharper lines between Ayurveda and Unani as the entire logic of balancing reflected the implicit belief that among 'indigenous' healing systems Ayurveda was for Hindus and Unani was for Muslims (see Berger, *Ayurveda Made Modern*, 108). Unfortunately, the Congress ministry, which came to power in 1937 in the United Provinces, carried the same faulty premise of communal affliations of healing practices while launching its ambitious scheme of opening subsidised dispensaries of 'indigenous' medicine in the rural areas.
78. 'Employment of Hakims and Baids by Local Bodies', F. No. 75-77, Medical Branch, Home Department, June 1907, NAI (emphasis added).
79. 'Legislative Assembly Proceedings—Unani and Ayurvedic Systems of Medicine', F. No. 53-104, Health Branch, Education, Health and Land Department, 1935, NAI.
80. 'Scheme for Grants to District Boards for Subsidies to Private Registered Medical Practitioners to Afford Medical Relief in Rural Areas', F. No. 522, Box No. 12, 1924, Medical Department, UPSA.
81. For detail on this scheme of establishing subsidised dispensaries of 'indigenous' medicine by the Congress ministry in the United Provinces, see Chapter 2 of the present book.

2

Indian National Congress and the Late Colonial Ayurvedic Movement

The official nationalist response to 'indigenous' medicine was largely constituted by the Indian National Congress and its leaders. Vaids and hakims often pushed their demands through their sympathisers like Hakim Ajmal Khan and Madan Mohan Malviya into the mainstream nationalist discourse of the Indian National Congress. Their broader argument was that '[I]f we want to take the administration of government into our own hands, we must right all national things, including the indigenous method of healing. Our real progress depends on these things. We fail in serving our country if we are dependent on outside things.'[1] In this regard, the formation of the Congress ministries in the provinces under the Government of India Act, 1935, was an important landmark. This was largely because health was the subject which appeared in the state list and hence the Congress ministries wielded effective powers in matters related to public health and in patronising healing systems. In the light of this, being basically a populist government, the Congress ministry in the United Provinces took several decisions which favoured the Ayurvedic practitioners and Ayurvedic pharmacies over Western system of healing. However, populist decisions at this front brought further challenges which have been delineated in this chapter in detail. Besides, this chapter also looks at the views expressed by some prominent nationalist figures—Hakim Ajmal Khan, Mahatma Gandhi and Govind Ballabh Pant—all of whom were associated with the Indian National Congress, on Ayurveda/'indigenous' medicine. The opinion of these individuals was significant keeping in mind both the short-term and the long-term impact of their ideas on the Congress-led nationalist movement.

THE INDIVIDUALS AND THEIR IDEAS ON AYURVEDA: AJMAL KHAN, MAHATMA GANDHI AND GOVIND BALLABH PANT

For nearly the first three decades of the twentieth century, Hakim Ajmal Khan was the chief torchbearer of the movement related to the revival of 'indigenous' medicine. Commenting on his pioneering contribution in the field of 'indigenous' medical movement, Barbara D. Metcalf states that he almost single-handedly made traditional medicine an integral part of the repertoire of nationalist political symbols.[2] Ajmal Khan was associated both with the Muslim League as well as the Congress, and was an influential figure in national politics. Going beyond the official line of the Congress party, which was focussing largely on the Indianisation of medical profession,[3] Ajmal Khan emphasised on the complete overhauling of the healing system. It was through the constant efforts of people like him that the Indian National Congress eventually recognised the claim of 'indigenous' systems of medicine and passed a resolution at its thirty-third session in December 1918, stating:

> Recognising the comparatively dominant prevalence of the Ayurvedic and Unani systems of medicine in India and their undeniable claims to usefulness this Congress strongly recommends to the Government of India the eminent desirability of taking definite steps to secure to them the advantages vouchsafed to the western system under the present administrative policy of the Government.[4]

Being himself a practitioner of 'indigenous' medicine, Ajmal Khan realised the importance of political associations as necessary for medical men to further their interests.[5] That is why he made constant attempts to bring all the practitioners of 'indigenous' medicine under one roof through organisations like the All India Ayurvedic and Unani Tibbi Conference.[6] However, as delineated in Chapter 1, the hakims of Lucknow disagreed with Hakim Ajmal Khan on various issues, particularly in his pursuit of aligning Unani with Ayurveda. Responding to them, at the second session of the All India Ayurvedic and Unani Tibbi Conference at Lucknow in November 1911, Ajmal Khan categorically stated:

> Whatever you wish to do for the country, nation or religion, you have to face the opposition. The Tibbi Conference also seems to be involved in it. You are perhaps, aware that the *Tabibs* and *Vaids* are desirous of functioning separately…but as you know the Conference aims at awakening both of them to work together…Both of you should, therefore, work together and work incessantly in this Conference which belongs to none but to your ownselves. I have firm faith that within a year or two your efforts will yield fruitful results.[7]

In fact, for Ajmal Khan, growing influence of Western system of medicine under the patronage of colonial state was the primary concern which required immediate attention of both vaids as well as hakims. Hence, he concentrated on waging a unified resistance against Western medicine. Here, his style of resistance matched the ideal moderate nationalist kind of politics, at least till 1910. However, in the later part of his life he drifted apart and openly came out against the colonial health policies, particularly in the wake of medical registration acts passed by various provincial governments in the second decade of the twentieth century.

Nevertheless, his anti-colonial stance nowhere made him the blind follower of orthodox traditional learning in the field of 'indigenous' medicine. Ajmal Khan was a firm advocate of modernising 'indigenous' healing systems so that they could provide effective remedies for curing the ills of the people. He, along with his brother Hakim Abdul Majeed Khan, had been making efforts in this regard since as early as 1892 when the Muhammedan Educational Conference met at Delhi. As the secretary of its reception committee, Ajmal Khan urged the patrons and practitioners of Unani system of medicine to respond to the changing needs of the time by making necessary changes.[8] Ajmal Khan also made a tour of Europe in 1911 whereby he visited important medical centres and hospitals of the West and met renowned physicians to learn the process of modernisation in the field of medicine.[9] The establishment of the Ayurvedic and Unani Tibbia College at Delhi in 1921 through diligent efforts of Ajmal Khan was a high point in this direction of modernising 'indigenous' healing systems in a collaborative fashion.

Unfortunately, in the 1920s, vaids and hakims throughout north India actively participated in communal polarisation of their respective professions and society at large. This was a serious blow to the efforts of leaders like Ajmal Khan who had been working to unite the 'indigenous' practitioners of both the religious camps in their fight against Western medical practice. 'Indigenous' healing practices which were envisaged by Ajmal Khan as the representatives of pluralistic culture of India eventually turned into symbols around which communal polarisation could take place.

Between the 1920s and the 1940s, Mahatma Gandhi also took keen interest in issues related to health and medicine. Interestingly, despite being champion of the cause of 'swadeshi' in every walk of life, Gandhi's critique of Western medicine or allopathy was mostly on ethical grounds,[10] otherwise on many occasions he found the Western system worthier than the contemporary state of 'indigenous' systems of healing—Ayurveda and Unani. In one of his letters, he even praised allopathy and considered it as an all-inclusive system.[11] He was of the opinion that '[I]f allopathy rids itself of the worship of mammon, which has overtaken most human activities and could *exclude vivisection and other (such) practices which I call black*, and liberally took advantage of the new methods discovered by lay people, it would become all-satisfying and quite inexpensive.'[12] Further, he went on to state: 'I am driven by the conclusion that allopathy, although it has great limitations and much superstition about it, is still the most *universal* and *justifiably* the most popular system.'[13] In another of his letters to the ailing Vallabhbhai Patel who had resorted to Ayurveda, Gandhi categorically stated: 'I have not much faith in Ayurveda. The vaids do not master their subject.'[14] Also, even if he criticised vivisection, vaccination, etc., all of which were an integral part of Western system of medicine, Gandhi always considered it as his 'individual' opinion. In fact, in some of his letters he even suggested people to get vaccinated if they did not have religious apprehensions about it.[15] Further, on certain occasions, Gandhi found himself obliged to use allopathic drugs instead of Ayurvedic as he found nothing so efficacious as quinine for malaria or iodine for simple pains or Condy's fluid as a disinfectant.[16]

However, all this is not to argue that Gandhi was the advocate of Western system of medicine and was antithetical to the Ayurvedic movement. In fact, Gandhi was critical of the Ayurvedic practitioner's lack of spirit of enquiry, a spirit which he found in the allopathic practitioners. Gandhi felt that although 'indigenous' medicine did accept a relationship between the body and soul, it lacked the spirit of enquiry which fired Western medicine to keep pace with the new challenges and gave it a contemporary relevance. That is why in his speech at the inauguration of the Ayurvedic and Unani Tibbia College[17] at Delhi in 1921, while he criticised modern medicine for the lack of humanitarian values, he equally condemned the Ayurvedic practitioner's apathy towards the spirit of enquiry:

> I would like to pay my humble tribute to the spirit of research that fires the modern scientists. My quarrel is not against that spirit. My complaint is against the direction that the spirit had taken. It has chiefly concerned itself with the exploration of laws and methods conducing to the merely material advancement of its clientele. But I have nothing but praise for the zeal, industry and sacrifice that have animated the modern scientists in the pursuit after truth. *I regret to have to record my opinion based on considerable experience that our hakims and vaids [do] not exhibit that spirit in any mentionable degree.* They follow without question formulas. They carry on little investigation. *The condition of indigenous medicine is truly deplorable.* Not having kept abreast of modern research, their profession has fallen largely into disrepute. I am hoping that this college will try to remedy this grave defect and restore Ayurvedic and Unani medical sciences to its pristine glory. *I am glad, therefore, that this institution has its western wing.*[18]

Gandhi reiterated similar viewpoints in his speeches at the Ayurvedic Pharmacy, Madras,[19] and the Ashtanga Ayurveda Vidyalaya, Calcutta. According to Gandhi, there was a time when he used to swear by Ayurvedic medicine and used to recommend it to all his friends, who had gone for Western medicine, to go to the Ayurvedic practitioners. But he soon got disillusioned by the sorry state of Ayurveda and Unani as physicians belonging to these systems lacked sanity and humility. He was severely critical of vaids' claim that mere feeling of the pulse could enable them to understand whether the patient was suffering from appendicitis or some such other disease. He found such diagnostic methods, as practised by vaids and hakims, false and incomplete in most of the cases.[20] In fact, in one of his letters to Vallabhram Vaidya, Gandhi went on to claim, 'Ayurveda has not yet become science. In a science there is always room for progress. Where is any progress here?'²¹

Such views of Gandhi on Ayurvedic practitioners attracted the ire of many prominent vaids of the time. In fact, Gananath Sen, the famous vaid from Bengal, sought clarification from Gandhi regarding his position vis-à-vis Ayurveda after his controversial speech at the Ashtanga Ayurveda Vidyalaya, Calcutta. Replying to him, Gandhi made it clear that he was not against Ayurveda as such, rather he was critical of the way Ayurvedic practitioners were conducting themselves, that is, their lack of humility and the absence of a spirit of enquiry.²² Thus, on several occasions Gandhi emerged as the 'internal critique' of the contemporary state of Ayurvedic system of healing. The very fact that he accepted the invitations to inaugurate and to deliver speeches at the institutions meant for propagating Ayurveda shows that he was not at all antithetical to the healing system itself, rather he found himself duty-bound to show the vaids and hakims the mirror regarding their limitations and shortcomings. Had he been absolutely hostile to the Ayurvedic movement, he would not have accepted these invitations.

Furthermore, Gandhi never endorsed the typical claim of the practitioners of 'indigenous' medicine, whereby they held the colonial regime responsible for the decline of 'indigenous' systems of medicine. According to Gandhi, Ayurveda could not be saved either by money or by the state. He believed that it was only through '*yajna*', which implied ceaseless selfless devotion and labour of vaids, that Ayurveda could be rescued. That is why Gandhi was critical of the exorbitant fees charged by eminent vaids like Gananath Sen.²³ Reiterating this, in his response to the letter of Brijlal Nehru who had condemned the colonial government and its lack of patronage for the decline of Ayurveda, Gandhi argued that

> I am unable to subscribe to the condemnation of the state for not providing institutions for research. I have always blamed the vaid's apathy in the matter of real research. The top ones are busy making money. The others are too ignorant to do so or are easily satisfied with what they find in the orthodox Ayurvedic books. I am sorry for this view. I come to it, in spite of my great regard for the Ayurvedic system and Unani which are suited to the soil.²⁴

In the same letter, Gandhi further stated that 'My love of nature cure and of indigenous systems does not blind me to advance that western medicine has made in spite of the fact that I have stigmatised it as black magic.'[25]

In fact, Gandhi was the advocate of bringing together the 'goods' of all the three systems—Ayurveda, Unani and Western medicine. He believed that such union of the three systems would result in a 'harmonious blending and in purging each of its special defects'.[26] Furthermore, it is interesting to look at the correspondence between Gandhi and Vallabhram Vaidya within whom he found his ideal of 'satyagarhi scientist' in the field of medicine. He wished Vallabhram to make Ayurveda as cheaper as possible through constant exploration and research. He even advised Vallabhram to tour the Himalayas and collect medicinal herbs.[27] In one of his letters guiding Vallabhram, Gandhi stated: 'You should show, if you can, that indigenous medicine is simple, inexpensive and capable of giving relief to 99 patients out of a hundred. If you feel that this cannot be done, then you should give up the profession.'[28] Meanwhile, keeping this in mind, Gandhi experimented with 'nature cure' as well. Actually, Gandhi wanted everybody to be his or her own doctor. In general, he was against the very profession of 'medical practitioner', be it of any system, as all of them in his opinion solely focussed on gaining money and neglected the 'soul' and 'self-control'.[29] That is why he continuously insisted on 'nature cure'. Nevertheless, frustrated by his attempts to develop a 'cohesive' and 'humane' system of healing and despite his advocacy and personal love for nature cure, Gandhi, on the eve of independence, in his letter to Sankaran, stated that 'Of course some harm has been done by allopathy, but the benefits are obvious. Otherwise there could never have been so many hospitals. *Allopathy suits well the present atmosphere.*'[30]

Another Congress leader whose stance on 'indigenous' medicine becomes significant especially in the context of the United Provinces is Govind Ballabh Pant. Born in present-day Uttarakhand, Pant was an influential figure in contemporary United Provinces. Unlike Ajmal Khan and Gandhi, Pant engaged with the issue of 'indigenous' medicine more pragmatically than ideologically. For him, medical relief was one of the fundamental requirements of the masses which needed to be fulfilled by the government. In this pursuit, he found 'indigenous' medicine handy in the Indian context on account of its inexpensiveness and easy availability, especially in the countryside. It was this pragmatic aspect which attracted Pant towards Ayurveda. While speaking at the Legislative Council of the United Provinces on the importance of 'indigenous' medicine, Pant clearly stated:

> Apart from other considerations I think the question of financial limitations is so very difficult to get over that we cannot do except by adopting these indigenous systems even for State purposes. The Board of my district, Naini Tal, had to replace two of the dispensaries this year, one by a *vaid* and the other by a *hakim*, simply because we could not find money to finance the dispensaries there if they were to run on allopathic lines, so the State ought to give every possible assistance to these systems.[31]

Besides the popular pressure of vaids and hakims, probably it was because of the cost-effectiveness of these systems, as envisaged by Pant, that the Congress ministry headed by him, in 1938, introduced the ambitious scheme to open subsidised dispensaries of 'indigenous' medicine throughout the province in order to extend the rural medical facilities.

Pant expressed similar opinion in his address to the Association of Surgeons in India in December 1952:

> Research in modern methods is no doubt very necessary for progress, but regard is also to be paid to very important factor of making the fruits inexpensive and available for the poorest in the land who stand in need of medical attention. *The indigenous system has this feature that attracts.* Research in perfecting this system that was founded on solid basis is also necessary, and I hope surgeons will also pay due attention to this aspect of the question.[32]

However, Pant at the same time never overlooked the shortcomings which shrouded the contemporary state of 'indigenous' medicine. In his speech at the legislative council, Pant stressed on the necessity of upgrading the texts/treatises used by the practitioners of these systems. According to Pant, 'it is necessary that we must revise the books on the subject and that they should be framed as to be more in line with the universally accepted views on anatomy, etc.'[33] Similarly, like Gandhi, Pant was also critical of tall and false claims made by the 'indigenous' practitioners of the time regarding their system of healing. As for instance, just like Gandhi, Pant also admonished the claims made by vaids that they could diagnose diseases merely by examining the pulse. Pant categorically stated:

> Whether there was any rational and scientific basis for such phenomena and whether there was invariable symptom of the disease discernible in the beat of the pulse I cannot say, but *if there was any such science at any time it has now disappeared and there is hardly any chance of it being rediscovered in the environment of a modern university*.[34]

Thus, Pant's views on medicine were more pragmatic and balanced. The significant feature of Pant's stance on medicine, which makes him different from other Congress leaders, was that he addressed the grievances of both the allopathic and 'indigenous' practitioners equally. That is why besides praising 'indigenous' medicine for its cost-effectiveness and easy availability, Pant kept on raising pertinent issues related to the 'native' practitioners of Western medicine as well. Time and again he voiced his position against the racial discrimination in medical services in India[35] and argued in favour of the need for more grants to mofussil hospitals,[36] etc. In other words, considering health and healing as a pragmatic necessity, Pant tried to overcome the prevailing contradictions among healing systems for the larger benefit of the masses.

PROMOTING AYURVEDIC PRACTITIONERS AND PHARMACIES: THE CONGRESS MINISTRY OF 1937–39

Following the withdrawal of the Civil Disobedience Movement, a major debate ensued amongst the Congress leadership regarding the future roadmap of the nationalist struggle. One of the contexts for the debate was provided by the Government of India Act, 1935, based on extended franchise. Although there was no dissension over the issue of fighting elections, it was the aftermath of the election that saw some contentious issues being raised. What was to be done if the Congress got a majority in a province? Should it accept the ministerial portfolios or not? Jawaharlal Nehru, Subhash Chandra Bose and the Congress socialists were opposed to the idea of 'office acceptance' as it might lead to the dilution of nationalist struggle by taking away its revolutionary zeal. For them it was 'surrender' before imperialism. However, the counter-strategy was in the line of the *Swarajists*, that is, entering the assemblies with a view of creating deadlocks and to make the working of the Act impossible. For them 'office acceptance' did not lead to co-option by the colonial regime, rather it was a way to defeat the colonial strategy. Nonetheless, for the time being, both the wings decided not to create split inside the Congress, and to fight the elections with full zeal, postponing the trickier decision on 'office acceptance' to the post-election period.[37]

After the elections in 1937, the Congress got an absolute majority in Madras, Orissa, Bihar, Central Provinces and United Provinces, and a near majority in Bombay. Such a massive mandate toned down the 'anti-ministerialists', including Nehru. The Gandhian strategy of Struggle–Truce–Struggle (S–T–S),[38] as envisaged by historians like Bipan Chandra, also favoured the formation of ministries by the Congress as it was not in a condition to raise another mass movement on a grand scale after the withdrawal of the Civil Disobedience Movement. Thus, as argued by Sumit Sarkar, electoral success strengthened and soon made irresistible pressures for ministry-formation by the Congress. This led to the defeat of Jayprakash Narayan's proposal of 'total rejection' of office, in favour of Rajendra Prasad and Vallabhbhai Patel's proposal of 'conditional acceptance' of office by 135 votes against 78 at the All India Congress Committee session of March 1937.[39] Under this scheme, a Congress ministry headed by Govind Ballabh Pant was formed in the United Provinces.

Interestingly, once the ministries were formed, they did not follow the older Swarajists' line of halting the progress of each and every legislation, thereby making the working of the Act almost impossible; rather the Congress ministries assumed more or less the shape of a 'populist government'. The Congress took it as an opportunity to show the masses glimpses of 'future India' under the Congress rule. Hence, it tried to win over each and every section/class often by making contradictory but popular decisions, thereby consolidating its mass base. From the very beginning, the Congress knew that the ministries were going to be a short-term affair and hence it did not have much problem in adjusting mutually contradictory class interests, as it never allowed the dust to settle down through the rapidity of its popular decisions.

The 28 months of Congress rule was quite a short period to put the Congress under any serious difficulty for its contradictory promises and decisions. However, towards the latter part of the Congress ministries, complications did emerge and the medical front was not an exception. Nonetheless, very soon the Congress ministries resigned, thereby shifting the focus of criticism again towards the colonial regime. Let us now examine the complications faced by the Congress ministry, with a special reference to the United Provinces, vis-à-vis the Ayurvedic revivalist movement and the long-term consequences of the 'populist decisions' taken by the Congress regime on this front.

In 1938, the Congress government of the United Provinces decided to promote 'indigenous' systems of healing. In this regard, S. P. Shah, secretary to government, United Provinces, issued a letter on 15 February 1938 to all the commissioners of divisions and to all the chairmen of district boards of the United Provinces. In order to bring medical aid by qualified practitioners of the Ayurvedic and Unani systems of medicine within easier reach of the rural population, in this letter the government proposed to introduce immediately a scheme designed to encourage the establishment of *aushadhalaya*s and *dawakhana*s (dispensaries pertaining to Ayurvedic and Unani systems of healing, respectively) and for settling vaids and hakims at suitable centres in the rural areas, both under a system of government subsidies.[40] This was reversal of the policy adopted by the colonial government during the 1920s which emphasised the encouragement of private medical practitioners of allopathy to settle down in villages for practice through the grant of medical subsidies and the supply of medicines from public funds in order to extend medical relief in the rural areas.[41]

The allotment made available for this scheme for the year 1938–39 was set at Rs 37,500 by the provincial government. Hence, it was unlikely that any district could be allotted more than Rs 2,000. However, once the district boards received this letter, they turned very enthusiastic towards the aforesaid proposal. District boards of Allahabad and Gorakhpur made an extravagant demand of 30 subsidised dispensaries (of 'indigenous' medicine) each of which was outside the budget allotted for each district. In fact, so overwhelming was the response that, according to an estimate, in order to fulfil all the demands the government needed more than thrice the money proposed in the budget. The total estimated annual expenditure on the basis of proposals received from various district boards was Rs 125,837 (Figure 2.1), whereas the proposed grant under the scheme was just Rs 37,500.

---

225 Ayurvedic and Unani dispensaries at Rs 450 each: Rs 101,250
17 'A' class vaids and hakims at Rs 405 each: Rs 6,885
36 'B' class vaids and hakims at Rs 270 each: Rs 9,720
Plus Rs 90 more in one case where district board could not meet even 1/4th of the cost (Jaunpur district): Rs 90

Lump sum demands from district boards:
Mainpuri: Rs 1,200
Hardoi: Rs 2,000
Jaunpur: Rs 4,692

Total: Rs 125,837

Figure 2.1: Estimated annual expenditure on the basis of proposals received from various District Boards[42]

This mismatch generated another inconclusive debate in the official circle, that is, whether the 400 to 500 centres, where the government proposed to start rural development work, were all to be provided with some form of medical relief and public health, or a smaller number of centres should be selected for this purpose.[43] Evidently, the government was in no position to meet all the demands. However, it proceeded with the scheme with whatever meagre funds it had at its disposal and provided subsidy to open several aushadahalayas and dawakhanas in different districts throughout the province.

Once the scheme was implemented, it brought several other complications which had long-term consequences for the ongoing movement for 'indigenous' medicine. To begin with, this very scheme further deepened the communalisation of healing systems in the United Provinces as the very first thing the government had to decide was the number of aushadhalayas (dispensaries pertaining to Ayurvedic healing system) and dawakhanas (dispensaries associated with Unani healing system) to be established under this scheme. At the same time, it was also to be determined at which place an aushadhalaya was to be established and where a dawakhana was to be founded. To resolve this issue, communities came to be identified as preferring a particular healing system. According to a report prepared by the local self government department, United Provinces, there were very few Hindus practising as hakims, while no Muslims were known to practise Ayurveda. The same report stated that 'in a few of the north-western districts and round about Lucknow both the systems are almost equally popular, but in the rest of the province *Hindus, especially in villages, take to Ayurvedic treatment, while Muslims go to hakims* if at all they are available.'[44]

Thus, by the late 1930s, the divide was not so much between 'indigenous' and allopathic practitioners;[45] rather it was more between 'Hindu' vaids and 'Muslim' hakims. Hindus and Muslims hardly availed themselves of training in 'opposite' system. Hence, suggestions were made during this time that since in the countryside population is mostly Hindu and people take more easily to Ayurvedic treatment, requirements of the locality should be taken into consideration and about 80 per cent of the subsidised rural dispensaries which had been proposed by the government (vide 15 February 1938 order) should be Ayurvedic dispensaries or aushadhalayas.[46] The government eventually sanctioned the opening of 146 Ayurvedic and only 46 Unani dispensaries in rural areas (a ratio of 3:1).

Consequently, in the official circles, communities were identified as preferring/belonging to a particular healing system, that is, Hindus with Ayurveda and Muslims with Unani. It should be noted that such implicit belief that Ayurveda was for Hindus and Unani was for Muslims first crept into the official health discourse of the province as early as the 1920s when, in response to the changing medical needs of the government personnel in post-dyarchic period (that is, after the instituialisation of the Montagu–Chelmsford reforms), the colonial government resorted to take into consideration the services of 'indigenous' medical practitioners. Sharper lines were drawn by the colonial government between vaids and hakims with insistence on balance while drafting its policy on 'indigenous' medicine. Subsequently, ramifications of the colonial politicisation of communal consciousness in the province impacted 'indigenous' medical discourse as well in the 1920s and the 1930s.[47]

Nevertheless, what is significant here is that this sort of communalisation of healing practices got deepened not only because of colonial policy of 'divide and rule'; rather it was also because of the decision taken by the government headed by the Indian National Congress to promote 'indigenous' medicine by opening subsidised aushadhalayas and dawakhanas. According to Rachel Berger, identification and association of the healing systems with specific communities in the official circle led to the dwindling of investment in Unani medicine throughout the 1940s as it was supposed to cater to only the minority community, that is, the Muslims.[48] While the number of schools, dispensaries and clinics staffed by vaids deploying Ayurveda mounted, the number of hakims and Unani institutions, even if they did not dwindle, certainly remained static. This, according to Berger, mirrored 'the growing disenfranchisement of Muslims in the province'.[49] Thus, Berger tries to link the marginalisation of Unani as a healing system with the broader marginalisation of the Muslim community on the whole in the province as 'second class' citizens in the communally charged atmosphere of the 1940s.

However, it is debatable whether the Indian National Congress really intended to deepen the communal division of healing systems under the majoritarian pressure of 'Hindu' vaids or it was just a negative consequence of the half-baked policy decision. In fact, pragmatically, the fewer number of registered Unani practitioners with the Board of Indian Medicine was also one of the reasons behind the imbalanced ratio of proposed aushadhalayas and dawakhanas. The number of registered hakims was far less than that of vaids.[50] In this situation, the officially sanctioned 3:1 ratio between aushadhalayas and dawakhanas seems a pragmatic compulsion and not a deliberate attempt to marginalise Unani/hakims/Muslims. Nevertheless, one thing is clear: the very idea of identification of a community open only to a particular healing system was faulty at its conception and was bound to deepen the communal division of healing systems in the long run, with the balance being tilted towards the majority community and its 'preferred' healing system.

Further, the above-mentioned government scheme to open subsidised dispensaries of 'indigenous' medicine required a proper list to be drawn of all the 'qualified' and 'genuine' vaids and hakims active in the United Provinces. This necessity eventually culminated in the United Provinces

Indian Medicine Act, 1939, which has been discussed in detail in Chapter 1. As argued, the clauses of this Act were such that it weaned out a large chunk of vaids and hakims who had received their training through non-institutional means, that is, through apprenticeship or family. In fact, this scheme created clear-cut distinctions not only between institutionally trained 'new' vaids/hakims and traditional hereditary practitioners of 'indigenous' medicine and folk healers, but also within 'new' vaids/hakims as well. The latter division was because of the decision to put institutionally trained vaids/hakims under two classes—Class 'A' and Class 'B'. According to the scheme, while those who passed out from the Ayurvedic College, Banaras Hindu University, Benares, and Tibbiya College, Muslim University, Aligarh, were supposed to be registered as Class 'A' vaids/hakims immediately after passing their respective degrees, the diploma holders of the Rishikul Ayurvedic College, Haridwar; State Aided Unani Medical School, Lucknow; and Unani Medical School, Allahabad were entitled to be registered as Class 'B' vaids/hakims.[51] Also, it was stated that those in 'A' category should be preferred in appointments under the extension of rural medical facilities scheme.

This categorisation bore discontent within the 'new' vaids/hakims later on. As for instance, in 1940, students of the Rishikul Ayurvedic College, Haridwar (who were entitled to Class 'B' registration), filed a petition against the preference given to the students of Ayurvedic College, Banaras Hindu University.[52] This added a new dimension to already variegated late colonial Ayurvedic movement.

Another pressing requirement which came on surface with the introduction of the above-mentioned scheme of extension of medical facilities in rural areas was the need for identifying 'genuine' pharmacies producing Ayurvedic and Unani drugs from where one could get supply of 'authentic' medicines and drugs for the proposed aushadhalayas and dawakhanas. This, in turn, brought forth the competition among the Ayurvedic pharmacies of the United Provinces on a new escalated level. In May 1938, the Congress government of the United Provinces directed the Board of Indian Medicine to draw a list of institutions and pharmacies which prepared Ayurvedic and Unani medicines for sale to the general public. In December 1938, the Board of Indian Medicine came up with the list of following six Ayurvedic and Unani institutions and pharmacies for the aforesaid purpose:[53]

- Ayurvedic Pharmacy, Hindu University, Benares
- Rishikul Ayurvedic College Pharmacy, Haridwar
- Ayurvedic Rasayanshala, Ayurvedic and Unani Tibbi College, Delhi
- Ayurvedic Pharmacy, Kashi Ras Shala, Gyanvapi, Benares
- Hindustani Dawakhana, Delhi
- Unani Dawakhana, Allahabad

It should be noted that two of the pharmacies in the list were from outside the province—Ayurvedic Rasayanshala and Hindustani Dawakhana. While the government for the time being accepted the claims of these two pharmacies from outside the province, it clearly stated to the Board of Indian Medicine that from now onwards no other Ayurvedic or Unani pharmacy situated outside the United Provinces should be considered for the present purpose.[54] Later on, the Board of Indian Medicine prepared an extensive district-wise list of 'genuine' Ayurvedic and Unani pharmacies, which has been given in Appendix 3.

Now, there were many pharmacies which failed to make an entry into this esteemed list of 'genuine' Ayurvedic and Unani pharmacies, including some really renowned ones such as Stri Aushadhalaya, Allahabad; Sudhanidhi Pharmacy, Daraganj, Allahabad; and Mahashakti Aushadhalya, Benares. In fact, in the archives, we do not have any correspondence of these renowned Ayurvedic pharmacies requesting to incorporate them into this 'esteemed' list of 'genuine' pharmacies. This was probably because these were already well-established pharmacies dispensing Ayurvedic medicine and had a large clientele on their own. In contrast, many small Ayurvedic pharmacies strived hard to get into this list often by supplying misleading information. Actually, there were cases when the Board of Indian Medicine had to strike off the names of some of the pharmacies as they failed to meet the demands placed before them; for example, the Indian Dawakhana (a Unani pharmacy) of Lucknow.[55]

Further, this scheme of drawing up the list of 'genuine' pharmacies led to several other problems as well. Pharmacies which failed to get into the list started questioning the wisdom of the government by wailing about those pharmacies that had been enlisted by it. In fact, on occasions where there were more than one pharmacy in the same area and while one of them managed to get into the list and the other(s) could not, this mutual rivalry became bitter. This often led to mutual defamation and demands of re-consideration. For example, in one such case, a vaid from Sitapur claimed that his pharmacy was better than the one enlisted.[56] In fact, there were a flood of applications, so much so that the government found it difficult to check the claims of all the applicants.

Further, when some of the renowned pharmacies were not placed in the initial list drawn by the Board of Indian Medicine, these pharmacies got offended. As for instance, Gurukul Kangri Pharmacy, whose name was missing in the first list, lamented over the government's decision and took it as a mark of disrespect for the institution and medicines produced by it. To quote the letter sent by the Gurukul Kangri Pharmacy:

> *Aap ko yeh gyat hi hai ki humare Ayurvedic College se sambaddha ek vrihat Ayurvedic Pharmacy hai jo pichhle pandrah varshon se desh bhar mein Ayurvedic aushadhiyon ka prachar va prasar karne mein lagi huyi hai. Humara toh yeh bhi daava hai ki Sanyukt Prant mein kisi sarvajanik sabha ki sab se unnat pharmacy hai jo vrihat pariman mein Ayurvedic aushadhi taiyar karti hai. Aap ko swayam bhi vyaktigat roop se humari is prasiddhi ka pata hai, kintu humein yeh jaan kar dukh hua hai ki pichhle dinon Sanyukt Prantiya sarkar ne apne dehati chikitsalayon ke liye jin pharmaciyon ke naam manjoor kiye hain un mein Gurukul ki pharmacy ka naam nahin hai. Is se na keval janata mein humari sanstha ka anadar hota hai apitu Ayurvediya aushadhiyon ke nirman mein humara jo utsah hai usey bhi dhakka pahunchta hai. In dinon dehat sudhar ke chikitsalayon mein Ayurvediya aushadhiyan kray ki ja rahi hain aur humein ummeed hi nahin nishchay hai ki aap dehat sudhar vibhag ke adhikariyon ko yeh spasht hidayat kar denge ki kam-se-kam is subey ke Merrut Rohilkhand, Agra aur Kumaon division ke chikitsalayon mein sab aushadhiyan Gurukul Kangri se hi mangayenge.*[57]

(Sir, as you know, we have an impressive Ayurvedic pharmacy, associated with the Ayurvedic College, which has been devoted to propagate Ayurvedic medicines since the last 15 years. We further claim that this is the most advanced public pharmacy producing Ayurvedic medicines at such a grand scale in the United Provinces. You are yourself aware of the popularity of our pharmacy; still we regret to find that the name of our pharmacy is missing from the list of the pharmacies drawn by the United Provinces government under the rural welfare scheme. This not only brings utter disrespect to our institution, but also demoralises us in our pursuit of manufacturing Ayurvedic medicines. We are not just hopeful but are assured that you would take a quick look into this matter and would order that at least the dispensaries located in Merrut Rohilkhand, Agra and Kumaon divisions would receive Ayurvedic medicines exclusively from the Gurukul Kangri Pharmacy.)

The Congress government was quick to recognise the substantial reputation of the Gurukul Kangri and immediately ordered to include its name in the subsequent list drawn for the aforesaid purpose.

Furthermore, there was also an ensuing struggle between the pharmacies on the 'permanent' and the 'provisional' lists. Those pharmacies which were placed in the 'provisional' list (drawn after preliminary enquiry) kept on sending letters to the government seeking place in the 'permanent' list so that they could have 'the same status as enjoyed by those associated with other affiliated institutions'.[58] In fact, after some time, a suggestion was made to drop the provisionally approved list altogether to stop the inflow of applications which were seeking entry into 'permanent' list merely based on 'subjective opinions' that they were better than the other pharmacies that were 'provisionally' approved. It was suggested that the government should prepare only one list after making extensive enquiries. However, the government found itself in a difficult position largely because, first, it did not have enough inspectors to make extensive surveys/enquiries, and second, dropping of 'provisional' list, it was felt, would lead to widespread discontent as some of the pharmacies enlisted in the 'provisional' list were quite well-known in their respective areas.[59]

However, the problem was not merely of listing. The actual problem started subsequent to this exercise. On 20 April 1940, in a letter sent to the director of public health, United Provinces, the Mool Chand Rastogi Trust Aushadhalaya of Lucknow (which was one of the entrants in the 'esteemed' list of 'genuine' pharmacies) lamented that

> [I]t appears that during the last year a number of firms have been brought on the approved list [of 'genuine' pharmacies]. Some of these firms have submitted tenders which are abnormally low. Without any desire to cast any reflections upon such firms, we may be permitted to submit that in the absence of common pharmacopoeia there is every probability of cheap and inefficacious medicine being supplied to the local bodies.[60]

This implies that there were instances where a particular pharmacy furnished extremely low figures in order to grab the tender of supplying Ayurvedic medicines to the subsidised dispensaries, thereby giving tough competition to the well-established pharmacies. The low bid could lead to supply of sub-standard medicines in the absence of any standard pharmacopoeia to reap profits. Hence, in order to ensure better control of the 'genuineness' of medicines to be supplied to local bodies, the Mool Chand Rastogi Trust Aushadhalaya came up with various suggestions such as compiling of a common pharmacopoeia, restricted use of patent medicines and devising some mechanism to check the 'genuineness' of the medicine supplied (for details, see Appendix 4).

Thus, enlisting of 'genuine' Ayurvedic and Unani pharmacies opened up a kind of Pandora's Box and the government did not have enough infrastructure and resources to resolve the consequent complications.

CONCLUDING REMARKS

Immediately after the Congress ministries resigned in October/November 1939, the colonial government passed certain orders that disappointed the vaids and hakims. For instance, in a government order issued by the medical department, United Provinces, vaids and hakims were restricted from issuing certificates of age, health and fitness or leave to the government servants. The same order also hampered the medico-legal works performed by vaids and hakims. They were no longer authorised to issue injury certificates in criminal cases or to tender expert's evidence in court. At the same time, vaids and hakims were told not to perform cholera and plague inoculations or vaccinate people.[61] In fact, when the Board of Indian Medicine Scholars' Association, Rishikul Ayurveda Mahavidyalaya, Haridwar, submitted a petition in this regard to Dr Panna Lal, advisor to the United Provinces Government, the government responded by stating:

> The question of permitting vaids and hakims to issue medical certificates to government servants was considered, and in connotation with the IGCH (Inspector general of civil hospitals) and DPH (department of public health) it was directed not to give them this right, nor the right of performing medico-legal work or inoculations of plague and cholera, as *the vaids and hakims,*

barring exceptions, are neither so well qualified nor so reliable as to be entrusted with these responsible duties.[62]

In fact, Schedule II of the Registration Rules for the practitioners of 'indigenous' medicine, which was passed by the Congress government, had imparted vaids and hakims the right to issue certificates to employees of local bodies. However, the colonial government believed that it should also be withdrawn as it had come to the notice of the government that persons with no qualification, and even boys of 14–19 years of age, had been issued registration certificates by the Board of Indian Medicine.[63] All this was taken by the colonial government as a handy pretext for denying vaids and hakims any extension of their privileges.

Thus, the entire issue of 'indigenous' medicine in the late 1930s and the 1940s got heavily politicised at the level of the health administration with the 'coming' and 'going' of the Congress government. It attracted multiple opinions ideologically, administratively and commercially. However, much before the era of the Congress ministry, at the level of discourse, the issue of 'indigenous' medicine had already got entangled in the larger biopolitics and discourses on caste, class, community and gender in the United Provinces, which has been dealt with in detail in the following two chapters.

NOTES

1. Hakim Ajmal Khan, writing in the Annual Report of the Tibbia College, 1920; cited in Barbara D. Metcalf, 'Nationalist Muslims in British India: The Case of Hakim Ajmal Khan', *Modern Asian Studies* 19, no. 1, 1985, 20.
2. Metcalf, 'Nationalist Muslims in British India', 4.
3. Being basically a party of urban professionals (at least until the beginning of the Gandhian phase of the nationalist struggle), the Indian National Congress in the initial phase raised its voice mostly against the 'apartheid' which was being followed in the medical profession in general and the IMS in particular. It should be noted that although the doors of IMS were thrown open to Indians ever since the introduction of competitive examinations for recruitment in the IMS (that is, from January 1855 onwards), by 1905 only 5 per cent of the IMS men were of Indian origin (see Jeffery, 'Recognising India's Doctors', 310). For further details on the nationalist demand for the Indianisation of

the IMS and subsequent reaction of the colonial officials and government, see Rai, 'Indianisation of the Indian Medical Service', 826–32.
4. See 'Memorandum', F. No. 174-175/B, August 1926, Health Branch, Education, Health and Land Department, NAI.
5. In fact, Metcalf views the political activities of Hakim Ajmal Khan as an inevitable outgrowth of his efforts devoted to reversing the tide of cultural decline in the field of medicine (Metcalf, 'Nationalist Muslims in British India', 4).
6. With the object of seeking widespread recognition for 'indigenous' healing practices and to forge unity among its practitioners, Hakim Ajmal Khan convened the first meeting of the All India Ayurvedic and Unani Tibbi Conference in Delhi in 1910 which was attended by as many as 300 vaids and hakims from different parts of the country. For detailed description of the conference, see Zafar Ahmad Nizami, *Hakim Ajmal Khan* (New Delhi: Publications Division, 1988), 33.
7. Cited in Nizami, *Hakim Ajmal Khan*, 33–34.
8. Ibid., 19.
9. Ibid., 34.
10. Gandhi's firm convictions regarding non-violence restricted him to accept Western system of healing in its contemporaneous form, largely because vivisection was the integral part of this system which did not go hand-in-hand with his idea of non-violence.
11. 'Letter to T. Titus, April 4, 1933', in *The Collected Works of Mahatma Gandhi* (hereafter *CWMG*), 3rd revised edn (New Delhi: Publication Division, 2000), 60: 270–72.
12. 'Letter to T. Titus', 271 (emphasis added).
13. Ibid. (emphasis added).
14. 'Letter to Vallabhbhai Patel, August 31, 1941', *CWMG*, 81: 43.
15. See 'Letter to Dudhbehn V. Desai, February 26, 1934', *CWMG*, 63: 225; and 'Letter to Satish Chandra Das Gupta, February 19, 1933', *CWMG*, 59: 325.
16. See 'Letter to Gangadhar Shastri Joshi, July 19, 1927', *CWMG*, 39: 253.
17. It was established through the efforts of Hakim Ajmal Khan.
18. 'Speech at Opening of Tibbi College, Delhi, February 13, 1921', *CWMG*, 22: 342 (emphasis added).
19. 'Speech at Ayurvedic Pharmacy, Madras, March 24, 1925', *CWMG*, 31: 33–34; 'Speech at Ashtanga Ayurveda Vidyalaya, Calcutta, May 6, 1925', *CWMG*, 31: 280–83.
20. 'Speech at Ashtanga Ayurveda Vidyalaya', 282.
21. 'Letter to Vallabhram Vaidya, June 28, 1942', *CWMG*, 83: 60.

22. 'Ayurvedic System, June 11, 1925', *CWMG*, 31: 460-62.
23. 'Letter to Vallabhram Vaidya', 60.
24. 'Doctors Criticised, Aug 4, 1946', *CWMG*, 91: 415.
25. 'Doctors Criticised', 415.
26. 'Speech at Opening of Tibbi College', 342.
27. 'Letter to Vallabhram Vaidya, March 20, 1941', *CWMG*, 80: 120.
28. 'Letter to Vallabhram Vaidya, May 28, 1942', *CWMG*, 82: 340.
29. See M. K. Gandhi, *Hind Swaraj*, 17th reprint (Ahmedabad: Navjivan Publishing House, September 2005), 50-52.
30. 'Letter to Sankaran, July 21, 1947', *CWMG*, 96: 98 (emphasis added).
31. Govind Ballabh Pant, 'On Indigenous System of Medicine, April 4, 1924', in *Selected Works of Govind Ballabh Pant* (hereafter *SWGBP*), ed. B. R. Nanda (Delhi: Oxford University Press, 1994), 2: 34-35.
32. Govind Ballabh Pant, 'Importance of Research in Medical Science, Dec. 1952', *SWGBP*, 2001, 14: 281 (emphasis added).
33. Pant, 'On Indigenous System of Medicine', 35.
34. Govind Ballabh Pant, 'On Suggestion for Synthesis of Allopathy and Ayurveda, 1948', *SWGBP*,2000, 13: 253 (emphasis added).
35. Govind Ballabh Pant, 'Racial Discrimination in Medical Service, March 15, 1928', *SWGBP*, 1995, 4: 257-60.
36. Govind Ballabh Pant, 'Need for More Grants to Mofussil Hospitals, March 21, 1925', *SWGBP*,1994, 2: 219-21.
37. Bipan Chandra, Mridula Mukherjee, Aditya Mukherjee, Sucheta Mahajan and K. N. Panikkar, *India's Struggle for Independence* (New Delhi: Penguin Books, 1989), 319-22.
38. Chandra et al., *India's Struggle for Independence*, 313.
39. Sumit Sarkar, *Modern India: 1885-1947* (Delhi: Macmillan, 1983), 350.
40. 'Payment of Grants for Subsidised 'Dawakhanas' and 'Aushadhalayas' during 1939-40', F. No. 155, Box No. 82, 1938, Medical Department, UPSA. For principal features of this scheme for establishing subsidised dispensaries of 'indigenous' medicine, see Appendix 2.
41. 'Scheme for Grants to District Boards for Subsidies to Private Registered Medical Practitioners to Afford Medical Relief in Rural Areas', F.No. 522, Box No. 12, 1924, Medical Department, UPSA.
42. 'Payment for Grants for Subsidised 'Dawakhanas' and 'Aushadhalayas',' UPSA.
43. See the letter by S. P. Shah, secretary to government, United Provinces; written to the minister, local self government, United Provinces, dated 10 June 1938, in 'Payment for Grants for Subsidised 'Dawakhanas' and 'Aushadhalayas'', UPSA.

44. 'Scheme for Medical Relief in Rural Areas', F. No. 337, Box No. 85, 1938, Medical Department, UPSA (emphasis added).
45. In fact, vaids and hakims by this time had started demanding supply of allopathic equipments and were also dispensing drugs pertaining to Western medicine besides the drugs belonging to their 'own' respective systems. Thus, the boundary between the 'indigenous' and allopathic systems of medicine was getting blurred on ground (For details, see 'Vaids and Hakims', F. No. 428, Box No. 99, 1940, Medical Department, UPSA).
46. 'Scheme for Medical Relief in Rural Areas', UPSA.
47. For details on this theme, see Berger, *Ayurveda Made Modern*, 106–27.
48. Rachel Berger, 'From the Biomoral to the Biopolitical: Ayurveda's Political History', *South Asian History and Culture* 4, no. 1, 2013, 61.
49. Berger, 'From the Biomoral to the Biopolitical', 61.
50. 'Vaids and Hakims', F. No. 428, Box No. 99, 1940, Medical Department, UPSA.
51. For details on how 'A' and 'B' class category was determined, see Schedule II of the Registration Rules, 1939, 'Vaids and Hakims', F. No. 428, Box No. 99, 1940, Medical Department, UPSA,.and/or the letter of secretary, Board of Indian Medicine, to superintendent, Medical Department, Civil Secretariat, United Provinces, in 'Scheme for Medical Relief in Rural Areas', UPSA.
52. 'Vaids and Hakims', UPSA.
53. 'List of Approved Ayurvedic and Unani Pharmacies in U.P.', F. No. 226, Box No. 83, 1938, Medical Department, UPSA.
54. Ibid.
55. See the letter from Sir Wazir Hasan, chairman, Board of Indian Medicine, United Provinces, to the under secretary to government, Medical Department, United Provinces (dated 30 December 1940), in 'List of Approved Ayurvedic and Unani Pharmacies in U.P.', UPSA.
56. 'List of Approved Ayurvedic and Unani Pharmacies in U.P.', UPSA.
57. Ibid.
58. See the letter sent by the secretary, Lalit Hari Ayurvedic College, Pilibhit, to the secretary to the United Provinces Government, Medical Department, Lucknow (dated 5 October 1942), in 'List of Approved Ayurvedic and Unani Pharmacies in U.P.', UPSA.
59. 'List of Approved Ayurvedic and Unani Pharmacies in U.P.', UPSA.
60. Ibid.
61. This is interesting as earlier whenever the government needed (such as during epidemics) it often enrolled vaids and hakims, keeping in mind their hold on the rural mass, to perform vaccination.
62. 'Vaids and Hakims', UPSA (emphasis added).

68. Three such cases from Meerut had been sent to the district magistrate for enquiry and report, whereas one such case was being sent separately to AGD with suggestions to punish the culprits and to make suitable amendments to the Registration Rules (for details, see 'Vaids and Hakims', UPSA).

3

Creating an Ayurvedic Discourse
Print, Organisation and Mobilisation

As argued earlier, by the late nineteenth and early twentieth century a substantial Ayurvedic discourse came up, propagating Ayurveda and its 'inherent' merits vis-à-vis the 'other' systems of healing. The present chapter delineates the ways and means through which this Ayurvedic discourse emerged in the public sphere in the specific context of the United Provinces. While doing so, this chapter also throws light on how the entire Ayurvedic discourse, right from its very beginning, got trapped into cynical tendencies exhibiting upper-caste/-class and community-oriented biases (to be discussed in greater detail in Chapter 4). At the same time, it also brings out the differences in terms of work ethics between the 'traditional' hereditary vaids and the 'new' vaids.

To begin with, print, organisation and mobilisation were the three crucial factors which created an Ayurvedic discourse in the late nineteenth and early twentieth century. Ayurveda and its utility were debated and discussed in public forums and attempts were made to obtain for it the 'due' place and the necessary patronage that it 'rightfully deserved'. Simultaneously, this drive also sought to 'standardise' and 'universalise' the Ayurvedic healing system by doing away with the extant differences of opinions over treatment methods, training and approach towards the subject. In this regard, desperate efforts were made to give all the practising vaids a 'corporate' 'unified' identity having uniformity of thought, opinions and ideals. Publication of several Ayurvedic journals and tracts, establishment of the All India Vaidya Sammelan and the United Provinces Vaidya Sammelan, institutionalisation of Dhanvantari Mahotsava, etc., were part and parcel of this pursuit of creating an Ayurvedic discourse having universalising tendencies.

AYURVEDA IN PRINT

Numerous Ayurvedic journals, magazines, books, advertisements and conference papers ran into print during this period. There were more than 25 Ayurvedic journals, published predominantly in Hindi, which came out from almost every part of the United Provinces during the first half of the twentieth century (see Appendix 5). Out of these, there were many which remained in print only for a few years or for one or two decades, but they contributed significantly in building the Ayurvedic discourse of the time. There were journals such as *Vaidya, Dhanvantari, Anubhoot Yogmala* and *Jeevan Shakti* which were mouthpiece journals of the related Ayurvedic dispensaries.[1] Besides, there were many journals which were launched by the 'new' vaids for the promotion of their own products. In other words, a whole lot of 'vaid-cum-editors' emerged in the United Provinces during this period.

Some of the representative figures of the aforesaid lot were Jagannath Sharma, Jagannath Prasad Shukla, Yashoda Devi, Pandit Kishori Dutt Shastri, and so on. Based in Allahabad, Rajvaidya Jagannath Sharma was a prolific writer and was founder of the *Prayag Samachar*. He also wrote various volumes of *Arogya Darpan* in the 1890s. Similarly, Jagannath Prasad Shukla started an Ayurvedic magazine in 1909 entitled *Sudhanidhi* and was also associated with the *Ayurveda Mahasammelan Patrika* (or *Vaidya Sammelan Patrika*). Yashoda Devi, the famous woman Ayurvedic practitioner from the United Provinces, also wrote and edited several volumes and journals on Ayurveda. She was the founder of Stri Shiksha Pustakalaya located in Allahabad and was editor of the only Ayurvedic journal devoted exclusively to women and children, entitled *Stri Chikitsak*. Pandit Kishori Dutt Shastri was the editor of the famous Ayurvedic journal *Chikitsak* which came from Kanpur. Shankar Lal Gupt (*Vaidya*), Shandilya Dwivedi (*Ayurveda Pracharak*), Rupendranath Shastri (*Rakesh*) and Rameshwar Mishra (*Ayurveda Keshari*)[2] were few other names in this long list of 'vaid-cum-editors' hailing from the United Provinces.

Besides these periodic journals, there were numerous books on Ayurveda which came into circulation in the late nineteenth and early twentieth century United Provinces. For example, different volumes of *Arogya Darpan* by Pandit Jagannath Sharma (Allahabad), *Vaidyak Sar* by Hazari Lal (Benares, 1910), *Arogya Mandir* by Pravasi Lal Verma (Benares, 1927), *Chikitsa Chandrodaya* by Babu Haridas Vaidya (Agra, 1935), *Auspargic Rog* by Ayurvedacharya Bhaskar Govind Ghanekar (Benares, 1937) and various books by Yashoda Devi. Some of the Ayurvedic texts were written in the verse form as well; for example, *Vaidya Priya* by Jawahir Singh Shrivastava (Naval Kishore Press, Lucknow, 1924). Some of the famous publishing houses of the United Provinces publishing Ayurvedic and health related tracts during this period were Ganga Granthagar (Lucknow), Stri Shiksha Pustakalaya (Allahabad), Naval Kishore Press (Lucknow), Mahashakti Sahitya Mandir (Benares) and Sudhanidhi Press (Allahabad).

Alongside, there were public polemics and conference papers of organisations like the All India Vaidya Sammelan (which held its various sessions in the United Provinces)[3] and the United Provinces Vaidya Sammelan which came to life during this period. These often contained the speeches and viewpoints of some of the renowned Ayurvedic professionals of their time. Supplementing this organised literary sphere, there were numerous advertisements and pamphlets by individual vaids and Ayurvedic medical stores appearing regularly in journals and newspapers like *Abhyudaya* (Allahabad), *Aj* (Benares) and *Saraswati* (Allahabad), and towards the end of the Ayurvedic tracts.

Rachel Berger has viewed this entire Ayurvedic print culture as an integral part of making of the urban middle class in north India in the first half of twentieth century.[4] Taking cue from Bayly[5] and Orsini,[6] who have talked about the assertion of the upper-caste/middle-class Hindu self through print creating a distinct community identity and assigning for themselves a culturally hegemonic role, Berger has argued that medical writings were crucial to identity formation in the United Provinces. 'Indigeneity' and 'Hinduness' of the Ayurvedic healing system provided a discrete identity to urban middle class of the province and Ayurveda became 'a banner heading for any non-allopathic medicine practised by Hindus'.[7]

In fact, as delineated by Charu Gupta, the number of printing presses in the United Provinces went up from 177 in 1878–79 to 568 in 1901–02 and 743 in 1925–26. Moreover, by 1925–26, the United Provinces had surpassed Bengal in the production of vernacular books.[8] Medical writings made up a large part of this thriving 'print public culture'. Interestingly, the authorship of these writings was not just confined to 'experts', rather the writers varied from Ayurvedic professionals to nationalist elites to antiquarian zealots to 'great patrons'[9] of 'indigenous' knowledge. Explaining this multiplicity of authorship which was widely prevalent in Ayurvedic print culture, Berger points out that '[D]espite the strict government control over who could and who could not practice, there was more flexibility in the publishing world to speak authoritatively about medicine; scientific information coupled with ideological leaning could construct authority'.[10]

However, this multiplicity of authorship eventually became an issue of concern for the universalising tendency which was unleashed with the establishment of the All India Vaidya Sammelan. The leaders of the Sammelan constantly advocated the publication of 'standardised' Ayurvedic tracts that were to be supervised by the Sammelan itself. The mushrooming of Ayurvedic tracts invoking Charaka and Sushruta was a serious challenge for this standardisation drive. Publication of a 'standard' and the 'most authentic' version of ancient *Samhitas* and Ayurvedic pharmacopoeia was one of the priorities of the Sammelan. In the Fatehpur session of the Sammelan (1928), Vaidya Yadavji Trikamji Acharya[11] went on to propose the establishment of an Ayurvedic publishing company to collect, amend, standardise and publish the Ayurvedic tracts and remedies.[12] Similarly, Gananath Sen Saraswati,[13] in his presidential address of the twenty-first session of the Sammelan at Mysore (1931), emphasised the need for publication of 'correct' and 'carefully revised' edition of *Charaka Samhita, Sushruta Samhita* and other standard works for restoration and development of Ayurveda. Simultaneously, he also suggested constitution of the Text Book Committee to publish new text books on Ayurveda in Sanskrit or in Hindi.[14] Nonetheless, the mushrooming of 'popular' Ayurvedic tracts continued. Most of them were short, easy to consult, affordable, neatly divided into sub-headings and reader-friendly, having simple language. Commercial incentives also drove many vaids and even non-vaids and book houses to publish such user-friendly Ayurvedic tracts.[15]

Actually, newly endorsed print culture in many ways embodied the changed ethos or working methods of the Ayurvedic practitioners. Earlier, the prevalent Ayurvedic practice was to personalise the knowledge system and subsequently hide it from other vaids. However, 'new' vaids found this practice detrimental in revival and spread of Ayurveda. They blatantly advocated sharing of knowledge not only within the circle of practitioners but also with the common populace. They believed that it was only through such sharing of knowledge that people could be made to realise the effectiveness of Ayurveda both in medical and pecuniary terms. Even G. Srinivasmurthy, president of the nineteenth session of the All India Vaidya Sammelan (Nasik, 1929), exhorted the vaids to hold conference from time to time to exchange knowledge and clear doubts. He also advised that any new useful findings by anyone should be circulated among the professionals by publication in *Vaidya Sammelan Patrika* and other journals.[16] In a similar vein, emphasising on the sharing of useful knowledge by vaids, *Anubhoot Yogmala*, an Ayurvedic journal published from Etawah (United Provinces), in one of its editions stated (in verse form):[17]

Vyasani vyasan chhipate apna,
Chor chhipate chori ko.
Lobhi sadah chhupa ke rakhte,
Apni maya punji ko.
Dharmachari sadah chhipate,
Apni dharma-bhrashtata ko.
Vaidya chhipave kyon faldayi,
Satvar siddha prayogon ko.

(It is the practice among the addicts to hide their addiction, thieves to conceal their theft, greedy to cover their wealth and religious crooks to mask their moral corruption; however, there is no point in hiding the useful testified knowledge by a vaid.)

It was in this context that numerous 'vaid-cum-editors' came up during the period under discussion. Praising the crucial role played by these vaid-cum-editors in the promotion of Ayurveda, Jagannath Prasad Shukla in his *Ayurvedic Patron ka Itihas* (History of Ayurvedic Journals) wrote:[18]

> *Lakhat gunat samujhat sadah rakhi sampadak drishti,*
> *Jagat bharan-poshan karat kari karuna ki vrishti.*
> *Punya paap bhalmand shubh ashubh adi kartavya,*
> *Dae alochak buddhi puni nirnay daet subhavya.*
> *Samay samay ki baat pae dae shubh gyan prakash,*
> *Andolan ki siddhi aru ruchir marg aabhas.*
> *Pragatat sakal jahan mein nij mahima vistar,*
> *Karein poorna 'jagdish' soi ayurvedoddhar.*

(A vaid-cum-editor should always keep an eye over several things determining inherent merit and shortcoming of all of them. It is his duty to induce critical faculty and to continuously show the correct path in the broader benefit of the movement. By doing so, he would not only earn fame for himself, but would also lead the path for Ayurvedic revivalism by the grace of God.)

STREAMLINING THE AYURVEDIC DISCOURSE: THE ALL INDIA VAIDYA SAMMELAN AND THE UNITED PROVINCES VAIDYA SAMMELAN

In 1907, at Nasik, the first All India Vaidya Sammelan was held with the twin objectives of 'streamlining' and 'standardising' the Ayurvedic discourse/movement and to bring all vaids under one roof, thereby giving them a collective corporate identity. It strived to cater support for Ayurvedic revivalism both from the government and the common public. It was found that despite the presence of so many eminent vaids in the country and a substantial population resorting to Ayurveda and related practices, the Ayurvedic healing system had been continuously losing its ground vis-à-vis Western medicine. The internal dissensions amongst the vaids on methods of treatment, lack of uniform curricula and training, absence of standardised books, etc., were held to be the primary causes behind this loss. Highlighting this phenomenon, Ranchhor Das Kirtikar in his presidential address of the fifth session of the All India Vaidya Sammelan (Mathura, 1913) stated:

Bharatvarsha mein aise Ayurveda pundit hain, jo chikitsa karne mein bhi nipun hain; durbhagyavash ek doosre ki sahmati se sahmat nahin hote. Uska karan samaan pathyakram pranali nahin hai; mudrit, amudrit, pramanit, apramanit pustakein padhte hain. Apni apni raag ki dafli bajate hain, jis se Ayurveda ki pramanikta mein sandeh ho jata hai.[19]

(In India, there are so many eminent vaids who are able to treat efficiently, but unfortunately they do not agree with each other. The primary reason behind this is the lack of uniform curricula and reading of various published, unpublished, standardised and unauthenticated texts. All of them keep dancing to their own tunes, thereby making the authenticity of Ayurveda ambiguous.)

The All India Vaidya Sammelan along with its provincial units such as the United Provinces Vaidya Sammelan resorted to address these issues of 'uniformity' and 'standardisation'. Through its annual sessions, the Sammelan came to develop a standard Ayurvedic discourse related to the hitherto evolution and merits of Ayurveda and things to be done for its revival. Delineating the hitherto evolution of Ayurveda, many presidents of the Sammelan began by considering Ayurveda as 'eternal' and of 'no human origin'.[20] The great assemblage of sages at the foot of the Himalayas to learn the 'Science of Life' from Lord Indra and its subsequent transfer and redaction by various saints constituted the set template in this story of Ayurveda. Simultaneously, Ayurveda was viewed as an integral part of 'divine' and 'eternal' Vedic corpus. From here they often passed on to describe the contribution of Ayurvedic theories in the development of Graeco-Roman healing system with the Egyptian world as mediator. Subsequently, they talked about the vicissitudes of fortune faced by Ayurveda owing to the 'attacks' of Alexander, Scythians and Huns. The brief revival took place under the Guptas and the rulers like Vikramaditya; however, the growing prominence of Buddhism and its excessive emphasis on non-violence led to the great loss of the surgical branch of Ayurveda. Then came the 'worst' with the arrival of 'Muslim aggressors' like Mahmud of Ghazni and Ghori who allegedly destroyed a large part of already thinned Ayurvedic manuscripts. Eventually, the reign of Aurangzeb and after him a period of rapine and anarchy thoroughly undermined the Ayurvedic healing system.[21]

Subsequently, interesting is the way the Sammelan approached the reign of the British. While the British were often condemned of patronising Western medical system, the presidents of the Sammelan fascinatingly viewed the British rule, unlike the rule of the Muslims, as the one having regenerative potentialities for Ayurveda. It was in this regard that the Sammelan presidents often used the terms like 'Pax Britannica',[22] 'kind-hearted rulers', 'enlightened' or 'benign government' for the British rule.[23] This was largely because the government still continued to be the primary source both for patronisation as well as legitimisation of healing practices/systems.

In this regard, the complexity of 'indigenous' resistance against Western medicine can be seen in the way 'indigenous' practitioners were trying to fight back the influence of Western medicine. On the one hand, they were thrashing the Western system of medicine for its 'alien-ness' and 'colonial' motives; on the other hand, they were trying to derive sanctity from the 'colonial' government to authenticate their newly discovered medicines. Consequently, the colonial government and the administrative authorities remained a vital source of legitimacy even for the practitioners of 'indigenous' medicine at least for the first two decades of the twentieth century. One can find numerous petitions by the practitioners of 'indigenous' medicine during this period praying that their medicine should be given a trial to cure the concerned disease.[24] Similarly, the advertisements of 'indigenous' medicine often carried testimonials of some men of authority such as headmaster of a school, policemen or civil servant to buttress its claim of efficacy.[25]

Moreover, the Sammelan tried to organise vaids and turn them into a corporate unit having similarity of opinions. Emphasising on the need for unity amongst vaids, Jagannath Prasad Shukla[26] in his presidential address of the seventeenth session of the Sammelan (Patna, 1927) urged them to come together and raise their voice in unison.[27] Similarly, Gananath Sen in his presidential address of the twenty-first session of the Sammelan (Mysore, 1931) advised the vaids to 'inculcate fellow feeling amongst them and make mutual relations more sweet and sincere' and to strictly avoid 'vilification of each other'.[28] Further, invoking the '*Kid mantra*' he appealed to the vaids to unite and know the minds of each other.[29] This unity of voice was essential to make the claims of the Sammelan influential in front of the government and the common populace.

However, the Sammelan always had a hard time dealing with dissenting voices. In fact, the very occasion of the annual *sammelan* or conference itself became one of the potential sites of embodying dissent. Commenting on this, Pandit Thakur Dutt Sharma Vaidya in one of his articles wrote:

> Over the time considerable successive meetings of the All India Vaidya Sammelan have been held so far; several Ayurvedic journals have marked their presence in every nook and corner of the country; many Ayurvedic tracts have been produced; various lectures have been arranged; still the kind of unity amongst the vaids, which is needed for the real progress of Ayurveda, is missing. Although the Sammelan somehow manages to hold its sessions in some city or other, it subsequently increases the tensions and dissensions amongst the vaids locally. Jealousy is deep seated in the hearts of vaids and there are only few of them who take delight in the praise of their fellow practitioners. Everyone considers himself as great as Lord Dhanvantari and belittle the achievements of others.[30]

Thakur Dutt Sharma then went on to give an advisory, which goes as follows:[31]

- Vaids should never condemn each other.
- They should consult each other while treating patients. In case any vaid is unable to treat a patient, he should readily seek the help of other vaid and should secretively tell him the mistakes, if any, committed by him during treatment. The other vaid should open-heartedly help his fellow vaid and should not treacherously try to win over the patient to his own side as the patient still belongs to the first vaid.
- Every city should time-to-time hold a vaid sammelan or conference of its own where vaids can share their experiences. They should organise public lectures and should distribute small tracts related to public health. This would increase the prestige of both the vaids as well as Ayurveda in the eyes of the common public.
- Vaids should administer medicines prepared or owned by their fellow vaids as well if the need arises. If there are 20 vaids in a locality and all of them possess, besides general medicines, 10 special medicines of their own respectively, then each vaid should be considered to have

200 special medicines at his disposal. There should be a proper list regarding the special medicines available with each vaid, so that in case of need one can take it from his fellow vaid.
- Vaids should attend the conferences with compassion and an open heart. They should consider it as their duty to help each other and share their respective knowledge. It has often been seen that vaids attend Ayurvedic conferences out of their self-interest such as for public honour or certificate, failing which they either stop attending such conferences or start criticising such gatherings. This attitude is absolutely wrong and defeats the purpose of holding such annual conferences.
- Every vaid should contemplate over the ways and means to secure the rights of the entire community. If the rights of vaids would keep depleting like this, then time is not far when nobody would like to be a vaid or a hakim.

The above advisory clearly reveals the prevalent differences of opinions among vaids despite the constant efforts of the Sammelan.

Incidentally, in order to unite the vaids, the Sammelan occasionally invoked the communal discourse of 'us' and 'them' vis-à-vis the Unani system of healing so that a 'false consciousness'[32] of belonging to one community could be forged amongst the vaids. The Sammelan claimed for itself the role of being the sole spokesperson of the interests of the 'Hindu' vaids, and emphasised the difference between the interests of 'Hindu' vaids and 'Muslim' hakims. Not only this, the Sammelan also attacked the All India Ayurvedic and Unani Tibbi Conference, established by Hakim Ajmal Khan, for favouring hakims over vaids. The Sammelan lamented the dominance of hakims in the All India Ayurvedic and Unani Tibbi Conference. In one of the circulars issued in the *Vaidya Sammelan Patrika*, it deplored the fact that despite much of the funding of the All India Ayurvedic and Unani Tibbi Conference coming from vaids, it exhibited dominance of hakims.[33] Further, the Sammelan and its presiding vaids kept raising controversial issues like the 'dying Hindu race', 'cow protection' and 'Ayurvedic origin of Unani system' from its different platforms.[34]

Incidentally, in its efforts to streamline the Ayurvedic discourse, not only were the practitioners of the 'other' systems targeted by the Sammelan, but alongside the Sammelan tried to purge a number of folk healers and lay practitioners ('subaltern vaids') as well from within its fold. It was believed that in due course of time many people had entered the field of Ayurveda who did not possess the 'required' wisdom for this Vedic knowledge. They were more interested in reaping pecuniary benefits by making some panacea or through patenting any useful Ayurvedic drug.[35] According to the established vaids, although such lay practitioners/subaltern vaids did help in making Ayurveda popular, eventually they were unable to understand the 'profound secrets' of Ayurveda and their 'uncontrolled' presence would harm the prospects of Ayurveda in long run.

In fact, Dr Mhaskar, in his article 'Ayurveda ki Sadyah Sthiti' (Contemporary State of Ayurveda), went on to group these lay practitioners of Ayurveda with *mali* (gardener), *chamar* (leather worker), *nai* (barber), *dhobi* (washerman) and *burhi vidhwa* (old widow) as 'practitioners of *Kali* age'.[36] According to Dr Mhaskar, these lay practitioners by flipping through some of the Ayurvedic texts and through advertisements had brought themselves and Ayurveda into limelight. In the opinion of Mhaskar, although they had made Ayurveda popular and accessible to common mass, they were actually 'enemies' created by the Ayurvedic movement itself. They had been referred by Mhaskar as '*teesra dal*' or 'third party' which was very vocal in the Ayurvedic movement.[37]

As suggested, the two significant ways to control the growth of these lay practitioners/subaltern vaids were standardisation or institutionalisation of Ayurvedic training/education and the registration of vaids. The Sammelan and its presidents constantly emphasised on the aforesaid two things. With the aim to standardise Ayurvedic training/education throughout India, the Sammelan, during its third annual session at Allahabad (1911), established an 'Ayurvedic Vidyapith' to promote Ayurvedic education and to prescribe the syllabus for the same. Incidentally, for the Sammelan, which was overtly dominated by the 'new' vaids, standardised and systematic institutional training was also an essential pre-requisite to bolster its claim for the launch of the scheme of registration of vaids and other 'indigenous' practitioners on similar lines as registration of the allopathic practitioners by the government.[38]

However, to what extent such efforts of the Sammelan to wean out the lay practitioners were successful is debatable. The medical market continued to have such 'subaltern vaids' in a large number. In a letter sent to the editor of *Vaidya Sammelan Patrika*, Krishna Dutt Gupt lamented that there were many members from places like Aligarh and Ajmer in the Katni branch of the Central Provinces Ayurveda Mandal[39] who by funding the organisation and by passing the designated exams got the high sounding titles of *Vaidya Bhushan, Vaidya Visharad, Bhisagacharya, Vaidya Shastri, Vaidyaratna, Chikitsa Chakravarti,* and so forth. Some of them, in fact, had received even honorary titles by giving fund of Rs 2 to the organisation. According to Gupt, many of these *Vaidyaratnas* were originally grocery merchants, and some of them were engaged in grinding mills till recently.[40]

In the United Provinces, the provincial unit of the Sammelan, that is, the United Provinces Vaidya Sammelan, was quite active. In fact, some of the key founding members of the All India Vaidya Sammelan such as Kunwar Saryu Prasad Narayan Singh[41] and Jagannath Prasad Shukla[42] hailed from the United Provinces and were equally active in the United Provinces Vaidya Sammelan as well. The United Provinces Vaidya Sammelan forwarded the task of its parent organisation in many ways. It came to design a uniform syllabus for the Ayurvedic schools affiliated through the Board of Indian Medicine (United Provinces) and strived to establish its control over the selection of representatives of vaids and teachers being sent to the Board. The presence of orthodox caste, class and community-oriented politics of the United Provinces also provided a fertile breeding ground for the realisation of the visions of the Sammelan. In fact, the Unted Provinces Vaidya Sammelan managed to bring together zamindars, civil surgeons and professionals such as lawyers, teachers and professors as well within the fold of its activities/conferences, thereby strengthening the claims of the Sammelan.[43]

Thus, the All India Vaidya Sammelan along with its provincial units made desperate efforts to streamline the Ayurvedic revivalist discourse by resorting to an organisation and standardisation drive. It tried to give vaids a corporate identity united by common interests and thoughts. In fact, Jagannath Prasad Shukla, in his presidential address of the seventeenth session of the Sammelan (Patna, 1927), went on to view the Sammelan as the 'parliament' (*sansad*) and 'central government' (*vaidyon ki sarkar*) of the vaids of whole India and the provincial units of the Sammelan as 'provincial governments' (*prantiya sarkar*). Not only this, he also visualised the Ayurvedic world as its 'territory/empire' (*samrajya*) and the acceptance of the glory of Ayurveda and its influence on other medical systems as its 'colony' (*upnivesh*).[44]

MOBILISING THE VAIDS: *DHANVANTARI MAHOTSAVA*

An integral part of creation of an Ayurvedic discourse in late colonial India was the celebration of Dhanvantari Mahotsava. This was the celebration especially popularised by the All India Vaidya Sammelan and its provincial units. Kavita Sivaramakrishnan views it as a kind of 'corporate' festival which projected Dhanvantari as a common professional deity of Ayurvedic practitioners.[45] There are references to Dhanvantari in ancient Ayurvedic tracts. For instance, *Sushruta Samhita* delineates that it was through Lord Dhanvantari who appeared on the earth as Divodasa, the king of Kashi, that the 'Science of Life' or Ayurveda was passed on to human beings.[46] Other ancient texts such as *Ramayana* and *Mahabharata* also talk about Dhanvantari. According to the grand narrative of the aforesaid epics, Dhanvantari first appeared as a consequence of the mythical churning of the celestial ocean ksheer-sagar. It was he who carried the 'nectar' in his hand, which eventually became a bone of contention between the gods and the demons, followed by the deceitful act of gods and their consequent immortality.[47]

Nevertheless, despite all such references, there is hardly any evidence of Dhanvantari being hailed as god of the Ayurvedic practitioners prior to twentieth century. As argued by Sivaramakrishnan, the initial popularity of Dhanvantari as a professional deity of vaids and related celebrations was clearly because of the support and publicity it received from popular Ayurvedic journals and the leaders of the Vaidya Sammelan.[48] In other words, Dhanvantari Mahotsava became a classic case of the 'invention of tradition'[49] in the Indian context where ancient materials were invoked to construct a unique tradition for quite novel purposes. It forged collective consciousness and identity amongst the vaids and gave their movement a sacred aura.[50] It was celebrated every year in the month of *Karthik* (thirteenth day of *krishna paksha*) as per the Hindu calendar. When this festival was first celebrated is difficult to ascertain; however, its dramatic rise, especially in various townships of the United Provinces, deems it fit well within the category of an 'invented tradition'.[51]

Pujan and *havan* (worship rituals) were used to be conducted publicly at numerous places every year on this occasion. Besides, display of Ayurvedic medicines and public lectures were organised to share Ayurvedic knowledge. Further, in order to attract the masses, at certain places cultural programmes were also held.[52] Thus, the occasion became a mass contact programme for the Ayurvedic practitioners to make Ayurveda popular. Commenting on the significance of Dhanvantari as lord and Dhanvantari Mahotsava, Jagannath Prasad Shukla in his presidential address during the second session of the United Provinces Vaidya Sammelan (Hardoi, 1919) stated:

> *Isht ke bina Isht-siddhi nahin hoti, isliye vaidyon mein apne abhisht dev ka Isht hone ke sivay Adivaidya Bhagwan Dhanvantari ka Isht hona avashyak hai, is se unki aushadhiyon mein vilakshan shakti avegi, unka piyushpanitva badhega. Prativarsha pratyek nagar mein Shri Dhanvantari Mahotsava hona chahiye aur sarva sadharan mein Dhanvantari puja ka mahatva pratibimbit karna chahiye. Is avsar mein jo sahayata mile usey Ayurveda Mahavidyalaya ki sahayata mein bhejna chahiye.*[53]

(There cannot be devotion without a deity; that is why, it is essential for vaids to have Lord Dhanvantari as their common deity along with their own personal deities. This would enhance the power of their medicine and knowledge of enhancing life. There should be celebration of Dhanvantari Mahotsava in every town and every year on a regular basis and attempts should be made to make common people realise the importance of worshipping Lord Dhanvantari, thereby popularising it. Donations received on this occasion should be sent to the Ayurveda Mahavidyalaya for its development.)

The above statement of Jagannath Prasad Shukla clearly manifests that deification of Dhanvantari and related celebrations was a recent phenomenon which was undertaken by vaid organisations out of some pragmatic concerns, that is, development of collective consciousness amongst vaids, popularising Ayurveda among the common populace and to collect funds for the Ayurvedic movement. This provides us a unique case study of worldly appropriation of religion and deification.

However, to what extent the Sammelan and its provincial units managed to accomplish the aforesaid pursuits through the deification of Dhanvantari and the celebrations of Dhanvantari Mahotsava is debatable. Lamenting on the gradually waning interest among vaids regarding the celebration of Dhanvantari Mahotsava, Govardhan Sharma Chhangani stated in 1931:

> Humare yahan prarambh mein kisi Mahotsava ke prarambh hote hi pehle uski baadh si aa jati hai, kintu baad mein veh utsah nahin rehta. Theek yahi avastha Shri Dhanvantari Mahotsava ki hai. Haan, kuch sthanon par Mahotsava manaya jata hai kintu uska parinam aaj tak kya hua hai, yeh hum keh nahin sakte. Dhanvantari Mahotsava manane se avashya kuchh labh hi hua hoga, kintu hum yeh keh sakte hain ki jaisa chahiye vaisa labh abhi is se nahin hone paya hai.[54]

(It has generally been seen that whenever some new Mahotsava appears on the scene, there comes a flood of celebrations. However, very soon the required enthusiasm wanes. Similar is the case with Dhanvantari Mahotsava. While it is true that at some places it is still being celebrated, we do not know the exact outcome of these celebrations. Of course, there must be some positive outcome of such celebrations, but we know they are still not enough.)

Nevertheless, as argued by Hobsbawm, appearance and establishment of an 'invented tradition' is more important than its chances of survival.[55] The fact that Dhanvantari was deified in the course of the late colonial Ayurvedic movement embodies the inherent duality of a revivalist movement in the colonial context where, on the one hand, vaids were attempting to claim the scientificity of their discipline and at the same time invoking the traditional ritual authority as well. This duality was inherent to nearly all the revivalist movements of the time and the Ayurvedic movement proved no exception to this norm.[56] In fact, the target audience for both the aspects of the Ayurvedic movement were different. While vaids were claiming 'scientific status' for their discipline to uphold the authenticity of Ayurveda as a legitimate healing system in the eyes of the 'modern' colonial regime, Lord Dhanvantari was invoked to establish a common meeting point and to develop a shared consciousness amongst vaids within the community. However, ritualisation of Ayurveda through such acts alienated the Muslims further from practising and consulting this particular healing system.

Regardless of the lack of enthusiasm reported above in celebrating Dhanvantari Mahotsava, the Sammelan succeeded in inculcating Dhanvantari as lord of the Ayurvedic practitioners. Numerous Ayurvedic journals carried the imprint of Lord Dhanvantari right in the beginning or on the cover page along with ritualistic hymns or *mantra* devoted to him. In the United Provinces, one very prominent Ayurvedic journal was established in the 1920s entitled *Dhanvantari*. Several Ayurvedic pharmacies also adopted the name Dhanvantari. Ayurvedic educational institutions came to set up the idol of Dhanvantari, where often collective prayers were offered.[57] Moreover, as pointed out by Madhuri Sharma, by the end of the 1940s each Ayurvedic practitioner used to keep an idol of Dhanvantari and began their daily routine only after praying to him.[58] Thus, Lord Dhanvantari and related worship/celebrations were utilised to streamline the Ayurvedic discourse by developing a shared belief system and associated nomenclature.

CONCLUDING REMARKS

Unity of thoughts and actions amongst the Ayurvedic practitioners was required in order to achieve the desired result of the revival of Ayurveda. Print, organisation and mobilisation were three ways in which this unity was attempted to be established. However, as shown above through various examples, differences of opinion continued to exist. Nevertheless, despite these differences, Ayurvedic discourse emerged as fallout of a hegemonic process. Debates and discussions over medical issues and Ayurveda reached the public forums whether in print, annual meetings or festive celebrations. This was, in itself, a fundamental change in traditional Indian medical discourse which was hitherto restricted to the families of practitioners. Dispersal of Ayurvedic knowledge and related discourse was one of the key features of the period under discussion.

Now, this Ayurvedic discourse was not just about the medical aspects of the healing system. Rather, a careful reading of the Ayurvedic journals, books/tracts, pamphlets, etc., of this period, an analysis of the Ayurvedic debates in the public sphere and an exploration of the activities of the All

India Vaidya Sammelan and its provincial units throw immense light on the socio-cultural and religious processes of the time. In other words, it gives us rich insights into the social history of the early twentieth century India. Incidentally, the kind of social culture which the early twentieth century Ayurvedic discourse (in the United Provinces) exhibits is highly casteist, communal, and gender- and class-biased in its colourings. We would examine this in the next chapter.

NOTES

1. Among these, *Dhanvantari*, published by the Ayurvedic pharmacy of the same name located at Aligarh, was particularly significant and was a widely circulated Ayurvedic journal. It commenced in the beginning of 1923 and was the first Ayurvedic journal to publish a special number in the same year. In 1926, it presented *Swapna-pramehank*, a special issue on one disease, first of its quality. In 1928, it came up with a *Praveshank* dealing especially with hysteria and also first large compilation of prescriptions. In the sixth, seventh, eighth and ninth years of its publications, more special numbers were presented, namely, *Grihasthank*, *Nari-rogank*, *Madhumehank* and *Siddhayogank*, respectively. It was registered under No. A 1215 and was the only medical journal approved for the school libraries by text-books committee of the education department of the Central Provinces and Berar.
2. The annual subscription of most of these journals ranged from Re 1 to Rs 4.
3. The third, fourth, fifth and fifteenth sessions of the All India Vaidya Sammelan were held in the United Provinces at Prayag (1911), Kanpur (1912), Mathura (1913) and Haridwar (1924) respectively. On the other hand, from 1918 onwards, meetings of the United Provinces Vaidya Sammelan were used to be organised at different places in the United Provinces on a regular basis.
4. Rachel Berger, 'Ayurveda and the Making of the Urban Middle Class in North India, 1900–1945', in *Modern and Global Ayurveda: Pluralism and Paradigms*, eds. Dagmar Wujastyk and Frederick M. Smith (Albany: State University of New York Press, 2008), 101–16.
5. C. A. Bayly, *Empire and information: Intelligence Gathering and Social Communication in India, 1780-1870* (Cambridge: Cambridge University Press, 1996).
6. Francesca Orsini, *The Hindi Public Sphere, 1920-1940: Language and Literature in the Age of Nationalism* (Oxford: Oxford University Press, 2002).
7. Berger, 'Ayurveda and the Making of Urban Middle Class', 112.

8. Charu Gupta, 'Procreation and Pleasure: Writings of a Woman Ayurvedic Practitioner in Colonial North India,' *Studies in History* 21, no. 1, 2005, 20.
9. Such as zamindars, princes and other such traditional elites along with merchants, officials (in administration) and other newly emerged elites.
10. Berger, 'Ayurveda and the Making of Urban Middle Class', 108.
11. Born in Porbandar in Gujarat in 1881, Yadavji Trikamji Acharya was one of the most influential members of the All India Vaidya Sammelan and was president of the twenty-second session of the Sammelan held in Gwalior in 1932. He was also the first director of the Ayurveda Mahavidyalaya at Banaras Hindu University. He authored numerous books on Ayurveda such as *Ayurveda Vyadhi Vijnana* (two volumes), *Dravyaguna Vijnana* (three volumes), *Rasamritam, Siddhayoga Samgraha, Rasa Prakash Sudhakar, Nadi Pariksha* and *Rasa Paddhati*.
12. *Vaidya Sammelan Patrika* 2, no. 1, January 1932, 18.
13. Born in 1877 in Varanasi, Gananath Sen Saraswati was a very renowned vaid of the twentieth century. Although trained in Western medicine, he later on turned into a staunch supporter of Ayurveda. In fact, he led the way of promoting 'mixed medical practice' for which he was often targeted by the 'purists'. In Calcutta, he founded 'Vishwanath Ayurveda Mahavidyalaya' for imparting training in mixed medical practice with Ayurvedic tilt. He also established 'Kalpataru Ayurveda Aushadhalaya' in Calcutta. From 1927 to 1938 he also headed the Ayurveda faculty of the Banaras Hindu University and was quite active in the Ayurvedic movement of the time. He was president of three sessions of the All India Vaidya Sammelan—Allahabad (1911), Indore (1920) and Mysore (1931).
14. 'Resume of Presidential Address of the 21st All India Ayurvedic Congress, Mysore', in *Akhil Bhartiya Ayurveda Mahasammelan ka Shatabdi Granth*, ed. A. K. Shrivastava (Delhi: All India Ayurvedic Congress, 2009), 75.
15. However, for someone like Yashoda Devi, publication of Ayurvedic tracts was not very encouraging, at least in the initial phase, from commercial viewpoint. She deplored the reading habits of the common populace which was more interested in sleazy novels, songs or the so-called 'dirty' literature. However, the very incentive of becoming 'one's own doctor' was the main driving force behind the sale and purchase of such 'popular' user-friendly Ayurvedic tracts (for further details on this theme, refer to Chapter 5 of the present work).
16. 'Resume of Presidential Address of the 19th All India Ayurvedic Congress, Nasik', in *Akhil Bhartiya Ayurveda Mahasammelan ka Shatabdi Granth*, 70.
17. 'Chhipane Yogya', *Anubhoot Yogmala*, Year 22, no. 7, July 1944.

18. Jagannath Prasad Shukla, *Ayurvedic Patron ka Itihas*, 2nd edn (Prayag: Sudhanidhi Press, 1953), 4. Its first edition was published in 1942.
19. 'Resume of Presidential Address of the 5th All India Ayurvedic Congress, Mathura', in *Akhil Bhartiya Ayurveda Mahasammelan ka Shatabdi Granth*, 40.
20. Talking about the 'divine' origin of Ayurveda, Kaviraj Jogindra Nath Sen of Calcutta in his presidential address at the fourteenth session of the All India Vaidya Sammelan (Colombo, 1924) stated that

    Orthodox Hindus as we are, gentleman would be presumptuous on our part to the beginning and date of Ayurveda. Ayurveda is *eternal* and of *no human origin*…Charaka, Vridha Vagbhata and others too, assert the Vedic origin of the Ayurveda and *it is not for us to question the origin of the Veda*. These are *eternal truths unlimited by time and space*; only they manifested themselves at different times in different forms.

    See Kaviraj Pratap Singh, *Nikhil Bharatvarshiya Ayurveda Mahamandal ka Rajat Jayanti Granth* (Benares: Mahashakti Press, 1936), 2: 34 (emphasis added).
21. Reference to this particular pattern of the history of evolution of Ayurveda can be found in bits and pieces in the successive presidential addresses at different sessions of the Sammelan. For a more compact embodiment of this template, see 'An Address on Hindu Medicine' by Gananath Sen (three times president of the All India Vaidya Sammelan) delivered at the foundation ceremony of Banaras Hindu University in 1916. See *Lectures of M.M. Gananath Sen Saraswati* (Varanasi: Chowkhambha Sanskrit Series Office, 2002), 1–32.
22. 'Pax Britannica' or the 'British Peace' was the concept used by the imperialist writers to refer to and subsequently justify the 'peaceful regime' and 'rule of law' ushered by the establishment of the British rule in the supposedly 'chaotic' Third World countries. Thus, colonialism was sanctified as a 'peace building mission'. The first president of the All India Vaidya Sammelan, Kunwar Saryu Prasad Narayan Singh, in his presidential address stated that the *'British shanti kaal'* (or the Pax Britannica) provides a congenial atmosphere for the revival and development of Ayurveda through constant efforts and research. See 'Resume of Presidential Address of the 1st All India Ayurvedic Congress, Nasik', in *Akhil Bhartiya Ayurveda Mahasammelan ka Shatabdi Granth*, 33.
23. See 'An Address on Hindu Medicine', in *Lectures of M.M. Gananath Sen Saraswati*, 1–32.
24. For example, 'Petition by Babu Satya Pado Banerji praying that his medicine for Cholera may be given trial in famine camps' (Home/Med/Sept 1900/2-3, NAI);

'Petition from Hakim Sayid Muhammad Ibrahim, submitting prescriptions for plague patients' (Home/Med/May 1900/138-39, NAI); 'Petition by Kaviraj Jogendra Chandra Sen Mullick, praying that certain medicines discovered by him may be experimentally treated and that he may be informed of result' (Home/Med/April 1901/42-43, NAI); 'Request that Messrs. Robindro Co's Malarial Pills known as '*Swarna Batika*' may be given a trial' (Home/Sanitary/Dec. 1909/193-96, NAI); 'Petition from Shaman praying that he may be granted a certificate regarding efficacy of his treatment of persons bitten by snakes and mad dogs' (Home/Med/Feb. 1910/13-4&7, NAI).

25. For detailed discussion on such usages of testimonials, see the section on 'Advertising Ayurveda' in Chapter 5.
26. Hailing from Fatehpur, United Provinces, Jagannath Prasad Shukla was the most prominent leader of the late colonial Ayurvedic movement. After the early demise of his father, he shifted to the Central Provinces to complete his study. In 1901, he came to Allahabad and became editor of *Prayag Samachar* (ran by Rajvaidya Pandit Jagannath Sharma). His closeness with Jagannath Sharma led to his interest in Ayurveda. He later on shifted to Bombay where he came in contact with Shankar Daji Shastri Pade. Shukla and Pade together worked out the plan to organise vaids and were the two key founders of the All India Vaidya Sammelan. Jagannath Prasad Shukla started an Ayurvedic magazine in 1909 entitled *Sudhanidhi* and was also associated with the mouthpiece journal of the Sammelan, *Vaidya Sammelan Patrika*. The numerous publications of Sudhanidhi Press of Allahabad were also handy works of Jagannath Prasad Shukla. He was also one-time president and twelve times prime minister of the All India Vaidya Sammelan.
27. 'Resume of Presidential Address of the 17th All India Ayurvedic Congress, Patna', in *Akhil Bhartiya Ayurveda Mahasammelan ka Shatabdi Granth*, 64.
28. 'Resume of Presidential Address of the 21st All India Ayurvedic Congress, Mysore', *Akhil Bhartiya Ayurveda Mahasammelan ka Shatabdi Granth*, 76.
29. *Kid mantra* states '*Sangachhdhvam sam vadadhvam sam vo manansi jantam*' (Move together; speak without discord; let your minds be in concord). *Rig Veda*, Mandala X, Sukta 191, https://vedicheritage.gov.in/hi/samhitas/rigveda/shakala-samhita/rigveda-shakala-samhita-mandal-10-sukta-191/ (accessed on 7 July 2023).
30. Pandit Thakur Dutt Sharma, 'Vaidyon ko Apas me Sangathit Hone ki Jaroorat Hai', *Vaidya Sammelan Patrika* 4, nos 7–9, July–September 1934, 200.
31. Sharma, 'Vaidyon ko Apas me Sangathit Hone ki Jaroorat Jai', 200.
32. For the idea of communalism being a 'false consciousness', see Bipan Chandra, *Communalism in Modern India* (New Delhi: Vikas Publishing House, 1984).

33. 'All India Ayurvedic and Unani Tibbi Conference', *Vaidya Sammelan Patrika* 2, no. 1, January 1932, 13. According to the circular, in the Lahore session (1931) of the All India Ayurvedic and Unani Tibbi Conference, the vaids of Lahore and Amritsar brought this to the notice of the then presiding officer Hakim Muhammad Iliyas Khan and Pandit Ramprasad and raised a demand to change the existing rules of the Conference. However, as per the circular, despite the assurances made, nothing concrete was achieved.
34. For further details on this communal aspect, refer to Chapter 4 of the present book.
35. Commenting on this trend, Pandit Shaligram Shastri of Lucknow stated:

> Now-a-days majority of people learn Ayurveda from the viewpoint of pecuniary benefits and many people have entered the profession who are unable to understand the classical texts of Ayurveda in their entirety. These people neither comprehend the secrets of Ayurveda nor do they have enough wisdom to accomplish that. Right from the beginning, they remain in hunt of some useful '*nuskha*' [formula] like that of *Amritdhara* and *Sudhanidhi*, so that they can patent it and become an abbot of some Ayurvedic establishment. These are self-proclaimed *kavirajs* or *vaids* who bring utter disrepute to Ayurveda.

See Pandit Shaligram Shastri, 'Vedon me Tri-dhatuvad', *Vaidya Sammelan Patrika* 3, nos 8–9, August–September 1933, 156.
36. Dr K. S. Mhaskar, 'Ayurveda ki Sadyah Sthiti', *Vaidya Sammelan Patrika* 1, no. 12, December 1931, 284. Here one can see the caste prejudices of the Ayurvedic practitioners as well. For further details on caste and class biases of the late colonial Ayurvedic discourse, refer to Chapter 4 of the present work.
37. Mhaskar, 'Ayurveda ki Sadyah Sthiti', 279. The other two parties were the established vaids and those practitioners of Western medicine who were recognising the merits of Ayurveda.
38. For details on politics of registration of medical practitioners by the government, refer to Chapter 1 of the present work.
39. There were various provincial units of the All India Vaidya Sammelan, each under the control of an Ayurveda mandal of its own. Organisationally, all the Ayurveda mandals used to function under the supervision of the Ayurveda Mahamandal which was a permanent standing committee and representative body of the All India Vaidya Sammelan. Ayurveda Mahamandal was founded during the third session of the Sammelan (Allahabad, 1911) to organise these annual gatherings, to formulate the norms of the profession and to keep an eye over Ayurvedic educational institutions.

40. 'Bhartiya Vaidya Sangh Sadasya Kaise Hone Chahiye', *Vaidya Sammelan Patrika* 5, no. 9, September 1935, 229.
41. Kunwar Saryu Prasad Narayan Singh was the first president of the All India Vaidya Sammelan held at Nasik in 1907. He belonged to the zamindari family of Baraon estate, Allahabad, and had keen interest in Ayurveda.
42. Jagannath Prasad Shukla was president of the seventeenth session of the All India Vaidya Sammelan (Patna, 1927) and was its prime minister for 12 years from 1909 to 1922.
43. As for instance, chairman of the reception committee of the second session of the United Provinces Vaidya Sammelan (Hardoi, 1919) was the civil surgeon Bankim Chandra Sanyal. Similarly, in the third session (Unnao, 1921) this post was held by the lawyer Vishwambhar Nath Vajpayee.
44. Kaviraj Pratap Singh, *Nikhil Bharatvarshiya Ayurveda Mahamandal ka Rajat Jayanti Granth* (Benares: Mahashakti Press, 1935), 1: 307–08. A noticeable point here is the admiration of the idea of its own brand of colonialism in the field of medicine by the Sammelan. The use of terms like *samrajya* and *upnivesh* clearly attests this.
45. Sivaramakrishnan, *Old Potions, New Bottles*, 117.
46. Bhishagratna, *Sushruta Samhita*, Sutra Sthana, Chapter 1, Verse 1–6.
47. Shastri, *Ramayana of Valmiki*, Chapter 41, verses 18, 19 and 21; Roy, *The Mahabharata*, Adiparva, Chapter 18, verses 38, 39 and 53.
48. In this regard, Sivaramakrishnan especially mentions the crucial role played by Jagannath Prasad Shukla and his journal *Sudhanidhi* in consolidating forms and rituals of Dhanvantari worship (see Sivaramakrishnan, *Old Potions, New Bottles*, 117).
49. Concept borrowed from the famous work of Eric Hobsbawm and Terrence Ranger by the same name. According to Hobsbawm, 'traditions' which appear or claim to be old are often quite 'recent in origin' and sometimes 'invented'. See Eric Hobsbawm and Terrence Ranger, eds, *The Invention of Tradition* (Cambridge: Cambridge University Press, 1983).
50. The All India Vaidya Sammelan made desperate efforts to provide the entire Ayurvedic movement a sacred aura right from the beginning. That is why when in Nasik, in 1907, the first session of the Sammelan was held, a *Sanatan Dharma Mahaparishad* was also organised side-by-side under the chairmanship of Raja Raghav Prasad Narayan Singh Bahadur (cousin of Kunwar Saryu Prasad Narayan Singh, president of the first session of the Sammelan).
51. According to Hobsbawm, 'The term 'invented traditions' includes both 'traditions' actually invented, constructed and formally instituted and those

emerging in a less easily traceable manner within a brief and debatable period—a matter of a few years perhaps—and establishing themselves with great rapidity' (Eric Hobsbawm, 'Introduction: Inventing Traditions', in Hobsbawm and Ranger, *The Invention of Tradition*, 1).

52. As, for instance, in Moradabad in 1929. For details, see 'News related to Shri Dhanvantari Mahotsava', *Vaidya Sammelan Patrika* 2, no. 7, November 1929, 31–33.
53. 'Presidential Address (Jagannath Prasad Shukla) of the Second Session of the United Provinces Vaidya Sammelan, Hardoi', in Singh, *Nikhil Bharatvarshiya Ayurveda Mahamandal ka Rajat Jayanti Granth*, 2: 564.
54. 'Dhanvantari Mahotsava', *Vaidya Sammelan Patrika* 1, no. 10, October 1931, 220–22.
55. Hobsbawm, 'Introduction', 1.
56. For a general description on duality of socio-religious reform/revivalist movements in the colonial context, see Kenneth W. Jones, *The New Cambridge History of India Vol. III.1: Socio-Religious Reform Movements in British India* (Cambridge: Cambridge University Press, 1989).
57. Later on, in the 1960s, when the permanent office of the All India Vaidya Sammelan and Ayurvedic Vidyapith was built in Punjabi Bagh, New Delhi, a temple of Lord Dhanvantari was erected inside the campus (see Appendix 7).
58. Sharma, *Indigenous and Western Medicine*, 81. Interestingly, Sharma discusses one very unique iconography of Dhanvantari, published in the monthly journal *Arogya Vigyan*, where he was shown pouring nectar to the people of all religions—Hindu, Muslim, Sikh and Christian—who were worshipping him. There might be nationalist influence at work behind such imagery of Dhanvantari, otherwise his general iconography is conspicuously that of a 'Hindu' male deity.

4

Healing the Society
Social Culture of the Late Colonial Ayurvedic Discourse

As delineated in the preceding chapters, by the late nineteenth and early twentieth century, against the growing dominance, and more so hegemony, of Western medicine, an entire discourse had come up in the public sphere to revive and restore the 'past glory' of Ayurvedic healing system. It was attempted through print, organisation and mobilisation which created a substantial Ayurvedic discourse. Now, a careful analysis of this discourse reveals that it was not just about the healing aspect of Ayurveda, rather it enthusiastically engaged with many of the contemporaneous socio-political debates. While reading many of the Ayurvedic tracts and conference proceedings published during the period under discussion, one can sense this engagement sometimes very explicitly and on other occasions implicitly. In other words, the Ayurvedic discourse of the time contains within itself varied social manifestations. Incidentally, such explicit and implicit social manifestations as reflected by the late colonial Ayurvedic discourse are highly casteist, communal, gender and class biased in their content. It was in this regard that most of the practitioners conceptualised the appropriate 'national body' not just as 'Hindu' but also as 'middle class' and 'twice born'.[1] Concerns and self-consciousness of the 'new' vaids were encapsulated within this overarching socially prejudiced frame wherein vaid publicists and ideologues of the late colonial Ayurvedic movement transcending their medical boundaries participated actively in the underlying social currents of the time.

The present chapter would one by one take up all such social biases/prejudices related to the late nineteenth and early twentieth century Ayurvedic discourse. Here the simultaneous effort is to delineate the social processes of the Hindi public sphere through the prism of Ayurvedic discourse. It would dissect the conscious/unconscious representations of vaid publicists and ideologues which were part and parcel of a broader upper-caste middle class–oriented discourse. Further, for the purpose of illustration, two of the issues—brahmacharya (or celibacy) and midwifery—widely discussed in the Ayurvedic tracts/proceedings of the period have been taken up in detail as case studies to provide a holistic picture of the aforesaid social engagement of a seemingly 'scientific' discourse.

CASTE/CLASS BIASES IN THE LATE COLONIAL AYURVEDIC DISCOURSE

The Ayurvedic discourse of the time (c. 1890–1950) was highly casteist and reflected upper-class biases. Lower castes and classes and their unclean habits were often held responsible for the spread of many of the diseases in contemporaneous Ayurvedic notions. For example, one of the texts entitled *Dadru-Chikitsa* (a text devoted to the cure of dermatophytosis or ringworm), while acknowledging the scientific basis of dermatophytosis (by recognising fungi as its causative agent), went on to blame the dirty habits of the barber, washerman, etc., for its spread.[2] In fact, barbers were attacked particularly in this text and they were held responsible for the spread not only of ringworm but also of leprosy. It went on to cite *Atharvaveda* to illustrate linkages between the barber and spread of skin diseases.

It should be noted that during this time the middle class–oriented health notions suspected servants and other lower classes of deliberately spreading skin diseases to their patrons (for an illustration, see Figure 4.1). These were the notions emulated by the Indian middle class from their colonial counterparts, who often articulated racial interpretations for the spread of disease.[3] The only shift was that the Indian middle class replaced racial interpretation with the one that emphasised caste

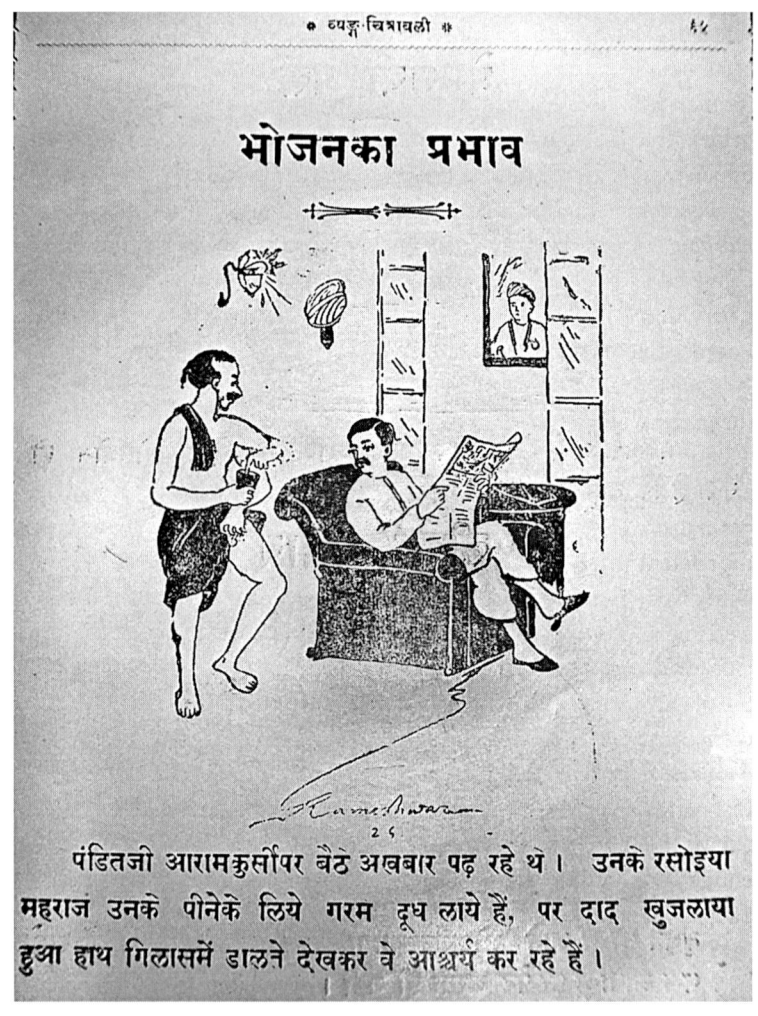

Figure 4.1: Effect of food: Pandit ji (patron) alarmed by the unexpected behaviour of his cook (servant), who after scratching his ring is putting his fingers in the milk he has brought for Pandit ji.[4]

and class.⁵ In the middle-class/upper-caste imagination, out of several other essentialised characterisations of a particular caste, sanitary sense became one of the characters on the basis of which a particular caste could be identified. Incidentally, lower castes and classes were indifferently seen as having unclean, insanitary, infectious and dirty habits. The Ayurvedic discourse often reflected these middle-class and upper-caste notions, as shown in the aforesaid example.

Following similar attitude, another Ayurvedic tract entitled *Plague Darpan* (1916), which was based on the speech of Rai Pooran Chand delivered at the All India Vaidya Sammelan in Kanpur,⁶ came up with a very unique theory related to the spread of plague. According to Rai Pooran Chand, plague was caused by a kind of poison termed by him as '*pad sangharshan vish*'. As articulated, this 'poison' was generated due to the friction between the 'bare feet' and the ground and entered the earth. When this 'poison' accumulated excessively inside the earth, the plague epidemics broke out.⁷ The point to be noted here is that this 'poison' was generated because of the friction between the 'bare feet' and the ground. In the contemporaneous society, Brahmins and the upper-caste people used either wooden sandals (called *kharaun*) or leather shoes while walking. It were the lower castes/class and women who usually walked bare-footed. Consequently, the indirect assumption was that these sections generated the plague-specific 'poison', although Rai Pooran Chand did not refer to them directly.⁸

Even some of the Ayurvedic tracts on child care published during this period clearly reflected caste, class and gender predilections in their conceptualisation of an ideal progeny. For example, one of the tracts entitled *Su-Santati Shastra* stated the need to encourage couples to give birth to '*deshodharak veer, sudharma pracharak mahant ya sadhu, vidvan Brahman, veer Kshatriya, dani Vaishya, sevabhawi Shudra, ek patni vrat-dhari purush aur pativrata striyan*' ('liberator of the nation, disseminator of the religion, scholarly Brahmin, brave Kshatriya, generous Vaishya, duty-bound/attending Shudra, monogamous men and chaste/faithful women').⁹

In fact, similar caste concerns in these child care tracts can be located if one examines the Ayurvedic discourse related to dhai (wet mother). One of the texts entitled *Santati Shastra* clearly stated that the wet mother or dhai should always be of one's own caste and should never be from 'menial' castes. According to it, a Brahmin family should always have a Brahmin, a Kshatriya family a Kshatriya, Vaishya family a Vaishya, and a Shudra family should have a Shudra woman as a wet mother.[10] In other words, it was believed that caste characteristics could be transferred through breastfeeding.[11]

Furthermore, even some of the advertisements of Ayurvedic medicines exhibited caste prejudices. For example, one of the advertisements of Ayurvedokt Aushadhalaya, Allahabad, stated: 'All kinds of medicines in this pharmacy are made *either by Brahmins or other superior castes* and instead of ordinary water we use nectar like water of the Ganges.'[12] It was an outright manifestation of the adoption of notions of purity/pollution underlying caste hierarchy by the aforesaid Ayurvedic pharmacy.[13]

Thus, the late nineteenth and early twentieth century Ayurvedic discourse clearly reflected the caste and class biases. Such caste and class prejudices of the Ayurvedic discourse were manifested even in its communal orientation, which would be discussed in the following sub-section. In fact, during this time we see the hinduisation or brahmanisation of Ayurvedic treatment. It was a complex process which saw, on the one hand, upper-caste vaids condemning the tribal and low-caste methods of treatment and, on the other hand, they were appropriating some of these methods by hinduising or brahmanising them. Here one needs to keep in mind that the caste and class leanings of the Ayurvedic discourse were part and parcel of this broader process of hinduisation or brahmanisation of the Ayurvedic treatment. One cannot look at the hinduisation of Ayurveda and its biases in isolation. As argued earlier (Chapter 1), the debate was not just over which healing system was worthiest for the claim of 'indigenous' healing system, but it was also over what were the practices which constituted that particular 'system of healing'. An integral part of this process was either deliberate silencing or ritual hijacking of the healing skills practised by people belonging to lower castes/class such as that of dais (midwives), bhagats (those healing snake bites) and potters (practising rhinoplasty).

For instance, while rhinoplastic operations had been mentioned in *Sushruta Samhita*,[14] evidence shows that they were actually practised by the low-caste potters. It is hard to ascertain that whether it was due to later demotion of the social status of those performing surgical operations or it was there right from the beginning;[15] however, this was certainly the case in the eighteenth century. *The Gentleman's Magazine* in October 1794 reported an instance of Cowasjee, a Maratha bullock cart driver employed in the English army in the Mysore war of 1792, who was captured by the soldiers of Tipu Sultan who cut off his nose and one of his hands. However, after remaining without a nose for 12 months, the *Magazine* reported, a new nose was put on his face by a man of 'brickmaker caste' near Poonah. The *Magazine* further claimed that such operation was not uncommon in India and had been practised from time immemorial. It then went on to describe how the whole operation was performed as witnessed by Mr Thomas Cruso and Mr James Trindlay, two of the medical gentlemen from Bombay presidency.[16]

Now, interestingly, the Ayurvedic tracts of the late nineteenth and early twentieth century, while boasting of the Ayurvedic knowledge of rhinoplasty as delineated in *Sushruta Samhita*, nowhere acknowledged the expertise that potters had over such operations. Similar was the case with the treatment of snake bites and midwifery. Bhagats and dais hardly figured in respectable terms in these tracts. So, while the Ayurvedic tracts made tall and often exaggerated claims of theoretical expertise in these areas of healing, the dominant practitioners of such areas were sidelined, invisibilised and often purged by ritually hijacking their healing skills.[17]

Thus, the Ayurvedic discourse of the period under discussion nowhere betrayed the social values/biases of the time; rather, it helped in consolidating them in many ways by providing scientific sanctity to such caste/class predilections. In fact, access to health care services was a luxury in colonial times and it was mostly the upper-caste/-class people who could avail proper treatment whether at the hands of Western medical practitioners or the vaids or hakims. In such conditions, healing systems were bound to acquire caste/class characteristics and hierarchies in order to protect the social sensibilities of their clientele/patrons.

Interestingly, one can draw this class perspective of access to healing practices from various writings of Premchand. As discussed by Madhuri Sharma, *Godan* offers numerous instances of it.[18] For example, it shows how illness becomes a luxury in the case of the upper classes, where they were never supposed to be suffering from ordinary illness and even the slightest sign of illness used to become a big issue for them:

> Raisaheb [the landlord] tells Hori [the peasant]: You know how it is, Hori! In a large family like mine, someone or the other is always falling ill. We are not expected to suffer from ordinary illness. If there is a slight temperature, we are treated for pneumonia; a pimple is always a carbuncle. Frenzied telegrams are sent to the assistant surgeon, the surgeon and the chief surgeon. Messengers rush to Delhi and Calcutta to bring hakims and vaidyas. In the family shrine Durga is invoked. The astrologers get busy on horoscopes. There is a tremendous activity to save the patient from the jaws of death. On the slightest sign of indisposition the doctors get ready to shake the pagoda tree.[19]

Commenting on this, Madhuri Sharma argues that '[I]t may be deduced that treatment from renowned doctors and vaidyas for a simple illness was a sort of status symbol for the landed gentry. It details the variety of treatments which the well-to-do could draw upon, ranging from Allopathic medicine to black magic and faith healing.'[20] On the other hand, in the same novel, Premchand mentions about the inaccessibility of medical care in the case of the lower classes. Out of the six children Hori and Dhania (the main characters of the novel *Godan*) had, three died because of the lack of proper medical treatment owing to their poverty. Thus, lack of economic resources was an important determining factor behind access to health facilities and even choice of healing system(s).

COMMUNAL ASPECTS OF THE LATE COLONIAL AYURVEDIC DISCOURSE

Besides being casteist, the Ayurvedic discourse of the time often also became communal in its orientation. The All India Vaidya Sammelan, which was very much active in the United Provinces, spearheaded the process of communalisation of the Ayurvedic discourse. Right from its inception, the Sammelan carried religious/communal symbols and overtones along with its pursuit of Ayurvedic revivalism and tried to bring them together. This is very much evident from the fact that the meeting of *Sanatan Dharma Mahaparishad* was held under the chairmanship of Raja Sahab[21] at the same venue as the first congress of the All India Vaidya Sammelan in Nasik in 1907. In fact, the founding members of the All India Vaidya Sammelan such as Shankar Daji Pade and Jagannath Prasad Shukla were also members of the Hindu Sabhas and the Hindi Sahitya Sammelan and were actively associated with Hindu communal politics.²²

As it has already been argued in Chapter 1, the Vaidya Sammelan often claimed itself to be the sole mouthpiece of the 'Hindu' vaid interests and stressed that the concerns and interests of the 'Hindu' vaids were not only different from but also antagonistic to those of the 'Muslim' hakims. This led to suspicion on the part of the Sammelan regarding the activities of the All India Ayurvedic and Unani Tibbi Conference which had been emphasising on the collaboration and cooperation among the 'indigenous' practitioners of both kinds. Incidentally, in the discourse of the Sammelan, the All India Ayurvedic and Unani Tibbi Conference was characterised as 'Vibhishana'²³ whose activities, no matter how righteous they might be, should always be handled with care.²⁴ Actually, the attitude of the Sammelan towards the Conference was similar to the attitude of the Hindu Mahasabha or the Rashtriya Swayamsevak Sangh towards the Indian National Congress. Thus, the Sammelan believed that the Conference was more inclined to appease the 'Muslim' hakims.²⁵

The Sammelan overwhelmingly used the popular templates of Hindu communal consciousness like 'Aryan heritage', 'ancient Hindu Sanskrit-based' learning of the sages and their 'sacred' writings, epics like *Ramayana* and *Mahabharata*, and 'Hindu science' in its discourse. In fact, the Sammelan made deliberate efforts to associate Ayurveda with the 'Sanskrit-based' textual tradition. Besides, it also believed firmly in the philosophy of going back to 'pristine' ancient texts. That is why it attempted to replace the vernacular and medieval medical anthologies which were popular among the vaids with the original Sanskrit texts of ancient period such as *Charaka*, *Sushruta* and *Vagbhata Samhitas*. In short, as argued by Kavita Sivaramakrishnan, the Sammelan attempted that '[t]he intellectual make-up of the Hindu vaid practitioner had to be anchored in its identification with a Sanskrit-based textual tradition'.²⁶ This particular aspect was clearly reflected in the following statement of Pandit Gananath Sen, president of the Vaidya Sammelan:

> Those who want to become vaids simply by reading *Lollambraj* or *Amritsagar* [vernacular medical texts popular among the vaids] needed to be warned against [such measures].... [for] if one *Amritsagar* and *Illajulgurba* could

make people into vaids then what was the need to take pains over Sushruta and Vagabhatta?[27]

A relatively more controversial communal template used by the Sammelan in its attempt to revive Ayurveda was the theory of 'dying or degenerating Hindu race'.[28] Invoking this imaginary theory of the 'dying Hindu race', Kaviraj Jogindra Nath Sen of Calcutta in his presidential address at the fourteenth session of the All India Vaidya Sammelan (Colombo, 1924) stated that the aim of Ayurveda was two-fold: first, the treatment of disease; second, the preservation of health. Taking reference of recent census reports, Sen argued of the 'terrible state of the health of the Hindus' of the time. Not only this, in his speech Sen frequently invoked the works of Sakharam Ganesh Deushkar, Colonel U. N. Mukherjee (*The Dying Race*), Kishorilal Sarkar (*Dying Race—How Dying?*) and Dr Kamakhy Charan Banerjea (*Hindu Dubila* or 'The Dying Hindu'). Sen further argued that in Bengal the number of Hindus in 1911 was 20,945,379; while in 1921, instead of increasing, it came down to 20,809,148, that is, fewer by about 136,000. At the same time, the Muslim population had been steadily increasing, and had come to represent more than one-half of the entire population of Bengal. According to Sen, 'the cause of this gradual decay is to be partially found in the utter disregard, on the part of the Hindus, of the general rules of hygiene as laid down in Ayurveda'.[29] Thus, links were sought to be established between the pursuit of revival of Ayurveda and a numerically preponderant Hindu race.

Further, from the 1920s onwards issues like 'Hindi *prachar*', 'cow protection' and the cause of 'Hindu education' often formed the subject of vaid campaigns.[30] One can cite here the example of Acharya Chandrashekhar Shastri who was a famous Ayurvedic practitioner as well as teacher at the Banaras Hindu University. While stressing the sanskritisation of Hindi language, Shastri argued that 'new words should only be generated when synonymous words are not available in our old Sanskritic repository. It is not only condemnable to use new words, leaving our old Sanskritic words; rather it also embodies our ignorance.'[31] Actually, while translating modern scientific technologies and concepts into Hindi, the vaids readily resorted to ancient Indian Sanskritic philosophies.[32] So, one can see cross linkages between science, language and cultural heritage in the discourse of the Ayurvedic practitioners.

Similarly, many of the Ayurvedic texts published from the United Provinces promoted the 'cow protection' movement. In fact, one of the texts by Yashoda Devi, the famous female Ayurvedic practitioner of Allahabad, contains an entire pamphlet entitled '*Gau Pukar*' (Cow's Calling) in which medicinal properties of cow products were enumerated in a lyrical form, and a call for protecting the cow was made to the people of all sects.[33] In another text, Yashoda Devi used the typical phraseology of the cow protection movement when she compared cow's milk and its properties with nectar (*amrit*). There is a couplet in this book:

> Amrit ka naam hi suna jata hai, kisi ne dekha na piya,
> Doodh hi amrit hai, doodh se hi sharir ka poshan hota hai.[34]

(We have only heard of nectar, but no one has actually tasted it. Milk is real nectar as it nourishes our body.)

A similar analogy between nectar and cow's milk was drawn by the famous Ayurvedic practitioner and activist Shankar Daji Pade in his pamphlet *Gorasadi Aushadhi*. In the pamphlet he argued that in ancient time people of all classes, whether rich or poor, were able-bodied, fit and strong as plenty of cow's milk was available to them. However, with the onset of the rule of '*go-bhakshak rajas*' (cow-devouring rulers)[35] the cow's population and subsequently cow products reported a steep decline owing to which the contemporaneous Indian populace became mostly short-statured, short-living, emaciated and less fertile. Hence, in the pamphlet he makes a call to both the government and the common people to protect the cow and its clan.[36]

In fact, cow's milk became an important ingredient of many of the suggested Ayurvedic remedies by this time. What is noticeable is that it was not just any milk; rather it was cow's milk which was of utmost importance for such remedies. Ironically, for some of the Ayurvedic practitioners even the colour of the cow mattered equally. For instance, Pandit Ramprasad Mishra, while suggesting the Ayurvedic remedy of infertility, stated that if an infertile woman takes the roots of herbs like *Mayurshikha* (Celosia Argentea) and *Jeevak* (Crepidium Acuminatum) along with the milk of *monochromatic* cow, she would certainly get pregnant.[37] Similarly, Shankar Daji Pade in the aforesaid pamphlet on

Gorasadi Aushadhi enumerates the specific benefits of the milk of yellow, white, red and spotted cows.[38]

The Ayurvedic practitioners also picked up the typical argument of Hindu communal consciousness which perceived all kinds of 'decline' being set in the medieval period. Pandit Gananath Sen in his presidential address at the third session of the All India Vaidya Sammelan (Allahabad, 1911) traced the downfall of Ayurveda to have commenced from the time of the 'external aggression' of Muhammad Ghori, Chengiz Khan and Taimur. As he saw it, this process of the decline of Ayurveda reached its climax during the reign of Aurangzeb—the favourite 'punching bag' of Hindu communalists. According to Sen, Aurangzeb not just demolished Hindu temples and desecrated Hindu religion, but also destroyed the ancient Hindu texts associated with science which was a fatal blow for Ayurveda.[39]

Furthermore, some of the Ayurvedic texts openly attacked 'Muslim rule' of the past for 'uncontrolled' and 'perverted' sexual behaviour leading to manifold diseases. For example, *Arogya Darpan*, Vol. 3 (published from Allahabad in 1898) while attacking anal sex or homosexuality, blamed 'Muslim rule' for it. It went on to claim that there was a verse in the *Quran* where Prophet Muhammad had 'advised' that if one's wife was pregnant, the husband could indulge in homosexual activities to satisfy himself.[40] Similarly, A. G. Vyas's *Su-Santati Shastra* does not mention any Muslim name in its exemplary list of 'ideal progeny' of India.[41] Incidentally, it contains the name of people like Maharana Pratap and Shivaji who fought against the Mughals and had emerged as 'freedom fighters' in the ongoing nationalist discourse of the early twentieth century. Following the same communal line, Vinayak Madhav Chingle, while stressing on brahmacharya, exhorted the Hindu youth to imagine the pain Maharana Pratap, Veer Shivaji and Maharaja Ranjit Singh would have to bear when they would see that the lioness (metaphor used for the earlier generation) had given birth to jackals (symbolising the early twentieth century youth) who could not defend their own religion.[42] Similarly, another author while stressing good health of the students, projected the physical weakness of the Hindu community to be the root cause of the prevailing communal tension, and advocated better health and virility of the Hindu youth as the solution.[43]

Moreover, the deification of Dhanvantari as the common 'professional deity' of Ayurvedic practitioners and related celebrations of Dhanvantari Mahotsava (as discussed in detail in the previous chapter) also gave a communal tilt to Ayurveda by ritualising many of the Ayurvedic practices. It became more and more a symbol of 'sacred' 'Hindu' science rather than just a healing system curing diseases. In fact, this ritualisation of healing practices/systems was another manifestation of intensified communal polarisation of Indian social landscape in the first half of the twentieth century.

There is need to look at this entire communalisation of the Ayurvedic discourse from another angle as well. Whenever we talk of communalisation in the Indian context, it immediately takes us towards the religious divide, conflicts, tensions, and so on. However, if we analyse closely the process of communalisation, besides creating religious dissensions, it also homogenises a community internally and purges 'unwanted' elements from within. In the colonial Indian context, communalisation often led to the brahmanisation or upper-caste/class control over the community. For example, when the Ayurvedic practitioners emphasised Sanskrit-based learning, it essentially purged those low-caste/class practitioners who were dependent on oral traditions and familial experiences (passed on from one generation to the next) for their skills. In other words, the emphasis on classical brahmanical texts in Ayurvedic learning was a strategy that worked to wean out the low-caste/class practices and influences.

Similarly, while condemning 'Muslim rule' for health related 'evil' practices, the attack was particularly directed against the Julahas. So, even among the Muslims, it was the lower classes which were targeted for their supposedly 'uncontrolled' sexual behaviour, prostitution, etc. In fact, Jagannath Sharma (the author of *Arogya Darpan*) went on to claim that it was precisely when the Muslims handed over their swords and shields to these 'sexually corrupt' Julahas, the Muslim rule tumbled and the Marathas and the English emerged as new forces in the subcontinent.[44] Consequently, communalisation, besides creating religious boundaries, also unleashed hegemonic upper-caste and class ideas that served to homogenise the communities.

GENDER BIASES IN THE LATE COLONIAL AYURVEDIC DISCOURSE

The Ayurvedic discourse of the time was heavily gender biased as well. Incidentally, the Ayurvedic practitioners often reinforced patriarchy. Even if this did not result out of a conscious effort, on many occasions they did help in reinforcing patriarchy. One can cite here Rai Pooran Chand's speech delivered at the All India Vaidya Sammelan in Kanpur in 1912.[45] Here he described an incident when he had gone to examine a female patient on the request of a reputed client. When he visited her for the first time, she was unconscious and unveiled. He examined her pulse and gave some medicine. When Rai Pooran Chand visited her the second time, she had regained her consciousness. And when he was examining her pulse this time, she veiled herself in modesty. To quote Rai Pooran Chand: '*Us din rogi ne apne se nadi dikhlaya. Mujhe dekh lajja prakash kar ghonghat de liya jabki barah ghante pehle ghar walon ke yatna karne par bhi tanik lajja na ki thi*' [That day the patient showed me the pulse on her own. She veiled herself in modesty, although twelve hours before (when she was unconscious) despite the attempts of the family members she had shown no such signs of modesty].[46] In this entire description, we find an indirect reinforcement of the purdah by a medical practitioner. In his speech, he very cleverly brought out the connection between purdah and its vital importance in so far as a conscious person was concerned. Thus, as the woman patient regained her consciousness, she found it obligatory to veil herself during the check-up.

Similarly, while discussing diseases related to women, texts like *Arogya Darpan* often assumed a didactic tone advising women how to conduct themselves in the social sphere. Even Yashoda Devi, the famous female Ayurvedic practitioner of Allahabad who had expertise on women-related diseases, cannot be cleared of this blame. Incidentally, Yashoda Devi claimed a larger status than a mere gynaecologist. She proclaimed herself as '*Stridharma Sikshak*'[47] (see Figure 4.2). This self-assumed title of Yashoda Devi reflects a coalescing of social and health concerns in the Ayurvedic discourse of the time where a gynaecologist/medical practitioner was assuming the title and role of a social mentor.

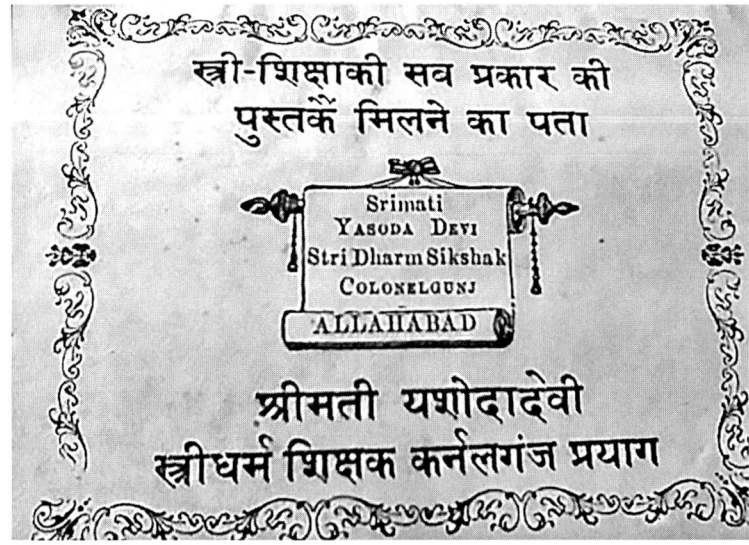

Figure 4.2: *Stridharma Sikshak*: One of the advertisements at the back of her book by Yashoda Devi.⁴⁸

In fact, the range of books published by Yashoda Devi clearly reflects her didactic concerns. Besides publishing books on Ayurveda, female health and child care, she also came up with the books like *Sugharh Grihani* (1924), *Pati-bhakti ki Shakti*, *Nari Dharma Shastra*, *Pak Shastra* (1924), *Sachcha Pati Prem* (1934), *Grihani Kartavya Shiksha* and *Nari Niti Shiksha*. Actually, she believed that the root cause of many of the health related problems of women was associated with their ignorance and troubled married life. That is why she emphasised on female education, but of a very different kind. She advocated heavy moral and ethical kind of education for women. She constantly underlined the necessity of *grihastha shiksha* (education related to domestic affairs) for a healthy life of the entire family. Here it is noticeable that while in case of males it was the 'brahmacharya ashram' which was the focal point of attention in the Ayurvedic discourse, in case of females it was the 'grihastha ashram' which was emphasised upon.⁴⁹ In fact, in one of the writings of Yashoda Devi, *Grihani Kartavya Shastra Arogyashastra Arthat Pakshastra*, cooking became intrinsic to the proper healthcare of family, responsibility of which was laid upon housewives.[50] As argued by Gyan Prakash, such prescriptive texts written by Yashoda Devi were in tandem with the typical middle-class imagery of Hindu wives who had to maintain the health of their families and thereby of the 'Hindu' nation through 'scientific' management within the household.[51]

Similarly, another female Ayurvedic practitioner from the United Provinces, Prakashvati Devi Jain[52] considered that the root cause of many of the diseases related to women was weakness of mind and heart. She believed that while treating bodily diseases of women it was important to know their mental disorders/problems first as women related diseases, in her opinion, were mostly the outward manifestations of their mental problems/fears. That is why she argued that normal methods of diagnosis like *nadi-parikshan* (pulse examination) did not precipitate desired results in case of women. Consequently, she argued the case of a soft-spoken female Ayurvedic practitioner to whom women could open up their mind and heart.[53] Inherent in her conceptualisation was the weakness of mind and heart of women which was perfectly in-tune with the contemporaneous patriarchal social perception of women, even as it touched upon the need for women to be able to share their suffering and agonies.

Further, if we look at the Ayurvedic tracts on child care (referred to as *Santati Shastra*) of the period under discussion, these tracts also reflected gender biases. For example, Yashoda Devi while talking of '*santan palan*' (that is, 'nurturing of progeny') focuses entirely on the healthy upbringing of the male child, and not of the female child. It should be noted that *santan* or progeny is a gender-neutral term. But in the text entitled *Santan Palan* she uses either the term '*ladka*' or '*bachcha*' and nowhere '*ladki*' or '*bachchi*'.[54] Similar is the case with another text of hers entitled *Shishu Raksha Vidhan*. *Shishu* is also a gender-neutral term but in the text she exclusively uses the term '*balak*'.[55] This aspect of Yashoda Devi's writings tells us something about the social culture of the Ayurvedic discourse of the period in relation to child care that was intimately associated with parenting. Thus, while the healthy upbringing of a male child was extremely significant, the female child's upbringing was virtually a non-issue.[56] In case of a female child or girl what was significant was only her proper social upbringing, which is evident from numerous didactic texts on this matter. Female health became a significant issue only once they acquired adolescence. This was largely because they were supposed to play significant social and familial roles—particularly the reproductive role—in their adulthood, which was not possible if they remained ill.[57]

Also one of the main areas of interest of the Ayurvedic texts of this period was to look at the possibilities of the birth of a male child. Many texts in this regard often contained a sub-section called '*Manmani or Manchahi Santan*' ('Desired Child'). Even Yashoda Devi talks about this in her *Dampati Arogyata Jeevanshastra* (Allahabad, 1927). In fact, one can also find texts devoted entirely to this theme and one can cite here *Manchahi Santan* (Allahabad, 1928) written by Rishilal Agarwal, as an example. Incidentally, *Vaidya Priya*, an Ayurvedic text written in verse form, came up with bizarre suggestions advocating the use of pigeon's shit, cannabis seeds, etc., in order to beget a male child.[58]

In fact, many pseudo-scientific theories regarding ways and appropriate timings of sexual intercourse were forwarded by several Ayurvedic tracts to realise the patriarchal desire of begetting a male child. Even well-established Ayurvedic journals like *Dhanvantari* could not escape this dominant template of the late colonial Ayurvedic discourse. Interestingly, one of the articles published in *Dhanvantari* (September 1934) by Vaidya Govind Prasad Varshaneya of Moradabad suggested a unique theory that it is the right testis and ovary of a man and a woman which produce sperm and ovum, respectively, fertilisation of which leads to birth of a male child. Contrastingly, fertilisation of sperm and ovum produced by left testis and ovary respectively begets a female child. Subsequently, Govind Prasad Varshaneya went on to suggest the ways in which the activities of the left testis or ovum could be suppressed such as by tying the left testis during copulation.[59]

Thus, in short, the contemporaneous Ayurvedic discourse emanating from the United Provinces clearly exhibited caste, class, community and gender biases. Let us now examine these biases in detail by taking some individual examples. Some of the issues which repeatedly appeared in the contemporaneous Ayurvedic discourse and had serious social underpinnings were the issues of brahmacharya, midwifery, purdah, wet mothers, female diseases, etc. One can find numerous Ayurvedic texts and health tracts devoted to these issues. They were significant for the Ayurvedic practitioners not only from the viewpoint of health but also in the broader interests of the 'community', 'society' and the 'nation'. Let us explore two of them—brahmacharya and midwifery—for the purpose of our illustration. It would be congenial to start with a discussion on brahmacharya or celibacy as this was the issue which gained tremendous public attention during the early twentieth century due to several reasons.

BRAHMACHARYA OR CELIBACY

In the late 1980s and 1990s, many historians, particularly feminist scholars, extensively analysed the discourses associated with the 'female body' and 'sexuality' and their linkages with the social reform projects and nationalist politics.[60] Although similar discussions over the 'male body' started around the same period,[61] this theme failed to attract ample historiographical attention. Nevertheless, it is a historical fact that 'female sexuality' was not the only thing which was attempted to be controlled and restricted during the late nineteenth and early twentieth century, since even 'male sexuality' came under scrutiny and restrictions were imposed on it as well.

The emphatic discourse over brahmacharya or sexual self-control became a key feature of nationalist as well as communal discourse of the period under discussion. Gandhi particularly brought the issue of brahmacharya to the forefront of nationalist politics.[62] According to Gandhi, those who wanted to perform national service, or to have a gleam of the real religious life, must lead a celibate life, whether married or unmarried.[63] Moreover, emphasising the necessity of continence, Gandhi argued:

> Many are the keys to health, and they are all quite essential; but the one thing needful, above all others is *brahmacharya*. Of course, pure air, pure water, and wholesome food do contribute to health. But how can we be healthy if *we expend all the health that we acquire*? How can we help being paupers if we spend all the money that we earn? There can be no doubt that men and women can never be *virile* or *strong* unless they observe true *brahmacharya*.'[64]

In fact, as shown by Joseph Alter, Mahatma Gandhi established an integral relationship among celibacy, non-violence and healthy body, each of them being contingent upon the other two. All the experiments of Gandhi pertaining to health, healing, dietetics, physical exercises, *pranayam*s and yoga *asana*s (physical postures) were ultimately aimed at and, in turn, based upon equilibrium of celibacy, non-violence and healthy body.[65]

Giving brahmacharya a more institutionalised shape, the Rashtriya Swayamsevak Sangh and its various affiliated organisations made sexual self-control the 'supreme characteristic' of a man. It projected brahmacharya as an essential trait for serving the nation and the society. In fact, only a '*brahmachari*' could ever rise to the status of the *sarsanghachalak*—the highest post in the Rashtriya Swayamsevak Sangh organisation. Thus, the communalisation of Indian politics in the early twentieth century gave brahmacharya a more institutionalised and militant form, both in the realm of politics as well as in the realm of public life in general.[66]

In short, by the early twentieth century, celibacy and sexual self-control came to be viewed as the most important ways to discipline one's own body and to make oneself 'healthy' and 'masculine' so that one could serve in the interest of the broader public and the nation. As a result, personal and public interests coalesced with each other in the discourse over brahmacharya. If we look at the Ayurvedic discourse of the time, it also reflected similar concerns regarding sexual self-control/restraint and brahmacharya. One can find endless guidelines for securing a celibate life in the Ayurvedic texts published from the United Provinces during this period. In this regard, some of the Ayurvedic texts identified eight kinds of sex ('*ashta-maithun*') leading to the loss of brahmacharya.[67] These were:

(i) *Smaran* (Remembrance): to recollect and remember a woman—heard of, read about or seen somewhere in a photograph
(ii) *Kirtan* (Eulogising): to narrate and praise the beauty, bodily attributes or manners of a woman and to involve in related 'dirty talk'
(iii) *Keli* (Fun and frolic): to play games such as Holi and cards with women or being waggish or humorous with them
(iv) *Prekshan* (Observation): to see a woman stealthily or to look at her with 'lustful eyes'
(v) *Guhya Bhasan* (Secret talk): to chat secretly with women, to read sleazy novels, stories, plays, etc., or to indulge in lustful talk with them
(vi) *Samkalp* (Determination): to try and get a woman by hook or by crook

(vii) *Adhyavasay* (Sexual enterprise): to come close to a woman with the desire for gratification or the actual sex

(viii) *Sambhog* (Copulation): to establish direct physical relationship with a woman

The Ayurvedic texts like the one written by Suryabali Singh claimed that in the case of an 'ideal' brahmachari, indulgence in any one of the above-mentioned activities would lead to the loss of brahmacharya. The logic behind it was that any activity which leads to ejaculation of semen comes in the category of sex. And, according to Suryabali Singh, due to indulgence in any of the activities enlisted above, semen moves from its 'proper' place and comes out of the body while urinating or sleeping.[68] Driven by the same logic, the text further suggested that a brahmachari should never ride a bicycle or a horse because this puts pressure on the vein between the scrotum and the rectum which leads to 'loss' of semen. Similarly, it also warned the brahmacharis against sleeping on soft and warm bedding.[69]

Thus, on the surface, the entire idea of brahmacharya or self-control appeared so fragile that it could be violated merely through engaging in fun and frolic with women or even through remembering them. Such Ayurvedic discourse reduced women in a misogynist manner as 'sexual objects' whose proximity and company could 'distract' men from the 'ideal' path of celibacy. This was in tune with the patriarchal conceptualisation of women's sexual behaviour.

The Ayurvedic texts also severely criticised masturbation and anal sex or homosexuality. In fact, these two were often regarded as 'horrendous' and 'immoral' forms of sex and, as discussed earlier, 'Muslim rule' was particularly held responsible for homosexuality.[70] Homosexuality/anal sex was attacked to such an extent that even sex with a prostitute and *niyog* (a conjugal practice according to which a childless widow could have sexual intercourse with her husband's younger brother in order to beget a child) were preferred over it, in case of extreme sexual desire.

However, by repeatedly attacking homosexuality, masturbation, etc., to such an extent, these Ayurvedic texts indirectly testify to the widespread prevalence of these seemingly 'immoral' sexual activities among the common public. In fact, the author of *Arogya Darpan* himself accepted that people engaging in anal sex and homosexuality were countless in places like Kashi (Benares) and Lucknow.[71] Similarly, one text which became particularly notorious in the United Provinces for the titillating stories which it contained on homosexual relationships was *Chaklet* written by Pandey Bechan Sharma 'Ugra' in 1927. Although at the end of each story it condemned such homosexual practices and brought out their negative outcomes, still, as argued by Charu Gupta, '[I]n the process of condemnation they also acknowledged the wide prevalence of such practices, especially in UP [the United Provinces], where the beautiful young boys were called 'chocolate', 'pocket-book' and 'money order".[72] Also, its commercial success despite all round criticisms testifies many things.[73] Then, there were colonial and native newspaper reports as well, which indicate the same thing.[74]

Nevertheless, brahmacharya and preservation of semen became essential both in personal as well as in the national interest. The Ayurvedic discourse of the period under discussion linked many diseases with the loss of semen (*virya*). For example, Yashoda Devi blamed the loss of semen as one of the causes behind constipation.[75] Similarly, attacking excessive sexual desire, masturbation and night-fall or wet dreams (*swapnadosh*), she stated that among per 1,000 tuberculosis patients, a large share was of those having uncontrolled sexual behaviour, then of those who masturbated and finally of those 'suffering' from night-fall or wet dreams.[76] Further, she argued that masturbation, anal sex, excessive uncontrolled sex, visits to prostitutes, etc., were responsible for male impotency as well.[77] The author of *Arogya Darpan* also emphasised on the preservation of semen for personal health, wealth, strength and intelligence. In fact, he opposed child marriage not because of its ill-effects on the girl's body, but largely because it was threat to brahmacharya and consequently a threat to healthy 'male body' and its future prospects.[78] It also blamed child marriage for arousing excessive inclination towards sex at a very early age and consequent visits to prostitutes.[79] Thus, one can see in the above arguments a male-centric perspective and raison d'être to oppose child marriage.

Furthermore, following the nationalist–communalist discourse, the Ayurvedic tracts stressed on the preservation of semen in broader interest of the 'nation' and 'community' as well. In fact, the basis of the British paramountcy was also seen in the preservation of semen by the English.

According to Jagannath Sharma, it was because of the valour associated with the preservation of semen that the English had been ruling India for more than 100 years.[80] Similarly, Suryabali Singh in his text argued that it was because of the loss of semen that 'we lost our independence and received all round disgrace'.[81] It was claimed that until and unless the youth of India recognised the significance of brahmacharya and tended to preserve semen, India could never regain its independence.

These texts eulogised Hanuman and Bhishma Pitamah for their lifelong brahmacharya and the associated courage. Brahmacharya was seen as the greatest asset of a young male and loss of semen was seen as synonymous with death.[82] Brahmacharya and ways and means to preserve semen (*viryarakshanopayah*) also figured as one of the topics of study in the syllabus of the Ayurvedic course conducted by the College of Ayurveda, Banaras Hindu University.[83] Interestingly, attempts were made to shun the popular romantic characterisation of Krishna as well and to retrieve a chaste, celibate deity. In this regard, a reinterpretation of Krishna's *raslila* (sensuous dancing) was attempted. It was argued that since Krishna was an ideal brahmachari having firm control over his senses, people of respected families allowed their daughters and sisters to play with him.[84]

One very remarkable feature of the Ayurvedic discourse on brahmacharya was that despite putting severe restrictions on male sexuality along with an uncompromising attack on the so-called 'wrong' sexual habits (such as masturbation, night-fall, anal sex and prostitution), the 'Hindu' male was rarely held responsible for indulgence in these 'wrong' sexual activities. In other words, the 'Hindu' male was often seen as an 'innocent entity' contaminated by some external agency—be it 'Muslim rule', modern civilisation and institutions, or immoral sexual behaviour of '*nautch* girls', prostitutes and the lower orders, etc. Thus, the onus of contaminating the 'Hindu' male was always on the 'Others'; and it often exhibited the caste, class, gender and communal prejudices. In other words, in such discourse, 'Hindu' male was mostly portrayed as a 'poor', 'innocent' and 'vulnerable' character who could easily be 'distracted'.

Pannalal Sharma in his text *Yuva-Rakshak* particularly attacked the 'nautch girls'/dancing girls, who used to perform in the countryside during wedding ceremonies, for promoting tendencies like masturbation, homosexuality and prostitution among the youth.[85] Similarly, the author of *Arogya Darpan* stated that '[I]t has often been seen that if a gorgeous, charming and extremely beautiful girl is born in the lower clan or in the poor's quarter, then she becomes sexually corrupt (*vyabhicharini*)'.[86] Adding to this caste/class attack, Chatursen Shastri argued that it was mostly the people of the low caste/class such as *kahar* (water or palanquin bearers), *dhiwar* (fisherman), *kochwan* (coachman) and *mali* (gardener) who instilled 'unnatural' sexual behaviour among small boys and exploited them sexually. Similarly, he blamed the low-caste women who frequented the homes of respected families as servants for sexually corrupting young girls, widows and daughters-in-law. Keeping all this in mind, Chatursen Shastri advised his readers to hire only aged kahar, dhiwar, kochwan, mali, dai, etc., and suggested that parents should always keep an eye over them and should never leave their children alone in the company of such people.[87] Thus, Ayurvedic tracts upheld caste/class boundaries as being vital, transgression of which could lead to serious sexual and health-related problems.

Here, one can clearly see a caste/class offensive which was launched by the proponents of brahmacharya. The accusation that 'Muslim rule' promoted homosexuality has already been discussed. Furthermore, attacking modern civilisation and institutions, Yashoda Devi in one of her texts supported the *gurukul* system over the modern system of education. This was largely because the gurukul system was able to safeguard brahmacharya, which she found almost impossible in the modern-day educational institutions.[88] Similarly, Chatursen Shastri also condemned the modern-day educational system and institutions for making the youth 'characterless', 'drunkards', 'smoke addicts', etc., because of which they ultimately fell in the trap of 'immoral' sexual activities (see Figure 4.3). Not only this, as caricatured in Figure 4.3, modern education was often seen as turning students effeminate, weak (with spectacles) and less virile. Incidentally, the most alarming feature which Shastri found in the modern educational institutes was the co-habitation of married and unmarried youths in the same hostel. He also believed that the kind of literature—full of romance and sensuality—that had become part of the syllabi of the modern-day educational institutions was dangerous from the brahmacharya point of view.[89] Following a similar line, Parshuram Shastri Vidyasagar of Ambala also, in his article on *prameha*,[90] hints

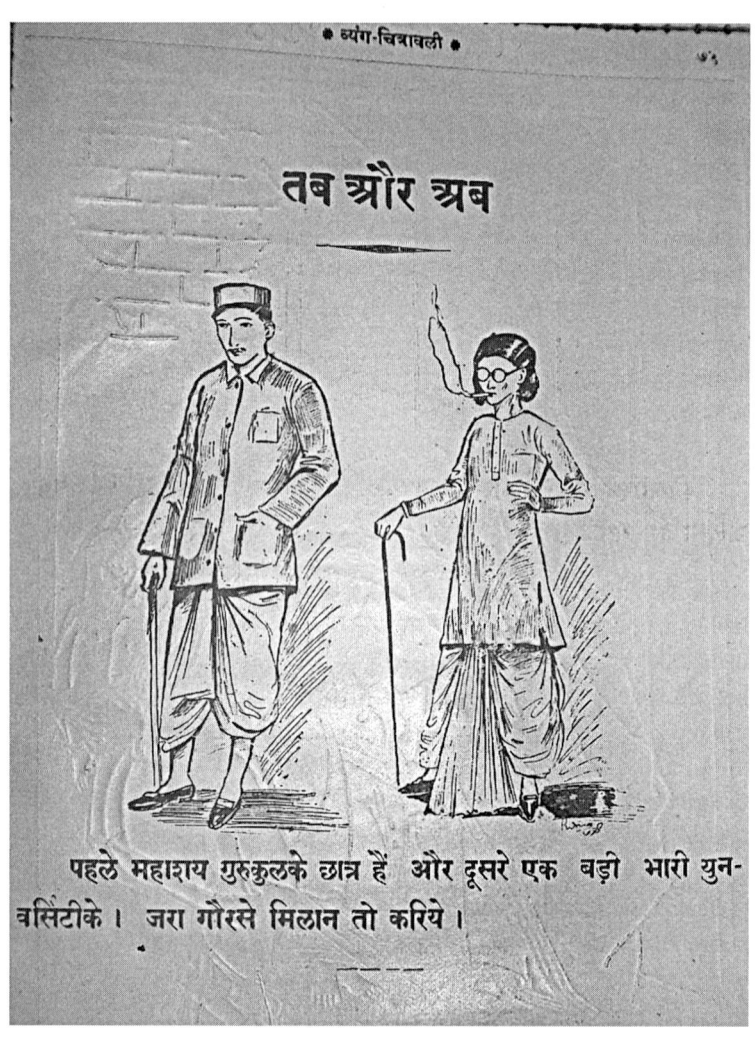

Figure 4.3: Then and now: Caricatured comparison between students belonging to *gurukul* and a modern educational institution.[91]

towards the extant 'unnatural' sexual bonds between students and teachers in schools.[92] In fact, in many of the health tracts of this period, schools, colleges, hostels, cinemas, theatres, social service organisations, parks, clubs, industrial townships and jails (all of which were, interestingly, products of colonialism and in a sense associated with the colonial modernity) were seen as potential sites for homosexual bonding and adultery. Modern way of living, diet (especially non-vegetarianism and drinking tea, coffee and alcohol) and Western medicine were also held responsible for adulterous sexual behaviour and subsequent loss of brahmacharya.[93] Thus, there were multiple explanations for the reasons behind the loss of brahmacharya, but none of them ever questioned the 'self-involvement' of (Hindu) male in it.

MIDWIFERY

The late nineteenth and early twentieth century Ayurvedic discourse on midwifery was equally casteist, communal, and gender- and class-biased. In India, the 'dais' were the ones who used to practice midwifery as a hereditary profession normally without any formal training. Due to the notions of 'ritual pollution' associated with birth, the dai was invariably a woman of low caste, often an untouchable or an adivasi (tribal). In the United Provinces, the dais belonged mostly to the Chamar caste; in Bengal they could be *Hadi*s or *Dom*s or tribals; in Punjab they were largely *Chuhrri*s; whereas in south India they often belonged to the *Barber* caste. At some places, they could be from among poor Muslim families (such as in Bengal and Punjab), but Muslim women generally did not perform the task of cutting the umbilical cord which was regarded as the uncleanest of all the jobs associated with midwifery, leaving it to the untouchable 'Hindu' midwife.[94] In fact, cutting of the umbilical cord was ritually so much polluting that '*Narketa*' (literally, 'one who cuts umbilical cord') was a term of abuse in most parts of north India, and even among Doms (an untouchable caste), the sub-caste which allowed its women to perform this task was regarded as inferior to other members of the same caste.[95] In other words, the dais, without any exception, came from among the untouchables and low castes/classes in most parts of India over the late nineteenth and early twentieth century.

Nonetheless, it was precisely during this period that we see a reformist middle-class and upper-caste discourse on midwifery which got its supporters from among the practitioners of 'indigenous' medicine as well. The Ayurvedic texts and pamphlets started advocating for 'refined' midwives belonging to 'respectable' castes and classes. The urge for professionalisation of midwifery became a handy tool in realising this process of purging the lower castes/class from the practices related to child birth. In other words, this discourse of professionalisation of the dais had many intricate dimensions, which included caste, class, gender and religious prejudices.

The demonisation of the Indian dais began in the latter half of the nineteenth century in colonial literature, when the colonial government sought to garner more and more ideological support for its presence in India in the wake of smothering resistance.[96] During the first half of the nineteenth century also the colonial government repeatedly highlighted issues like *sati* and the poor conditions of widows as being the indicator of the 'civilisational backwardness' of India, and posed itself as the liberator of India's 'suffering daughters'. Following this, the high maternal and infant mortality of India became a handy pretext of the 'civilising mission' in the second half of the nineteenth century. This took a formal shape through the establishment of the *Countess of Dufferin's Fund* in 1885 with the avowed aim of providing better medical facilities to India's 'suffering women', especially the pregnant women. An interesting apocryphal story behind the establishment of this fund was that Queen Victoria was moved by the touching message of the Maharani of Panna (via the medical missionary Elizabeth Bielby), who begged the Queen to 'do something' for her 'daughters in India' who suffered so much of pain during child birth. That is why, when Lady Dufferin was leaving for India along with her Viceroy husband in 1883, the Queen commanded her to initiate some plan to relieve the 'suffering daughters of India'.[97] This royal command became a kind of symbolic guideline for future vicereines as well. Beginning from Lady Harriet Dufferin, vicereines such as Lady Curzon, Lady Hardinge, Lady Chelmsford and Lady Reading came up with their own schemes of maternity and child care in India.

However, all this was not without a cultural baggage. Most of these schemes shared the demonisation of the traditional midwives in India.

Actually, in the twentieth century, while responding to the prevalence of high maternal and infant mortality rate in India, despite its 'civilising presence' for the last 150 years, the colonial government often blamed dais for this phenomenon. They were portrayed as the real 'demons' of the story. Here is the portrayal by Mary Frances Billington (a journalist working for the *Daily Graphic* who visited India in the 1890s and wrote as many as 28 articles on women's lives in India) of a traditional Indian dai, wherein a connection was established between the ways and methods of a dai and the high infant mortality rate of India:

> That infant mortality is very high is not on account of evil intent, but is due to the appalling ignorance of the *dais*, the professional class of midwives or monthly nurses whose methods of treatment are simply *barbarous*, and, indeed, viewed in the light of our scientific knowledge, seem as if they would be *enough to kill every unfortunate victim upon whom they practised.*[98]

It was in this overall context that the colonial government pushed for the professionalisation of dais and their training in Western methods of child birth. Thus, in colonial perception the professional training of the dais was not just an issue of public health, but also a civilisational and social one.

Although it was the colonial government which initiated the process of demonisation of the dais and their subsequent replacement by professional midwives trained in Western methods, the Indian upper-caste/middle-class reformist elites provided the catalytic force to this entire project. This was reflected in the Ayurvedic discourse and popular health tracts of the time. Pandit Kishori Dutt Shastri in his presidential address at the sixth United Provinces Vaidya Sammelan (Haridwar) stressed on the necessity of having trained midwives.[99] Despite being engaged in a head-to-head fight against the Western system of medicine, the Ayurvedic practitioners cherished the idea of the *sarkari* training of the dais. In fact, being part of the upper-caste/middle-class elite, these Ayurvedic practitioners had many reasons to support the process of the professionalisation of dais. First, the newly emerging reformist elite had imbibed the Western parameters of civilisational advancement to such an extent that they found the untrained dais really 'embarrassing'. The reformist elite were desperate to pose themselves as a champion of women's cause both in their collaboration with and fight against the colonial regime; hence, eradication of suffering in child birth was an issue significant to them, at least in public polemics and debates. That is why we see princes, zamindars, business class, professionals, etc., donating handsomely to Dufferin's fund and other maternity and child care schemes launched by the vicereines and the colonial authorities.[100]

Second, there were political underpinnings as well. It should be noted that the colonial linkages between treatment towards women and civilisational status, which first came to be established in the early nineteenth century, continued to be there throughout the colonial rule as an important parameter to judge the progress of India, and more so of the Indians. That is why, Katherine Mayo, writing as late as in 1927, argued in her much controversial *Mother India* that a nation incapable of treating its women better was unfit for self-government.[101] Furthermore, the issue of maternal health and pronatalism got inextricably linked with the health of the 'nation' both in inter-War Europe and the colonial world. A 'healthy progeny' and a 'healthy mother' became symbols of a 'healthy nation' and its bright future. In this regard, the traditional dais were seen as enemies of the 'health of the nation' as they were blamed for the high infant and maternal mortality of India.

Besides these overtly political reasons, the reformist urge regarding the professionalisation of dais had caste/class dimensions as well. As argued earlier, the entire project to recast 'indigenous' medicine, which was going on in the late nineteenth and early twentieth century, cannot be studied by ignoring the paradigm of caste/class. While the newly emerging vaids and hakims were contesting the dominance of Western medicine, they were also trying to purge the tribal and lower-caste healing practices and influences out of the fold of Ayurveda and Unani methods of healing. In other words, the upper-caste/middle-class elite (which commanded the Ayurvedic discourse of the time) attempted to draw clear-cut boundaries in terms of lower- and upper-caste/class healing practices. It was also a significant part of identity formation for the reformist middle class and for that it invoked traditional notions of 'purity' and 'pollution' related to caste.[102]

In the United Provinces, the early twentieth century vernacular medical texts condemned the dais for their alleged 'unclean and polluting' habits and behaviour, not just physically but also morally and sexually. It is noticeable that in the United Provinces the dais belonged mostly to the

Chamar caste, which made them appear as people of 'doubtful decency and of being dirty and unsanitary' in middle-class imagination.[103] *Grihastha Jeevan*, a text written by Keshavkumar Thakur in 1932, emphasised the rich and well-cultured surroundings and found it dirty and unhygienic to have people of lower castes in close proximity.[104] Interestingly, when the colonial government pushed for the professionalisation of dais, it tried to train the same hereditary low-caste dais in Western methods of child birth and convert them into professional dais. In contrast, the upper-caste/middle-class reformists wished 'refined' and 'respectable' women to enter this profession. The call was made especially to the widows of 'good families' to take up this job.[105]

There was an effort to safeguard the newly born babies from the 'unhealthy' and 'immoral' influences of the low-caste dais. It should be noted that the dai in pre-colonial Indian society commanded huge authority over child birth. She was the sole companion of pregnant women during their most troublesome days, especially in *sutika griha* or *antur ghar*.[106] She was the first one to come in contact with the newly born baby, sometimes even before the mother (in cases when the mother fell unconscious after delivery). Also, she was the first one to report to the rest of the family members whether the newly arrived member of the family was a son or a daughter, which had great significance in a patriarchal society. In such a situation, the upper-caste/middle-class elite which was trying to demarcate the caste and class boundaries found it awkward as well as embarrassing to have a low-caste person whose morality and cleanliness (both in the physical and the sexual sense) was 'doubtful'.

Even though it was impossible to replace all the dais, the urban upper-caste/middle-class of the United Provinces often shunned the services of these 'lowly' dais, thereby asserting their caste and class superiority.[107] At the national level, in 1934, the All India Women's Conference (AIWC), an organisation dominated by the reformist middle-class Indian women, passed a resolution requiring 'compulsory registration' of all the dais and midwives, and argued in favour of the dais and midwives trained in Western medicine and hygiene and supervised by approved medical personnel in place of the traditional neighbourhood dais.[108]

The gender aspect was also involved in this reformist urge for the professionalisation of dais. As argued by the feminist scholars, every public debate around women's issues in colonial India in a way ended up by 'recasting patriarchy'.[109] Even those scholars who argue strongly in favour of 'women's agency' involved in these debates and see women as not being 'passive victims' of the reformist forces[110] cannot completely discard the fact that patriarchy in the middle-class discourse found multiple camouflaged techniques to assert itself. The issue of child birth prior to the twentieth century in India was an exclusively woman-dominated sphere. Men were excluded completely from sutika griha or antur ghar and they hardly had any say in birth rituals and activities. However, the professionalisation of midwifery was supposed to open up this sphere even for males, as it did in Europe. Queen Victoria had herself been delivered by a male surgeon.[111] In fact, controlling women's reproductive health was central to securing a middle-class life in the metropolitan world as well as in colonial India. Exclusive women's spheres were looked upon with a lot of suspicion and disdain by the male members of the reformist middle class and they attacked these spheres which were associated directly with women under some pretext or the other. Sometimes the language of this attack was communal (such as in the case of attack on women's practice of visiting the *pirs*),[112] whereas sometimes it was casteist (as in the case of the dai), but a hidden gendered agenda of exercising control and regulating these relatively 'semi-autonomous' spheres was always there.

Last but not least, communal perceptions also determined the demand for the professionalisation of dais, especially in Bengal and Punjab, where poor Muslim women were engaged in midwifery. In the era of communal polarisation, the Muslim dais were blamed for the 'degenerating' Hindu race. For example, a pamphlet by Bibi Mahindra Kaur (an upper-caste midwife from Punjab) entitled *Murakh Daian* (1930) claimed that the Muslim dais used to read the *kalima* (Muslim sacred utterance) instead of whispering *nam* (name of God) and *shabad* (sacred word) in the ears of new-born babies, thereby making them perverts.[113]

However, despite all this upper-caste/middle-class discourse to professionalise midwifery, little could be achieved on the ground, especially in the rural areas. The traditional dais did not disappear from the scene all of a sudden. According to the Bhore Committee Report, as late as in 1946, there were only 10,856 certified midwives and 662 assistant midwives registered by the provincial councils. Even these figures, according to the Report itself, were probably in excess of the correct number. It speculated the correct number of trained midwives to be somewhere around 5,000. Further, as delineated, in order to provide one (trained) midwife for every 100 births, 100,000 midwives were required.[114] This shows that even as late as the mid-twentieth century, a huge population of India had still been resorting to the services of traditional 'untrained' hereditary midwives.[115] Incidentally, Premchand also acknowledges this ground reality in his short story 'Doodh ka Daam' as follows:

> Ab bade-bade shehron mein daiyan, nursein aur lady doctor, sabhi paida ho gayi hain; lekin dehaton mein jachchekhanon par abhi tak bhanginon ka hi prabhutva hai aur nikat bhavishya mein is mein koi tabdili hone ki asha nahin.[116]

(Now-a-days there are trained midwives, nurses and lady doctors in the big cities; still in the rural areas the dominance of *Bhangin*s has remained unchallenged in case of delivery of a child and there is no hope of change in this situation in near future.)

Thus, the continuing dominance of traditional low-caste dais posed a real challenge to the rural upper caste/middle class. As, on the one hand, they were trying to purge these 'lowly' dais out of the fold of maternal health care, but at the same time they required their services. This ambiguity of the rural middle class has been brought out wonderfully by Premchand in the aforesaid story where he shows how the village zamindar, being unable to pay the exorbitant fees of the trained midwives and nurses, had to resort to the services of a traditional dai called Bhungi, who was from an untouchable caste. Bhungi also stepped into the role of a dhai (wet mother) and fed the newly born baby of the zamindar as his wife failed to provide sufficient milk for the infant. According to Premchand, for almost a year Bhungi was the mistress of the entire household and exercised commanding authority over other servants.

> Ghar mein Malkin ke baad Bhungi ka rajya tha. Mehriyan, maharajin, naukar-chakar sab uska roab mante the. Yahan tak ki khud Bahu ji bhi us se dab jati thin.[117]

(After the landlady, Bhungi was second-in-command of the entire household. All the servants of the household obeyed her. In fact, on occasions even the landlady had to accept her sayings.)

At this juncture of need, nobody objected to the perks enjoyed by Bhungi. However, as soon as the baby grew up and no longer needed to be fed by a lactating woman, the *pundit*s of the village came onto the scene and objected to the continuation of the services of Bhungi on the basis of her being a low/untouchable caste. To quote Premchand:

> Bhungi ka shasan kaal saal bhar se aage na chal saka. Devtaon ne balak ke Bhangin ka doodh peene par apatti ki, Moteram Shastri toh prayashchit ka prastav kar baithe.[118]

(The reign of Bhungi could not continue for more than a year. The Gods objected on the milk of a Bhangin. Not only this, Moteram Shastri even suggested for repentance.)

Thus, Premchand brings out the contradictions exhibited by the rural landowning class/upper castes on the issue of midwifery as the ideological concerns and pragmatic necessities were pulling them into two opposite directions. At the same time, he also suggests the extreme pragmatism of the rural propertied class in this regard.

CONCLUDING REMARKS

The Ayurvedic discourse of the late nineteenth and early twentieth century in the United Provinces while, on the one hand, condemned the popular vernacular and medieval medical anthologies, on the other hand, it was very selective in its adoption of the Ayurvedic norms, concepts and treatment methods from ancient Indian health treatises like *Charaka*, *Sushruta* and *Vagbhata Samhitas*. There was a selective reading of such ancient health treatises by the 'new' vaids who reinforced the prevalent social—particularly brahmanical—norms. For example, many of the Ayurvedic texts during this time emphasised vegetarianism. In fact, one of the grounds on which the system of Western medicine was attacked by the Ayurvedic practitioners was that allopathic medicines often contained animal flesh and alcohol, both having 'polluting' effects from the religious point of view.[119] However, if we look at the ancient health treatises, many of them have praised non-vegetarianism from the health perspective. Incidentally, '*mansa-rasa*' or meat soup has been deemed by most of these texts as the best medicine in case of extreme emaciation. For example, Charaka has enumerated the following benefits of 'mansa-rasa' in curing *pitta*-imbalance, in improving voice strength, skin quality, immunity, etc.:

> For all living beings, meat soup is nourishing and refreshing. This is regarded as nectar for the dehydrated, during convalescence, for the emaciated, and for those desirous of strength and lustre. Meat soup prepared accordingly alleviates many diseases. It promotes voice, youth, intelligence, power of the sense organs and longevity. The persons who are indulged in physical exercise, sex and wine do not fall ill or become weak if they take a diet with meat soup regularly.[120]

Suggesting almost the same thing, the *Vagbhata Samhita* states that 'nothing in this world is more invigorating than meat'.[121] Furthermore, the *Sushruta Samhita* provides an extensive catalogue of meats and their therapeutic linkages. In totality, Sushruta lists 168 types of meats (of different animals) in his catalogue of meats impacting the designated humor[122] or disorder either by 'calming' it or 'exciting' it.[123]

Similarly, Charaka has suggested the non-restriction of any of the 'natural flow' coming out of the body ('*na vegan dharye dhimanah*'),[124] as this may lead to various kinds of diseases. Interestingly, the 13 'natural outflows' of the body listed by him include the ejaculation of semen as well. In other words, the rigorous preservation of semen, which the early twentieth century Ayurvedic texts were emphasising, was not suggested in the ancient health treatises but was a modern invention. Thus, the socio-political context in which the late colonial Ayurvedic discourse unfolded had huge bearings on its social content/texture.

Now, as will be seen, the market and its dynamics also played a major role in shaping this socially prejudiced Ayurvedic discourse of the late nineteenth and early twentieth century, and was crucial in determining the course of the late colonial Ayurvedic movement. The next chapter analyses the salient features of the Ayurvedic print as well as drug market to assess the impact both of them generated on the late colonial Ayurvedic movement/discourse.

NOTES

1. Berger, *Ayurveda Made Modern*, 89.
2. Pandit Ganesh Dutt Sharma, *Dadru-Chikitsa*, 1st edn (Benares, 1932), 3.
3. For such kind of racial interpretation of diseases and sanitary habits by the colonial authorities and its effect on the Indian populace, on their lifestyle and on their dwelling places, especially in the aftermath of the 1857 uprisings, see Veena Oldenburg, *The Making of Colonial Lucknow: 1856–77* (Princeton: Princeton University Press, 1984). Tremendous stereotyping was carried out regarding the sanitary habits, cleanliness and dwelling places of Indians in the post-1857 Lucknow which, in turn, paved the way for racial division of space as well.
4. Baijnath Kedia, *Vyang Chitravali* (Calcutta and Benares: Hindi Pustak Academy, 1932), 65. Interestingly, the servant/cook caricatured here appears to be an upper-caste servant as evident from his *shikha* (tuft of hair). This is largely because cooks in a Hindu household mostly belonged to the upper caste owing to the fact that the brahmanical order differentiates between the 'cooked' and the 'uncooked' food as carriers of pollution. Cooked food is liable to pass on pollution, while uncooked food is not. So, while uncooked food may be received from members of any caste, cooked food cannot be accepted from the member of a lower caste. For details on such distinctive characterisitics of cooked/uncooked food, see Mary Douglas, *Purity and Danger: An Analysis of Concepts of Pollution and Taboo* (London: Routledge, 1966), 34. However, in terms of class status, even an upper-caste servant or cook belonged to the lower class and was subjected to similar class prejudices as can be seen in the caricature.
5. It is noticeable that naturalisation of caste hierarchy by superimposing it over racial differences was one of the characteristic features of colonial construction of caste as exhibited through the writings of H. H. Risley, the British census commissioner. Risley emphatically argued that caste distinctions had a racial basis. According to him, upper castes were basically from superior races whereas lower castes were racially inferior. The Indian middle class that comprised primarily of people drawn from upper castes was quick to endorse this newly constructed racial interpretation of caste. In this regard, H. H. Risley's decision to arrange the castes in terms of their social precedence in the census of 1901 gave further fillip to racialised notions of caste and subsequent formation of caste groups competing with each other to pose themselves higher in the caste ladder and agitating for the same.
6. Rai Pooran Chand was a member of the All India Vaidyak Vidyapith and a member of the commission appointed by the All India Vaidya Sammelan to

enquire into plague, cholera, malaria and other epidemic diseases of India and their remedies. Plague, in fact, attracted the fantasy of many of the Ayurvedic practitioners towards the end of the nineteenth and early twentieth century due to frequently occurring epidemics. The Ayurvedic practitioners acknowledged the utility of a curative prophylactic developed by W. M. Haffkine in diminishing the incidence of plague attacks on the inoculated population, but they never considered this remedy absolute. In fact, in the world view of the Ayurvedic practitioners, there were several other factors creating congenial conditions for plague infection such as indigestion, overfeeding, fasting, irregular diet, uncleanliness, constipation, and even sleeping late hours at night and too much sleeping during the day. For some interesting insights on the Ayurvedic response to plague, see Natasha Sarkar, 'Fleas, Faith and Politics: Anatomy of an Indian Epidemic, 1890–1925' (PhD diss., Department of History, National University of Singapore, 2011), 182–86.

7. Rai Pooran Chand, *Plague Darpan* (Patna City: Satya Sudhakar Press, 1916).
8. Bimal Roy in his cult movie *Sujata* (1959) also portrayed an interesting corollary related to prevailing pseudo-scientific social notions regarding the linkage between the lower castes/untouchables and spread of disease or polluting substance. In this movie, a Brahmin pundit has been shown advising one of the main characters that he should abandon the untouchable child (that is, Sujata), whom he had adopted, as soon as possible as it was a 'proven scientific fact' that there comes out a kind of gas from the body of the untouchables which pollutes the body, mind and soul of the 'noble' people.
9. A. G. Vyas, *Su-Santati Shastra* (Mathura, 1929), 5.
10. Bhargava, *Santati Shastra*, 252–54.
11. Incidentally, by the late nineteenth and early twentieth century, both colonial and 'indigenous' representations of child maternity and infant feeding fused with issues related to the health, strength and well-being of the caste, community and nation. For a recent intervention in this regard, see Ranjana Saha, 'Infant Feeding: Child Marriage and 'Immature Maternity' in Colonial Bengal, 1890s–1920s', *Proceedings of the Indian History Congress*, 75th session, New Delhi, 2014, 708–15. Saha has shown how during the particular time span of 1890s–1920s, breastfeeding and artificial feeding of infants got entangled with broader discussions on the body, age of consent for sexual intercourse, conjugality, maternity, nutrition, midwifery, and high infant and maternal mortality rates in colonial Bengal.
12. See page 16 of the pamphlet titled 'Bharat ki Unnati ka Vaidyak Pratham Anga Hai', in Pandit Jagannath Sharma, *Arogya Darpan*, Vol. 3 (Prayag, 1898) (emphasis added).

13. One of the fundamental ideas underlying caste hierarchy is the notion of 'purity' and 'pollution'. The brahmanical idea of dualism suggests that everything in this world is either the manifestation of 'purity' or 'pollution'. Correspondingly, within caste hierarchy, Brahmins represent the 'purest' (and hence are at the top of the hierarchy) and the untouchables or the outcastes represent the 'most polluted' beings. All other castes lie in between these two extremes in purity/pollution scale. For details on this theme, see Louis Dumont, *Homo Hierarchicus: The Caste System and Its Implications*, trans Mark Sanisbury, Louis Dumont and Basia Gulati (Chicago: University of Chicago Press, 1980).
14. 'Sutrasthana, Chapter XVI', in Bhishagratna, *Sushruta Samhita*, 1: 152–54.
15. Referring to such demotion of the social status of a medical practitioner from that of a royal surgeon to a barber and potter in the latter period, Susmita Basu Majumdar, on the basis of the study of epigraphs, argues that most of the physicians performing surgical operations had to look for alternative professions for subsistence and they mostly took the professions of barbers (as they already had surgical instruments which sufficed the requirements of the barbers' art) and potters (as besides making pottery the art of a potter also includes making clay models and the surgeons having a thorough knowledge of human anatomy could easily shape such models). See Susmita Basu Majumdar, 'Medical Practitioners and Medical Institutions: Gleanings from Epigraphs', *Proceedings of the Indian History Congress*, 69th session, Kannur, 2008, 196–210.
16. *The Gentleman's Magazine* 64, Part 2, October 1794, 891–92.
17. This ritual hijacking by adding Sanskritic chants to already extant practice was very much evident in the case of treatment of snake bite as discussed in Chapter 1 of the present work.
18. Sharma, *Indigenous and Western Medicine*, 43–44.
19. Premchand, *Godan: A Novel of Peasant India*, tr. Jai Ratan and P. Lal, 16th enlarged edn (Bombay: Jaico Publishing House, 2002), 12.
20. Sharma, *Indigenous and Western Medicine*, 4.
21. Raghava Prasad Narayan Singh alias 'Raja Sahab' was the chieftain of Baraon estate of Allahabad and was elder cousin brother of Kunwar Saryu Prasad Narayan Singh—the first president of the All India Vaidya Sammelan.
22. *Sudhanidhi* 17, no. 1, 1928, 8–14.
23. A mythical character of the legendary epic *Ramayana* who went on to become a symbol of fratricide.
24. *Sudhanidhi* 2, no. 3, 1913, 168.
25. *Sudhanidhi* 7, no. 3, 1918, 13–14.

26. Sivaramakrishnan, *Old Potions, New Bottles*, 145.
27. Cited in Sivaramakrishnan, *Old Potions, New Bottles*, 145.
28. For a detailed discussion on the various aspects of the aforesaid theory of the 'dying Hindu race' and its socio-political and communal significance and repercussions in colonial period, see P. K. Datta, *Carving Blocs: Communal Ideology in Early Twentieth Century Bengal* (Delhi: Oxford University Press, 1999), 21–63.
29. Singh, *Nikhil Bharatvarshiya Ayurveda Mahamandal ka Rajat Jayanti Granth*, 2: 43.
30. In case of Punjab, Kavita Sivaramakrishnan has clearly shown this thing by looking at the writings of Bhai Mohan Singh Vaid. See Kavita Sivaramakrishnan, 'The Use of Past in a Public Campaign: Ayurvedic *prachar* in the Writings of Bhai Mohan Singh Vaid', in *Invoking the Past: The Uses of History in South Asia*, ed. Daud Ali (New Delhi: Oxford University Press, 1999), 178–91. Similar trends can be seen in the late nineteenth and early twentieth century Ayurvedic discourse emanating from the United Provinces as well.
31. Acharya Chandrashekhar Shastri, *Sharir Vigyan* (Delhi: 1937), 13.
32. For example, Acharya Chandrashekhar Shastri, while translating modern scientific terms like 'microbes', 'protoplasm' and 'matter' in Hindi, borrows the words from Jaina philosophy and Nyaya darshan (see Shastri, *Sharir Vigyan*, 11).
33. Yashoda Devi, *Ghar ka Vaid* (Allahabad, 1914), 42–48.
34. Yashoda Devi, *Dehati Chikitsa* (Allahabad, n.d.), 22.
35. It indirectly refers to the Muslim rulers of India.
36. Shankar Daji Shastri Pade, *Gorasadi Aushadhi* (Allahabad: Sudhanidhi Granthavali, n.d.), 1.
37. Pandit Ramprasad Mishra 'Rajvaidya', *Kuchimartantram*, 4th edn (Aligrah: Dhanvantari Press, 1965), 38. Its first edition was published in 1925.
38. Pade, *Gorasadi Aushadhi*, 2.
39. Presidential address by Pandit Gananath Sen at the third All India Vaidya Sammelan, Allahabad, 1911 (for the speech, see Singh, *Nikhil Bharatvarshiya Ayurveda Mahamandal ka Rajat Jayanti Granth*, 1: 45–86).
40. Sharma, *Arogya Darpan*, 3: 9.
41. Vyas, *Su-Santati Shastra*, 4.
42. Vinayak Madhav Chingle, 'Brahmacharya', in *Arogya Mandir*, ed. Pravasi Lal Verma (Benares, 1927), 145–46.
43. Verma, *Arogya Mandir*, 72–73.
44. Sharma, *Arogya Darpan*, 3: 1.

45. Published in the form of a booklet by Rai Pooran Chand, entitled *Plague Darpan*.
46. Rai Pooran Chand, *Plague Darpan*, 138.
47. Literally, it translates as: 'A Guide to Proper Code of Conduct of Women'.
48. Yashoda Devi, *Santan Palan*.
49. As per Hindu scriptures, an individual's life passes through four different but sequential stages or *ashramas* namely Brahmacharya (student), Gṛihastha (householder), *Vanaprastha* (forest walker/forest dweller), and *Sanyasa* (renunciate).
50. Interestingly, as argued by Rachel Berger, by referring to her cookbooks as *pakshastra*s (literally, 'the written scriptures of nutrition'), Yashoda Devi gave historic gravitas to her writings as textually authoritative and backed by the sense of 'timeless wisdom' as delineated in classical texts of the Hindu tradition. For detailed discussion on cookbooks belonging to the early twentieth century Hindi print culture and how they reflected and shaped middle class sensibilities and notions, see Rachel Berger, 'Between Digestion and Desire: Genealogies of Food in Nationalist North India', *Modern Asian Studies* 47, no. 5, September 2013, 1622–43.
51. Prakash, *Another Reason*, 148–49. However, all this is not to undermine the 'unique' position that Yashoda Devi held in the field of a healing system (that is, Ayurveda) which was dominated almost exclusively by male practitioners. While patriarchy was rearticulated and reinforced through her medical discourse, her writings in many ways, through their focus on relatively tabooed subjects like women's sexual pleasure and non-consensual sex, offered a critique of male sexual behaviour and occasionally gender hierarchies. In fact, as argued by Charu Gupta, Yashoda Devi's discourse is 'ambiguous and fractured at various levels' and it is difficult 'to enframe her within any fixed category'. According to Gupta, her writings simultaneously reiterated gender hierarchies and also questioned them (see Gupta, 'Procreation and Pleasure', 38).
52. Very little is known about Prakashvati Devi Jain. However, unlike Yashoda Devi who did not have any formal training in Ayurveda and had received her training and education from her father (Gupta, 'Procreation and Pleasure', 26), Prakashvati Devi used the title of '*Vaidya Visharada*'—a title used generally by the vaids having some sort of institutional training or having passed some kind of qualifying examination conducted by an institute/organisation devoted to the cause of promotion of Ayurveda. Also, Prakashvati Devi Jain was the president of the women's department of Amrit Karyalaya located in Agra.

53. Prakashvati Devi Jain, 'Mahila Prayog', in *Anubhoot Yogmala*, Year 22, no. 7, July 1944, 227–30.
54. Yashoda Devi, *Santan Palan* (Allahabad, 1913).
55. Yashoda Devi, *Shishu Raksha Vidhan arthat Balrog Chikitsa* (Allahabd, 1912).
56. Also see Mahendranath Pandey, *Hamare Bachche* (Prayag, 1931), and Jagannath Sharma, *Santan Palan* (Benares, 1933).
57. Incidentally, as Shalini Shah argues, even the seminal Ayurvedic texts like *Charaka Samhita*, *Vagbhata Samhita* and *Madhavanidana* marginalise, if not exclude, women in their discussion of diseases. The only discussions on female body in these texts are in connection with the diseases of uterus (*garbhavyapta*) and genital area (*yonivyapta*) largely because, as argued by Shah, it was only the uterus and genital area of women which was of some significance to a patriarchal male society and related health discourse. Thus, even the discussion on garbhavyapta and yonivyapta was not because of the concern for women's health per se, but because a healthy uterus was crucial for healthy child birth. In all other cases, men's health and virility take an upper hand over that of women in these texts, reducing them as mere 'sex woman'. See Shalini Shah, 'Representation of Female Sexuality in the Ayurvedic Discourse of the Early Medieval Period,' *Studies in History* 22, no. 1, 2006, 45–58.
58. Jawahir Singh Shrivastava, *Vaidya Priya* (Lucknow: Naval Kishore Press, 1924), 241–42. The text suggested applying the paste of pigeon's shit and borax (*suhaga*) on the penis before copulation in order to beget a male child. Similarly, it advised pregnant woman to eat cannabis seeds to fulfil their desire of a male child.
59. Vaidyabhushan Govind Prasad Varshaneya, 'Ichchanusar Putra ya Kanya Hona', *Dhanvantari* 10, no. 4, September 1934, 388–90.
60. Exemplary works in this regard were those of Partha Chatterjee, *Nationalist and the Colonial World: A Derivative Discourse* (London: Zed Books, 1986); Partha Chatterjee, 'Colonialism, Nationalism and Colonised Women: The Contest in India', *American Ethnologist* 16, no. 4, 1989, 622–33; Partha Chatterjee, 'The Nationalist Resolution of the Women's Question', in *Recasting Women: Essays in Indian Colonial History*, eds Kumkum Sangari and Sudesh Vaid (New Brunswick: Rutgers University Press, 1990), 233–53; Lata Mani, 'Contentious Traditions: The Debate on Sati in Colonial India', *Cultural Critique* 7, 1987, 119–56; Uma Chakravarti, 'Whatever Happened to the Vedic Dasi? Orientalism, Nationalism and a Script for the Past', in Sangari and Vaid, *Recasting Women*, 27–87; Susie Tharu, 'Tracing Savitri's Pedigree: Victorian Racism and the Image of Women in Indo-Anglican Literature', in Sangari and Vaid, *Recasting Women*, 254–68.

61. Some noticeable works on this theme are Rosselli John, 'The Self-Image of Effeteness: Physical Education and Nationalism in Nineteenth Century Bengal', *Past and Present* 86, 1980, 121–48; Joseph S. Alter, 'Celibacy, Sexuality and the Transformation of Gender into Nationalism in North India', *The Journal of Asian Studies* 53, no. 1, February 1994, 45–66; Gupta, *Sexuality, Obscenity, Community*.
62. Pat Caplan, 'Celibacy as a Solution? Mahatma Gandhi and Brahmacharya', in *The Cultural Construction of Sexuality*, ed. Pat Caplan (London: Routledge, 1987), 271–95; Alter, 'Celibacy, Sexuality and the Transformation of Gender'.
63. This, in fact, constituted one of the vows drawn up by Gandhi for those seeking the membership of his ashram at Sabarmati. For the vows, see Charles F. Andrews, *Mahatma Gandhi's Ideas* (London: Allen and Unwin, 1929), 101–11.
64. M. K. Gandhi, *A Guide to Health*, trans. A. Rama Iyer (Madras: S. Ganesan Publisher, 1921), 70 (emphases added). Noticeable is the link established between brahmacharya, wealth and virility or health in the aforesaid statement.
65. For details on this integral linkage among celibacy, non-violence and healthy body in Gandhian philosophy, see Joseph S. Alter, *Gandhi's Body: Sex, Diet, and the Politics of Nationalism* (Philadelphia: University of Pennsylvania Press, 2000).
66. Walter K. Anderson and S. D. Damle, *The Brotherhood in Saffron: The Rashtriya Swayamsevak Sangh and Hindu Revivalism* (Boulder: Westview Press, 1987); Philip H. Ashby, *Modern Trends in Hinduism* (New York: Columbia University Press, 1974); Joseph S. Alter, 'Somatic Nationalism: Indian Wrestling and Militant Hinduism', *Modern Asian Studies* 28, no. 3, 1994, 557–88.
67. See Suryabali Singh, *Brahmacharya ki Mahima* (Benares, 1931), 23–24; Yashoda Devi, *Dampati Arogyata Jeevanshastra* (Allahabad, 1927), 30; Chatursen Shastri, *Brahmacharya Sadhan* (Lucknow: Ganga Granthagar, 1928), 58–64.
68. Singh, *Brahmacharya ki Mahima*, 23–24.
69. Ibid., 145.
70. Sharma, *Arogya Darpan*, 3: 9.
71. Ibid.
72. Charu Gupta, 'Dirty Hindi Literature: Contests about Obscenity in Late Colonial North India', *South Asia Research* 20, no. 2, 2000, 114–15. Incidentally, it also hints towards the possibility of male child prostitution where small boys were coerced into this practice, especially at pilgrim centres.
73. According to Charu Gupta, '[T]he book (*Chaklet*) proved to be a commercial sensation, and within six weeks of its publication two editions were sold out' (Gupta, 'Dirty Hindi Literature', 115).

74. For details, see Gupta, 'Dirty Hindi Literature', 116–17.
75. Devi, *Dampati Arogyata Jeevanshastra*, 49.
76. Ibid., 20.
77. Ibid., 66.
78. Sharma, *Arogya Darpan*, 3: 2; also see Babu Kedarnath Gupt, *Swasthya aur Jal Chikitsa* (Allahabad: Chhatra Hitkari Pustakmala, 1933), 1.
79. Sharma, *Arogya Darpan*, 3: 2.
80. Ibid., 1.
81. Singh, *Brahmacharya ki Mahima*, 4.
82. '*Marnam bindu paten jeevanam bindu dharnat*' (Loss of semen is death-like and its preservation is essential for life). For such emphasis on preservation of semen, see Srikrishna Dev Tripathi, 'Dhatu-ksheenata, Virya-srava, Prameha', *Dhanvantari* 10, no. 3, August 1934, 321–22.
83. 'Prospectus of Studies for Examinations of the College of Ayurveda, Benares Hindu University, 1935', in Singh, *Nikhil Bharatvarshiya Ayurveda Mahamandal ka Rajat Jayanti Granth*, 2: 201–30.
84. Shastri, *Brahmacharya Sadhan*, 27–28.
85. Pannalal Sharma, *Yuva-Rakshak* (Agra, 1908). A similar tract was *Jawaan ke Kaan mein Upyogi Vyakhyan* (Mathura, 1916) which attacked '*nautch* girls'.
86. Sharma, *Arogya Darpan*, 3: 29. Thus, 'beauty' of a girl belonging to the lower caste often inflated caste insecurities at the upper echelons leading to character assassination of the girl.
87. Shastri, *Brahmacharya Sadhan*, 74–75.
88. Devi, *Dampati Arogyata Jeevanshastra*, 33–34.
89. Shastri, *Brahmacharya Sadhan*, 77–78.
90. *Prameha* is a generic Ayurvedic term for metabolic disorders in which the person suffers from passage in urine of one or more products of metabolism, which may or may not be a normal constituent of urine, in large amount. For example, *madhumeha* (diabetes mellitus) and *shukrameha* (nightfall).
91. Baijnath Kedia, *Vyang Chitravali* (Calcutta and Benares: Hindi Pustak Academy, 1932), 75.
92. Parshuram Shastri Vidyasagar, 'Prameha', *Anubhoot Yogmala*, Year 6, nos 7–8, April 1928, 187.
93. Vidyasagar, 'Prameha', 187.
94. Supriya Guha, 'From Dais to Doctors: The Medicalisation of Childbirth in Colonial India', in *Understanding Women's Health Issues: A Reader*, ed. Lakshmi Lingam (New Delhi: Kali for Women, 1998), 153.
95. Guha, 'From Dais to Doctors', 153. It shows the prevalence of purity/pollution-based hierarchy even among the untouchables.

96. One very popular idea used by the colonial administration in this regard was that of 'civilising mission'. James Mill in his *The History of British India* (first published in 1817) had propounded that women's position in a society was one of the indicators of its advancement. The colonial government was quick to grab this theory to show India's 'civilisational backwardness'.
97. Geraldine Forbes, 'Managing Midwifery in India', in *Contesting Colonial Hegemony: State and Society in Africa and India*, eds Dagmar Engels and Shula Marks (London: British Academy Press, 1994), 159.
98. M. F. Billington, *Woman in India* (first published, 1895; New Delhi: Amarko Book Agency, 1973, reprint), 2; also cited in Forbes, 'Managing Midwifery in India', 160 (emphasis added).
99. 'Presidential Address of Kishori Dutt Shastri at the 6th United Provinces Vaidya Sammelan, Haridwar', in Singh, *Nikhil Bharatvarshiya Ayurveda Mahamandal ka Rajat Jayanti Granth*, Vol. 2.
100. Related to this was the 'politics of donation'. Donation to such schemes was a handy tool to garner official patronage. Shirish N. Kavadi, 'Philanthropy, Medicine, and Health in Colonial India', in *Encyclopaedia of the History of Science, Technology, and Medicine in Non-Western Cultures*, ed. Helaine Selin (Dordrecht: Springer, 2016).
101. Katherine Mayo, *Mother India* (New York: Blue Ribbon Books, 1927).
102. Anshu Malhotra, 'Of Dais and Midwives: 'Middle Class' Interventions in the Management of Women's Reproductive Health in Colonial Punjab', in *Reproductive Health in India: History, Politics, Controversies*, ed. Sarah Hodges (Delhi: Orient Longman, 2006), 199–226.
103. Gupta, *Sexuality, Obscenity, Community*, 181–82.
104. Keshavkumar Thakur, *Grihastha Jeevan* (Prayag, 1932), 70–71.
105. Ishwaridutt Sharma, 'Atm-tyag', *Saraswati* 17, nos 2–3, September 1916; Prasadilal Jha, 'Achchi Daiyon ki Avashyakta', *Stri Darpan* 29, no. 3, September 1923.
106. *Sutika griha* or *antur ghar* was a dark unventilated small room or hut generally built outside the main quarters, where the woman used to spend last few days of her pregnancy, just before the beginning of labouring activity, and also 10–12 days after giving birth to baby for ritual cleansing. All the routine activities of the pregnant woman during this period of confinement such as from cleaning her clothes to feeding her and all the menial jobs were used to be performed by a dai as only the birthing mother and dai were allowed inside the sutika griha.
107. Gupta, *Sexuality, Obscenity, Community*, 183–84.
108. All India Women's Conference, *All India Women's Conference: Annual Report* (Calcutta, 1934), 150.

109. For example, see the early feminist writings: Lata Mani, 'Contentious Traditions'; Sangari and Vaid, eds, *Recasting Women*; Mrinalini Sinha, *Colonial Masculinity: The 'Manly Englishman' and the 'Effeminate Bengali' in the Late Nineteenth Century* (Manchester: Manchester University Press, 1995).
110. For example, see Douglas E. Haynes and Gyan Prakash, eds, *Contesting Power: Resistance and Everyday Social Relations in South Asia* (Berkeley: University of California Press, 1992); Anindita Ghosh, *Power in Print: Popular Publishing and the Politics of Language and Culture in a Colonial Society, 1778–1905* (New Delhi: Oxford University Press, 2006).
111. Guha, 'From Dais to Doctors', 146.
112. For details, see Anshu Malhotra, *Gender, Caste, and Religious Identities: Restructuring Caste in Colonial Punjab* (New Delhi: Oxford University Press, 2002), 164–99; Gupta, *Sexuality, Obscenity, Community*, 268–320.
113. Malhotra, 'Of Dais and Midwives', 221.
114. *Report of the Health Survey and Development Committee* (New Delhi: Government of India Press, 1946), 2: 397.
115. The *Bhore Committee Report* took into cognisance the kind of influence enjoyed by these hereditary dais over a considerable section of the population and categorically stated that any attempt to professionalise midwifery was futile without taking the traditional hereditary dais into confidence (*Report of the Health Survey and Development Committee*, 2: 399).
116. Premchand, 'Doodh ka Daam', in *Naya Mansarovar*, ed. Kamal Kishore Goenka (New Delhi: Sasta Sahitya Mandal Prakashan, 2017), 8: 68. This story was first published in *Hans*, July 1934.
117. Premchand, 'Doodh ka Daam', 71.
118. Ibid., 71.
119. See the pamphlet entitled 'Bharat ke Unnati ka Vaidyak Pratham Anga Hai', in Sharma, *Arogya Darpan*, Vol. 3.
120. Gupt, *Charaka Samhita*, Sutra Sthana, Chapter 27, Verse 312–315 (author's translation).
121. '*Nahin mansa samah kinchit anyadeh brihatvakrit.*' Brahmanand Tripathi, *Ashtang Hridayam of Srimad Vagbhata* (Delhi: Chaukhamba Sanskrit Pratisthan, 2014), 196.
122. The concept of '*tridosha*' or the three humors is central to the Ayurvedic treatment. According to the Ayurvedic philosophy, all the bio-elements responsible for proper functioning of body can be categorised into three types of humors: *vata* (or the airy elements), *pitta* (or the fiery element) and *kapha* (or the watery element). A healthy body exhibits the proper balance of all the three types of humors inside it. However, these humors by nature

are highly unstable and change with day and night and with food. Hence, proper daily routine and dietary habits are essential to maintain humoral equilibrium. Disease is nothing but expression of either excess or deficiency of one or more types of humors at a particular point of time, thereby distorting the equilibrium. As per the Ayurvedic philosophy, health can be restored by mitigating such excesses or deficiency by advising respective diet and routine. Consequently, Ayurvedic treatises categorise the nature of diseases and food also under the three categories of aforesaid humors. Sushruta, in this regard, goes on to place different types of meats also under the aforesaid humoral categories.

123. For an interesting analysis of Sushruta's catalogue of meats, see Francis Zimmerman, *The Jungle and the Aroma of Meats* (Delhi: Motilal Banarsidas, 1999). However, as shown in a recent PhD thesis by Shankar Kumar, even in these classical medical treatises such empirical observations are usually hidden beneath value-laden brahmanical norms, thereby deviating from its secular and empiric rootedness. In other words, extra-medical concerns including semantic proliferation owing to the meter requirements of the stanzas can often be found in the list of meats and plants and their therapeutic usages provided in the classical Ayurvedic treatises. See Shankar Kumar, 'Ancient Indian Medicine in the work of Charaka, Sushruta and Vagbhata—A Textual and Historical Study', (PhD diss., Department of History, University of Delhi, 2013). Nevertheless, as I argued in the 'Introduction' of the present work, in ancient Indian context such deviations were normal keeping in mind that juxtaposition of essential and useful knowledge with prevailing belief system and religious faiths was an integral part of pre-modern knowledge systems throughout the world.

124. Gupt, *Charaka Samhita*, Sutra Sthana, Chapter 7, Verse 3.

5

Ayurveda in the Market

Economic Underpinnings of the Late Colonial Ayurvedic Movement

Dynamics of the market (print as well as drug market) considerably shaped the late colonial Ayurvedic movement in multiple ways. In fact, the kind of socio-political manifestations which we see in the late colonial Ayurvedic discourse had an economic logic as well, besides being 'merely social' and 'political'. In this regard the present chapter explores the ways in which the late colonial Ayurvedic movement in India tactfully used as well as succumbed to the market forces to fight back the growing influence of the Western system of healing. This interactive relationship shared between the Ayurvedic movement and the market forces eventually laid down the characteristic features of Ayurvedic pharmacies and drug manufacturing in India. It is interesting to note that the 'new' vaids of the late nineteenth and early twentieth century India particularly focussed on those aspects of the medical market which were either spared or overlooked by the practitioners of Western medicine such as production of tonics and vitalisers, all-encompassing drugs or panacea, and aphrodisiacs—a trend which continues till today. These 'new' vaids were very well aware of the fact that the Ayurvedic movement could not sustain itself without proving its market potential and utility for the masses. That is why they often resorted to techniques which were alien to the classical system of Ayurveda in order to meet the demands of the consumer market. After all, unlike nationalism, Ayurveda was not an abstract ideology; it was a healing system producing consumable goods. Hence, it had to create its own market and 'consumers' out of the 'users', besides the ideological and emotional mobilisation of the masses.

However, the earlier works on 'indigenous' medical movement only tangentially touched this dynamic relationship shared between the market forces and the late nineteenth and early twentieth century movement to revive Ayurveda as 'indigenous' system of healing. Scholars like Brahmanand Gupta and K. N. Panikkar did talk about the entrepreneurial ventures of the late nineteenth century Ayurvedic practitioners and sympathisers, but they discussed it as being an integral part of the evolution of a broader Ayurvedic movement.[1] In these earlier works the market and its economics hardly found an independent space in shaping the characteristics and different dimensions of the Ayurvedic movement. Nonetheless, recently historians working on the social history of health and medicine have realised the transformative powers of the market and have begun to fill the hitherto extant gap in the historiography of 'indigenous' medicine.[2]

The areas which have primarily attracted the attention of historians include the mass production of Ayurvedic medicines (that is, the study of pharmaceuticalisation of Ayurvedic medicines) and the study of Ayurvedic advertisements. Incidentally, both these areas of study deal only with the marketing of Ayurvedic drugs. One aspect of the market-Ayurveda relationship which is still largely unexplored is the Ayurvedic print market which was crucial to the late colonial Ayurvedic movement to establish its claims. The present chapter analyses various features of both—the Ayurvedic print market as well as the market of Ayurvedic drugs—with special reference to the United Provinces. In the course of it I would establish the link between prevailing social ideas/practices and marketing techniques as well.

However, before going into the details of the aforesaid themes it is essential to understand why the market became such an important factor in shaping the late nineteenth and early twentieth century Ayurvedic movement. It is noticeable that by this time the traditional structure of courtly patronage which was hitherto enjoyed by various forms of art, science and culture had almost collapsed. Although some of the big zamindars (landed elites) and princely states tried to uphold the traditional structure of patronage, they had their own limitations in a colonial context. No ruler or zamindar was ready to enter into direct conflict with the mighty colonial government in order to promote 'indigenous' art, culture or medicine. This was the reason why some of the princes and zamindars who donated substantially to promote Ayurveda simultaneously provided land and money for the setting up of Western hospitals and dispensaries as well. In such a situation, where Ayurveda was not just devoid of state patronage but also facing a hostile regime, the proponents of the Ayurvedic revivalism had to shift their support base from a few zamindars and princes to a larger clientele in order to fight back the influence of Western medicine. And here the market forces gained significance as it was through the market that the Ayurvedic ideas penetrated and consolidated themselves in society. Alongside, the market also served to procure the necessary funding to keep the Ayurvedic movement alive. Of course, the enhanced commercialisation of the Indian economy under colonialism also made the market crucial for the spread of the Ayurvedic movement. Once the Ayurvedic movement went into the lap of the market, it had to continuously engage with its dynamics. This engagement was very well reflected in the Ayurvedic print culture and the drug market. Let us begin by analysing various dimensions of the Ayurvedic print market which is hitherto a neglected area of research so far as economic aspect of the movement to revive Ayurveda as 'indigenous' medicine is concerned.

THE AYURVEDIC PRINT MARKET

Agar ek adbhut baat koi gyat mujhko ho gayi,
Toh haaye! Mere sath hi samsar se voh kho gayi.
Us ko chhipa rakhun na main toh, kaun puchhega mujhe,
Kitne prayog pradeep, is anudarta se hain bujhe.[3]

– Maithilisharan Gupt

(Countless lamps of knowledge have got extinguished owing to the tendency of concealment of the newly acquired knowledge by the researchers in order to maintain their esteemed status in the society.)

The 'new' vaids often held the hiding of 'useful knowledge' by the vaids of earlier generations as one of the causes responsible for the 'decline' of Ayurveda. Prior to the period of our study, Ayurvedic knowledge was highly personalised in nature. There were texts dealing with the broader concepts of Ayurveda (such as various Sanskrit *samhitas*), but the Ayurvedic practitioners often used their own experience and skills to prepare the desired medicine. In this situation, if an Ayurvedic practitioner discovered some new medicine or useful herb, the tendency was to conceal it from the rest of the world and to make that particular medicine the 'pride possession' of the family (*khandani vishesta*). Such discoveries were personalised to such an extent that, many a time, the methodology of preparing a particular medicine disappeared with the death of the particular practitioner. The above-mentioned verse of Maithilisharan Gupt indicates this tendency of concealment and its repercussions in the field of 'traditional' Indian sciences.

However, the late nineteenth and early twentieth century witnessed a new development in the field of Ayurvedic treatment. The 'new' vaids believed that one way of countering the growing influence of Western medicine (which was incidentally backed by the colonial public health policy) was to disseminate the 'useful' Ayurvedic knowledge among the lay public. The idea was to simplify the complex Sanskritic Ayurvedic knowledge and to make it available to the general public in its own language. These 'new' vaids had the conviction that once people would learn about the cheaper, home-made and more effective Ayurvedic treatments of the common diseases, they would naturally turn away from the expensive system of Western medicine. In this context, David Arnold goes on to argue that in the East–West encounter, Ayurveda and its textual tradition played an important role in 'establishing claims for the validity and rationality of Hindu science as a whole'.[4]

In the above-mentioned pursuit, the 'new' vaids received overwhelming support of some of the renowned publishing houses of the United Provinces. The first such big publishing house that came in support of the 'new' vaids was the Naval Kishore Press of Lucknow (established in 1858), the largest Indian-owned printing press and publishing house of the subcontinent in the nineteenth century. According to one estimate, the Naval Kishore Press published around 39 Ayurvedic texts, 15 of them in Sanskrit and 24 in Hindi/Hindusatni language.[5] The story began with *Vaidyajivan* (an immensely popular sixteenth-century text by Lolimbaraja) which was published by Naval Kishore in 1868. It contained both Sanskrit verses with Hindi translation. However, it was *Amritsagar* which sensationalised the Ayurvedic print market. The first edition of *Amritsagar* was published from Agra in 1864 in the Marwari dialect. Realising its market potential, Naval Kishore commissioned Pandit Kalicharan to translate it into 'standard' Hindi.[6] After the completion of translation, when its second edition (published this time by the Naval Kishore Press) came out in 1869, it recorded an exceptionally high print-run of 5,500 copies.[7] By 1878, four editions of *Amritsagar* had already gone into print, and keeping in mind its commercial success Naval Kishore decided to bring out its Urdu translation as well.[8]

Afterwards, the Naval Kishore Press came up with many other Ayurvedic texts both in Hindi (such as *Ramvinod* in 1874, *Vaidyamanotsav* in 1874, *Aushadhi Sangrah* in 1875, *Rasayan Prakash* and *Vaidya Darpan*) as well as in Sanskrit (suc as *Nighant-ratnakar* in 1892, *Sushruta Samhita* in 1891 and *Bhaisajya-ratnavali* in 1892). In 1924, the Naval Kishore Press also published an Ayurvedic text in verse form: *Vaidya Priya*. The inspiration for it was drawn from *Kavi-priya*—the renowned anthology of poems by Keshavdas. The author of *Vaidya Priya* claimed that this text was like the '*nayika*' (lead heroine) of Vaidyak-shastra, which is adorned with all the 16 adornments (*solah shringar*) of a Hindu bride as manifested in the form of its 16 chapters.[9] The basic idea behind bringing an Ayurvedic text in verse form was that it was easy to memorise which in turn was handy in the dissemination of Ayurvedic principles/remedies.

Besides the Naval Kishore Press, there were many other publishing houses which helped in the dissemination of Ayurvedic texts. For example, Ganga Granthagar of Lucknow, Stri Shiksha Pustakalaya of Allahabad, Mahashakti Sahitya Mandir of Benares and Sudhanidhi Press of Allahabad. Out of these, many were owned by some famous Ayurvedic practitioners of the United Provinces. For instance, Stri Shiksha Pustakalaya was owned by the famous female Ayurvedic practitioner of Allahabad, Yashoda Devi. Further, many Ayurvedic practitioners were frequently commissioned by these publishing houses either to translate any classical Ayurvedic text or to edit a new one. Supplementing the publications of Ayurvedic texts, a huge number of vernacular Ayurvedic journals came to life during this period.[10] These journals played an equally significant role in the dissemination of Ayurvedic knowledge.

Advertisements and Strategies of Marketing Ayurvedic Texts

Strategies of marketing books are the least explored aspects of the early history of print culture in the Indian subcontinent.[11] Nonetheless, an exploratory analysis of this aspect of print culture provides some interesting insights into the Ayurvedic print market. The best way to advertise an Ayurvedic text was through newspapers. Publishers like Naval Kishore advertised their forthcoming publications regularly in the much acclaimed Urdu newspaper *Awadh Akhbar*.[12] Other publishing houses also resorted to such techniques since newspapers and journals had the widest circulation among the printed materials. However, keeping in mind the cost of advertisement, the more convenient and cost-effective way to advertise the existing and forthcoming Ayurvedic texts was the books themselves. One can often find a book list (see Figure 5.1) or announcements of forthcoming publications at the beginning or end of

ब्रह्मचर्य तथा स्वास्थ्य-संबंधी

बेजोड़ पुस्तकें

ब्रह्मचर्य-विज्ञान	।॥-)	ज्ञाचा	॥=), १=)
ब्रह्मचर्य की महिमा	१)	तात्कालिक चिकित्सा	१), १॥)
ब्रह्मचर्य ही जीवन है	॥)	प्रसूति-तंत्र	२॥), ३)
ब्रह्मचर्य	।)	संक्षिप्त शरीर-विज्ञान	॥=), ॥।)
ब्रह्मचर्य	१।)	संक्षिप्त स्वास्थ्य-रक्षा	॥=), ॥।)
हम सौ वर्ष कैसे जिएँ	१)	सरल व्यायाम	।=)
स्वप्न-दोष	१॥)	शीघ्रपतन	।=)॥
स्वास्थ्य	≡)	वीर्य	॥=)
स्वास्थ्य-दीर्घजीवन	॥=)	मैं नीरोग हूँ या रोगी	।)
स्वास्थ्य-रक्षक	२॥)	स्वास्थ्य की कुंजी	१), १॥।)
स्वास्थ्य-रक्षा	३।), ३॥।)	प्राणायाम	।॥=), १।=)
स्वास्थ्य-विज्ञान	२॥), ३)	हठयोग	१।=), १॥।=)
स्वास्थ्य-साधन	२)	दीर्घायु	२॥)
धात्री-शिक्षा	२), २॥)	जल-चिकित्सा	३॥)
गुप्त संदेश	१)	आरोग्य-साधन	।=)
स्वास्थ्य और योगासन	१)	आरोग्य-प्रदीप	१।=)
स्वास्थ्य के १० नियम	॥=)	आसन	२)
स्वस्थ शरीर	४)	स्वास्थ्य और व्यायाम	१॥)

हिंदुस्थान-भर की हिंदी-पुस्तकें मिलने का पता—

गंगा-ग्रंथागार, लखनऊ

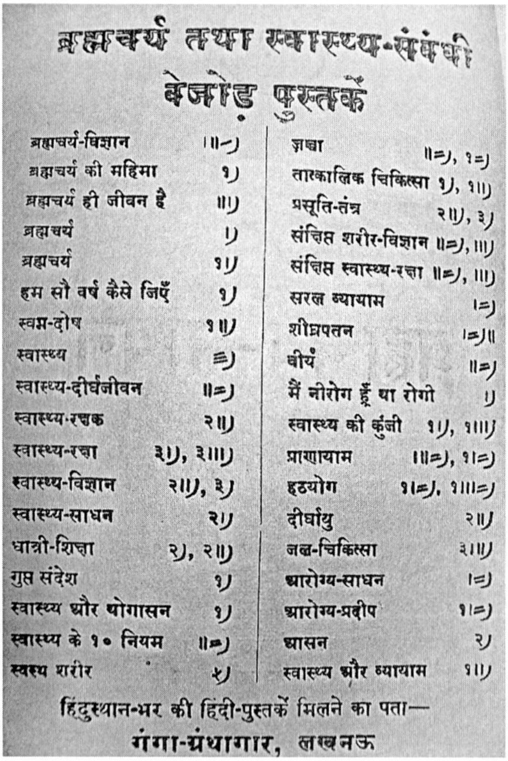

Figure 5.1: Book list at the beginning of an Ayurvedic text; Ganga Granthagar, Lucknow.[13]

an Ayurvedic text. Some of the publishing houses also offered detailed catalogues (*suchi-patra*) that provided the names, prices and the basic content of the books published by them. One could order these catalogues through post as well.

Such advertisements of Ayurvedic texts often carried eye-catching phrases in bold letters to attract the readers and to arouse their interest in the text. The author (who was simultaneously an Ayurvedic practitioner as well) often eulogised his/her achievements in order to convince the reader about the effectiveness of the treatment offered in the text. Some of the publishing houses also adopted the strategy of free-of-cost advance booking of the forthcoming Ayurvedic texts. For this, the reader had to simply write a postcard to the publisher showing his/her interest in the forthcoming book (Figure 5.2). This helped publishers to gauge the mood

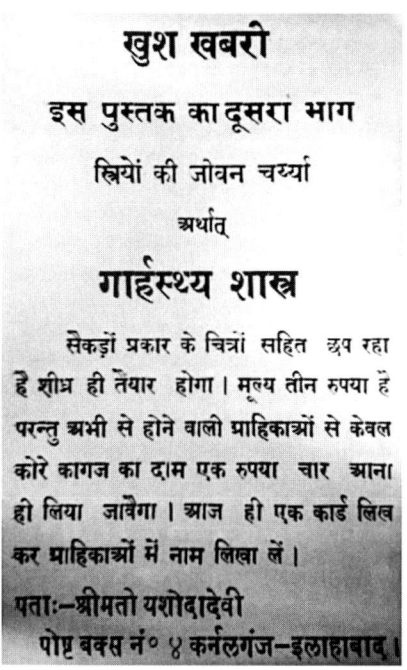

Figure 5.2: An illustration of advance booking of forthcoming text by Yashoda Devi.[14]

of the market and to estimate the possible readership of the forthcoming publication which, in turn, was helpful in deciding the number of copies that had to be published in the first round. Also, it was helpful in deciding its commercial viability.

In fact, the vernacular Ayurvedic texts had tremendous commercial potential as they were targeting the non-specialist lay readership market which was really huge. These tracts were not just for practising vaids but, as was often claimed, also for the common householder or *grihastha* (see Figure 5.3). In fact, the very prospect of becoming 'one's own doctor', which these texts were offering, was really attractive.[15] Some of these texts claimed that they have been written in such an 'easy language' and 'lucid manner' that even a 'fool' could understand them and get benefits from them (for an illustration, see the advertisement by Yashoda Devi, Figure 5.4). Further, the economic incentive was also there as these texts contained mostly household remedies for common as well as complicated diseases.

However, despite all this, the journey of the vernacular Ayurvedic texts was not that easy. Since these texts were targeting the reading habit of the lay public, they had to compete with a wide range of reading material available in the print market that targeted the same clientele. If we look at the testimonial of Ayurvedic practitioners like Yashoda Devi, then it appears that the outcome was not very enthusiastic for them, at least in the initial phase. Complaining about the reading habits of the lay readers (especially women), Yashoda Devi in one of her books lamented the fact that she failed to meet even the cost of putting a stall at the *Magh Mela*,[16] while at the same time stalls selling sleazy novels, songs, etc., recorded a robust sale.[17] Further, she complained that the literate women were so fond of such 'dirty' literature that one could easily find one or two of them in their trunk. According to Yashoda Devi, she used to receive several letters daily demanding such sleazy literature.[18] In other words, the competition of the vernacular Ayurvedic texts was not just with other medical texts and manuals produced by the practitioners of Unani, Homeopathy and Western system of healing; rather, in their quest for readership, they also competed with the utterly 'unscientific' fictions and novels.[19]

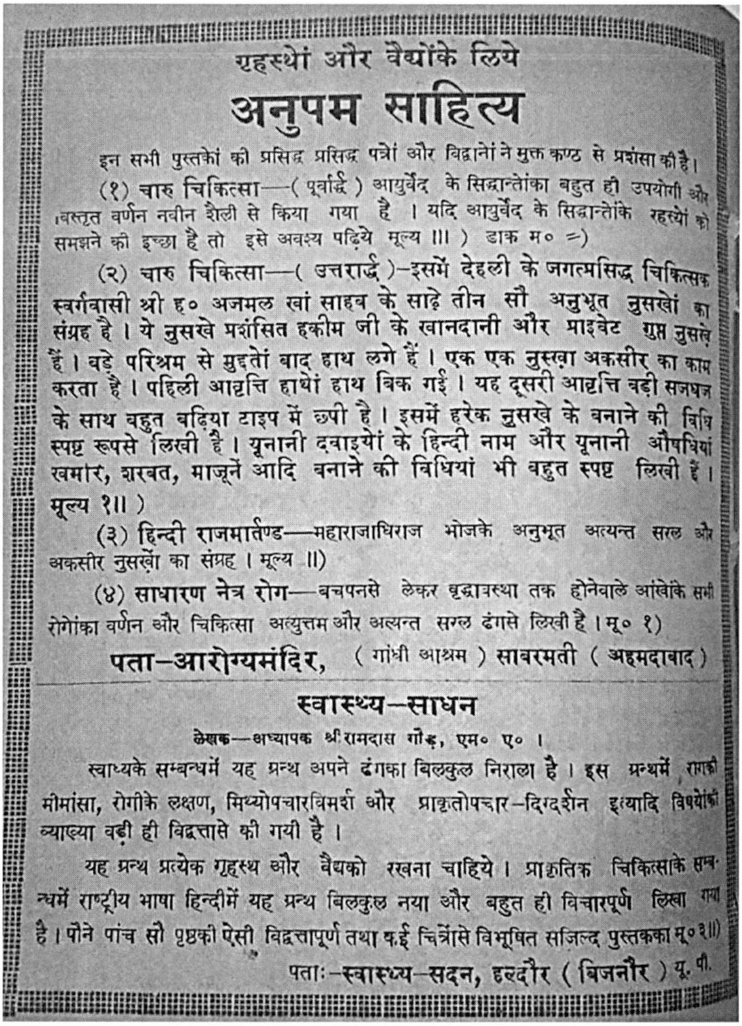

Figure 5.3: *Anupam Sahitya*: For Common Householders and Vaids.[20]

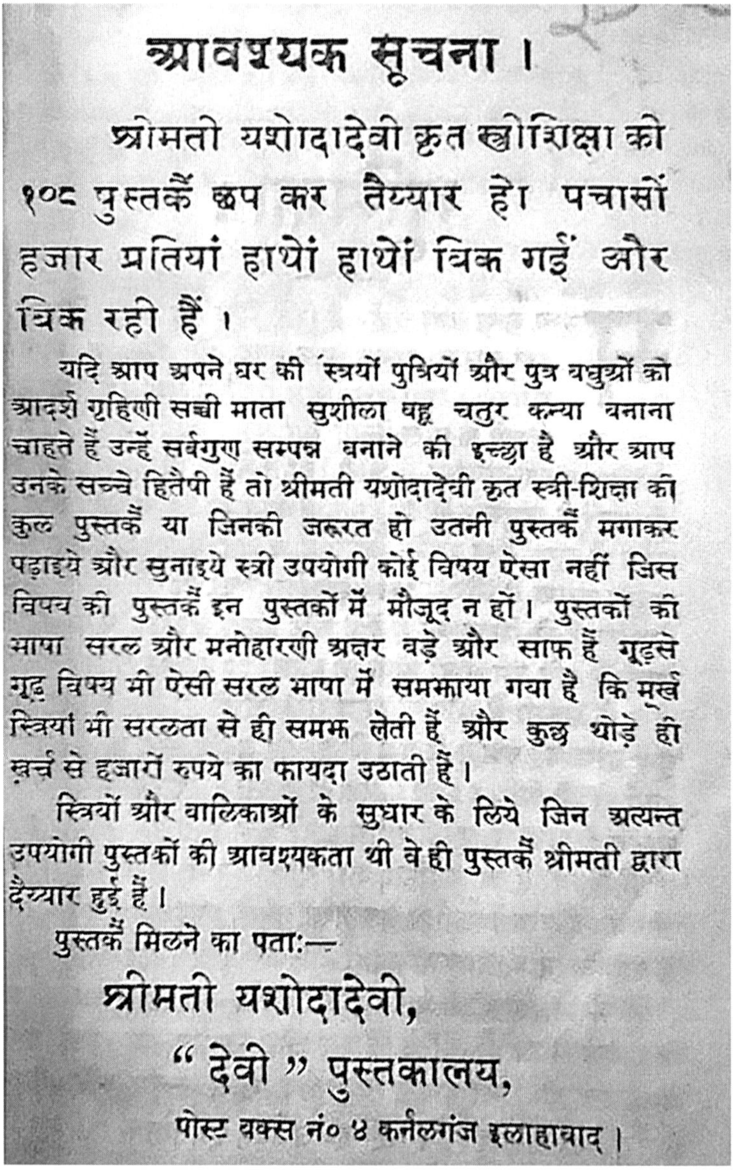

आवश्यक सूचना ।

श्रीमती यशोदादेवी कृत स्त्रीशिक्षा की १०८ पुस्तकैं छप कर तैय्यार हो पचासों हजार प्रतियां हाथों हाथों बिक गईं और बिक रही हैं ।

यदि आप अपने घर की स्त्रियों पुत्रियों और पुत्र बधुओं को आदर्श गृहिणी सच्ची माता सुशीला बहू चतुर कन्या बनाना चाहते हैं उन्हें सर्वगुण सम्पन्न बनाने की इच्छा है और आप उनके सच्चे हितैषी हैं तो श्रीमती यशोदादेवी कृत स्त्री-शिक्षा की कुल पुस्तकैं या जिनकी जरूरत हो उतनी पुस्तकैं मगाकर पढ़ाइये और सुनाइये स्त्री उपयोगी कोई विषय ऐसा नहीं जिस विषय की पुस्तकैं इन पुस्तकों में मौजूद न हों । पुस्तकों की भाषा सरल और मनोहारणी अक्षर बड़े और साफ हैं गूढ़से गूढ़ विषय भी ऐसी सरल भाषा में समझाया गया है कि मूर्ख स्त्रियां भी सरलता से ही समझ लेती हैं और कुछ थोड़े ही खर्च से हजारों रुपये का फायदा उठाती हैं ।

स्त्रियों और बालिकाओं के सुधार के लिये जिन अत्यन्त उपयोगी पुस्तकों की आवश्यकता थी वे ही पुस्तकैं श्रीमती द्वारा तैय्यार हुई हैं ।

पुस्तकैं मिलने का पता:—

श्रीमती यशोदादेवी,
" देवी " पुस्तकालय,
पोस्ट बक्स नं० ४ कनेलगंज इलाहाबाद ।

Figure 5.4: An advertisement by Yashoda Devi's Devi Pustakalaya, Allahabad.[21]

The Social Context of Ayurvedic Print Culture

Incidentally, in the context of the late nineteenth and early twentieth century, the Ayurvedic texts reproduced and reinforced the upper-caste/middle-class norms both directly or indirectly (as discussed in Chapter 4) through the dynamics of the print market. In this regard, in his influential theory of contextualising the literary sphere, Pierre Bourdieu talks about two categories of literary production—'restricted production' (small-scale production of artistic, aesthetic and scientific works emphasising on the excellence of print culture) and 'large-scale production' (commercially oriented mass-scale production of saleable texts with exclusive focus on financial gains).[22] However, while both kinds of literary production may conform to the existing social norms of their clientele, the chances of doing that is greater in the case of large-scale production. After all, in order to become a commercial success, a book has to conform to the existing social norms. Such books, moreover, were not supposed to hurt the sentiments of its readership. Following this line, the market-oriented mass-scale production of the early twentieth century Ayurvedic texts did respect the social sensitivity of its readership, that is, the upper-caste/middle-class population.

In fact, it is very important to notice one major shift in the patronage structure related to the production of literary works which has been hinted at in the beginning of this chapter. Prior to the period of our study, literary works were often patronised by the royal houses, wealthy zamindars/princes and sometimes by the colonial institutions (Asiatic Societies, educational institutions, etc.). In such a milieu, the author often took care only of the needs and viewpoints of his patron and a select audience of connoisseurs. However, by the early twentieth century, with the beginning of mass production of literary works, a new class of consumer emerged. Although private patronage continued, the main focus now shifted towards a larger audience and the publishing houses, by and large, came to be dependent on the lay reader for their commercial success. With the gradual transformation of books into a saleable commodity, literary production succumbed to the dynamics of the market for the first time. Now, the fate of a book and its author came to be inextricably linked to the reception and saleability of his/her work in the market.[23]

Furthermore, as argued by Pierre Bourdieu, although the literary field is a 'relatively autonomous' structured space and has its own 'laws of operation', it is always embedded within and subject to the indirect influences of a larger field of socio-political and economic power.[24] In fact, drawing upon the conceptual framework of Peter Hohendahl,[25] Francesca Orsini has shown that the educated Indians often advanced their political and social agendas through 'literary institutions' (publishing houses) active in the Hindi public sphere over the phase 1920–40.[26] In such a situation, these socio-political interventionist forces also impacted the production of the Ayurvedic texts. In fact, many of the Ayurvedic practitioners were themselves active socially and politically as well. For example, Yashoda Devi considered herself as someone working for the broader social welfare of women; Jagannath Prasad Shukla was active in the Hindu politics of the United Provinces; and nearly all of them had firm conviction that they had been working in the direction of attaining '*swaraj*'. That is why while writing Ayurvedic texts the socio-political ideas of the authors/practitioners indirectly entered these texts. After all, an Ayurvedic practitioner, howsoever professional he/she might be, could not escape his/her immediate socio-political surroundings and pressures exerted by them on his/her 'scientific' thinking.

However, one may argue that in a largely illiterate colonial society, print culture might not be such a major factor in carving social identities and shaping public culture. This argument has already been posed while criticising the theory of Benedict Anderson regarding the formation of 'national' communities, especially in the context of the illiterate colonial societies of Asia and Africa.[27] Nevertheless, it is not so easy to assess the impact of print culture simply by looking at the literacy figures in colonial India due to the tendency of 'secondary reading' of the texts. Especially in the case of Ayurvedic texts, 'secondary reading' was very popular. Someone having a text on Ayurveda often read it out or told people close to him about the remedies and Ayurvedic concepts it mentioned. This aspect of 'secondary reading' of the Ayurvedic texts can be seen even in the latter half of the twentieth century. In short, the Ayurvedic print culture facilitated the extant practice of self-medication among the Indian masses. In fact, the practice of self-medication was now backed by these 'scientific' texts.

THE AYURVEDIC DRUG MARKET

Standardisation and Pharmaceuticalisation

The period under discussion also witnessed the standardisation and pharmaceuticalisation of the Ayurvedic drug market. Earlier vaids and hakims did not merely prescribe the medicines; rather they themselves prepared and gave those medicines as well. In other words, the same person assumed three different roles—of a doctor, a pharmacist and a chemist. However, colonialism fundamentally altered this unified set up of the Ayurvedic healing system where all the three identities (that is, of the doctor, pharmacist and chemist) were merged into one person. In its effort to fight back the influences of the Western healing system, the Ayurvedic practitioners decided to expand their horizon by directly reaching to the masses. This was not possible without standardisation and pharmaceuticalisation of the Ayurvedic drugs. In this regard, as Madhulika Banerjee argues, 'when many petitions and exhortations for their medical and scientific value failed to elicit any substantial response and invited ridicule instead, they had to explore alternative avenues of expression for the purpose—and this was provided by the market'.[28]

In fact, as pointed out by Banerjee, the pharmaceuticalisation process serves as an inevitable link between the development of 'modern medical knowledge' and the 'momentous developments' of the economy and society. Hence, according to her, the birth of the Ayurvedic pharmaceuticals was something inevitable if Ayurveda were to find a place in the rapid socio-economic changes of the late nineteenth and early twentieth century India.[29] Here the hint is towards the 'capitalist enterprise' that had started developing roots in the Indian society by this time.

One should not forget that this was the same period when the Indian economy and society had been witnessing a level of development of industrial capitalism—a process which reached its peak during the First World War. The forced closure of the Indian market due to disruption of international trade routes, the enhanced War demands, the decline in foreign competition, the price differential between agricultural and industrial products, and the stagnation or decline in real wages were some of the factors which created a short War-time boom in Indian industries during 1914–19.[30] However, Anil Kumar argues that in case of the industrial evolution and promotion of Ayurvedic and Unani drugs, state protection or the 'forced protection' of the War period had absolutely no role to play. According to Kumar, the Ayurvedic and Unani drug industry owed its growth and expansion to individual enterprise, the support of its admirers and the quality of their products.[31]

Nevertheless, Kumar seems to contradict his own conclusion by saying that during the War years the government bought nearly 95 per cent of the total produce of Bengal Chemicals and Pharmaceutical Works, which was one of the leading pharmaceutical company manufacturing Ayurvedic drugs.[32] As far as the question of lack of state initiative is concerned, this holds true for many other industries as well which grew and developed in India through indigenous efforts. In fact, the real transforming potential of colonialism was that it brought with itself the culture of mass-scale production of goods through industrial capital.

During the period of our discussion, even Ayurveda was sought to be 'formatted' and 'co-opted' by this capitalist culture which led to the standardisation and pharmaceuticalisation of Ayurvedic drugs.[33] The 'new' vaids were highly critical of the personalised character of Ayurvedic drug manufacturing. Pandit Yadavji Trikamji Acharya, while delivering his presidential speech at the fifteenth All India Vaidya Sammelan held at Haridwar (United Provinces), particularly stressed on this issue.[34] He argued that one of the major reasons behind the success of Western medicine was its easy availability even in the remote towns. Consequently, he urged for the opening up of Ayurvedic pharmacies and stores along the same lines, even in rural areas, to extend the clientele of Ayurvedic medicines.[35] He also emphasised on the practice of labelling the Ayurvedic drugs. The inspiration for this was drawn from the Western medicine manufacturing system, where drugs carried the label of BP, which meant that the given medicine was manufactured in accordance with the standards of British Pharmacopoeia. This was a clear manifestation of textual authority gaining prominence over the experiential and personalised knowledge of the vaids.

Related to this was the concern over the production of substandard and adulterated Ayurvedic drugs in the market. It was believed that such substandard/adulterated drugs produced by some 'greedy businessmen' had grossly damaged the image of Ayurveda in the eyes of the common public and the government. Consequently, it was argued that there has to be a close vigilance over the production of Ayurvedic drugs. Ayurvedic journals such as *Dhanvantari* also launched a campaign against the production of such substandard drugs, urging people to be more alert and watchful (see Figure 5.5). Nevertheless, as argued by Nandini Bhattacharya, in the absence of a standard pharmacopoeia, a huge unregulated 'indigenous' drug market continued to flourish in India and the debates on standardisation and adulteration were fused. Until the active principles of 'indigenous' drugs were identified and tested 'scientifically', it was difficult

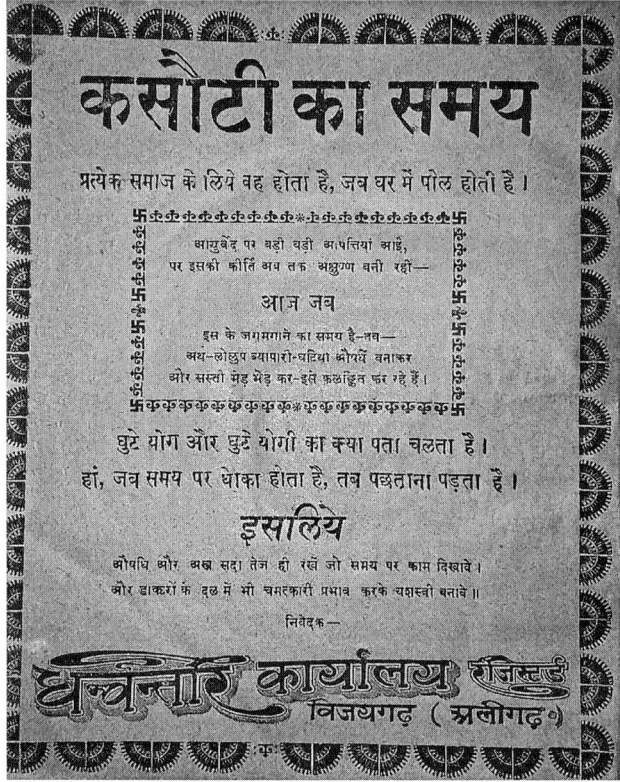

Figure 5.5: Testing times: An advertisement cautioning people against the substandard Ayurvedic drugs available in the market.[36]

to bring them within a regulated market producing standardised drugs, thereby creating scope for adulteration. Further, presence of multiple and diverse layers of manufacturers, agents and distributors also facilitated availability of the same Ayurvedic medicine in varying potencies in the drug market.[37]

Ayurvedic Pharmacies and Stores

Due to the standardisation and pharmaceuticalisation drive of the Ayurvedic drug market, India witnessed a vibrant growth of Ayurvedic pharmacies manufacturing Ayurvedic drugs and Ayurvedic stores selling the mass-produced Ayurvedic drugs in most part of the subcontinent. Some of the renowned Ayurvedic pharmacies of the period have been enlisted in Table 5.1. In the United Provinces also there was no dearth of such Ayurvedic pharmacies. One can find many such pharmacies coming up in different parts of the province. In fact, some of them (for instance, the Dhanvantari Aushadhalaya, the Sudhanidhi Aushadhalaya, the Ayurvedic Pharmacy (BHU), etc.) were famous at the national level as well (see Table 5.2). Most of these pharmacies were often owned by famous Ayurvedic practitioners of the time who were actively engaged in the late colonial Ayurvedic revivalist movement as well.

Table 5.1: Ayurvedic Pharmacies in the Late Nineteenth and Early Twentieth Century India[38]

S. No.	Pharmacy	Place	Year of Establishment
1.	Kalpataru Ayurvedic Works	Calcutta	1884
2.	Dabur India Limited	Calcutta	Founded in 1884, but mass production started in 1896
3.	C. K. Sen & Company	Calcutta	Established in 1878, but started large-scale production from 1898 onwards
4.	Dhoot Papeshwar	Bombay	1888
5.	Shadhona Aushadhalaya	Dhaka	1888
6.	N. N. Sen & Company	Bengal	1898

S. No.	Pharmacy	Place	Year of Establishment
7.	Arya Vaidyasala	Kottakal (Kerala)	1901
8.	Shakti Aushadhalaya	Dacca	1901
9.	Bengal Chemist and Pharmaceutical Works Limited	Calcutta	1901
10.	Arya Vaidya Pharmacy	Coimbatore (Tamil Nadu)	1902
11.	Zandu Pharmaceutical Works	Bombay	1910
12.	Andhra Ayurvedic Pharmacy	Madras	1920
13.	Ayurvedashram Pharmacy Limited	Ahmadnagar	—
14.	Ayurvedic Pharmaceutical Company Limited	Lahore	—

Table 5.2: Popular Ayurvedic Pharmacies of the United Provinces in the First Half of the Twentieth Century[39]

S. No.	Pharmacy	Place	Manager
1.	Dhanvantari Aushadhalaya	Aligarh	Vaidya Bankelal
2.	Gurukul Ayurvedic Pharmacy	Haridwar	Gurukul Kangri
3.	Ayurvedic Pharmacy (BHU)	Benares	Kaviraj Pratap Singh
4.	Mahashakti Aushadhalaya	Benares	—
5.	Stri Aushadhalaya	Prayag	Yashoda Devi
6.	Sudhanidhi Aushadhalaya	Prayag	Jagannath Prasad Shukla
7.	Mrityunjaya Aushadhalaya	Lucknow	Pandit Shalgram Shastri
8.	Jain Aushadhalaya	Kanpur	Kanhaiyalal Jain
9.	Prakash Aushadhalaya	Kanpur	Pandit Shivnarayan Mishra
10.	Jagadbhaskar Aushadhalaya	Kanpur	Kishori Dutt Shastri
11.	Sukhsancharak Company	Mathura	Pandit Kshetrapal Sharma
12.	G. A. Mishra Ayurvedic Pharmacy	Jhansi	—

The economic strength and giant stature of these Ayurvedic pharmaceutical companies in the market can be perceived from the fact that by 1924 Zandu Pharmaceutical Works Limited was paying an impressive sum of Rs 5,960 annually as income tax to the Government of India.[40] Similarly, the sales of P. S. Varier's medicines rose from Rs 14,000 in 1902–06 to Rs 170,000 during 1914–18.[41] In fact, P. S. Varier, the founder of the famous Arya Vaidyasala of Kottakal (Kerala) in 1901, was the first major Ayurvedic practitioner to realise the significance of the market-based 'packaging' of Ayurvedic medicines, instead of focussing solely on teaching and research to combat the influence of Western medicine. Varier, as pointed out by Deepak Kumar, believed that Western medicine appeared more attractive to people because it was tastier, gave quick relief and came without any restriction on food, all of which made Western medicine a very good 'package' for an ailing person.[42] On a similar line, the Ayurvedic pharmaceutical companies of the early twentieth century sought to overhaul Ayurveda, making it more appealing, engaging and a kind of 'swadeshi package' for the potential consumers.[43]

However, the beginning of most of these Ayurvedic pharmacies was very humble. They not only had to face stiff competition from the imported Western medicine, but also had to fight the personalised set-up of the Ayurvedic drug manufacturing. In fact, as pointed out by Anil Kumar, '[S]elling Ayurvedic drugs proved more difficult than the BP (British Pharmacopoeia) drugs. *Masik Vasumati* reported that P.C. Ray himself hawked them in the streets of Calcutta carrying in his folio, sample phials of the syrup of vasak and ajowan water.'[44] Similarly, Dr S. K. Burman, the founder of Dabur India Limited, made a humble beginning in the bylanes of Calcutta.

The Ayurvedic pharmacies resorted to several techniques and strategies to establish themselves in the market. Free postal assistance and medical advice to the patient were offered by many of them along with the pre-paid delivery of medicines through post (see Figure 5.6). Furthermore, most of them offered various incentives to the retailers. Small shopkeepers were promised generous commission on the sale of Ayurvedic drugs by the concerned pharmacies.[45] Established pharmacies also offered sale of agencies in order to increase the circulation of Ayurvedic drugs produced by them. Various items such as posters, handbills, calendars and pads were given free of cost to such agents to advertise their drugs in a more organised fashion [see Figure 5.7(a) and Figure 5.7(b)]. Besides this, social networks were exploited by these Ayurvedic pharmacies effectively to increase their sale. Often the advertisements of Ayurvedic drugs by these pharmacies used to carry testimonials by prominent personalities of the locality and the country and even colonial officials.[46]

The popularity of these Ayurvedic pharmacies can be assessed from the following inspection notes of R. B. B. Ghanshyam Dass, deputy commissioner of Sitapur, who visited one such pharmacy named as

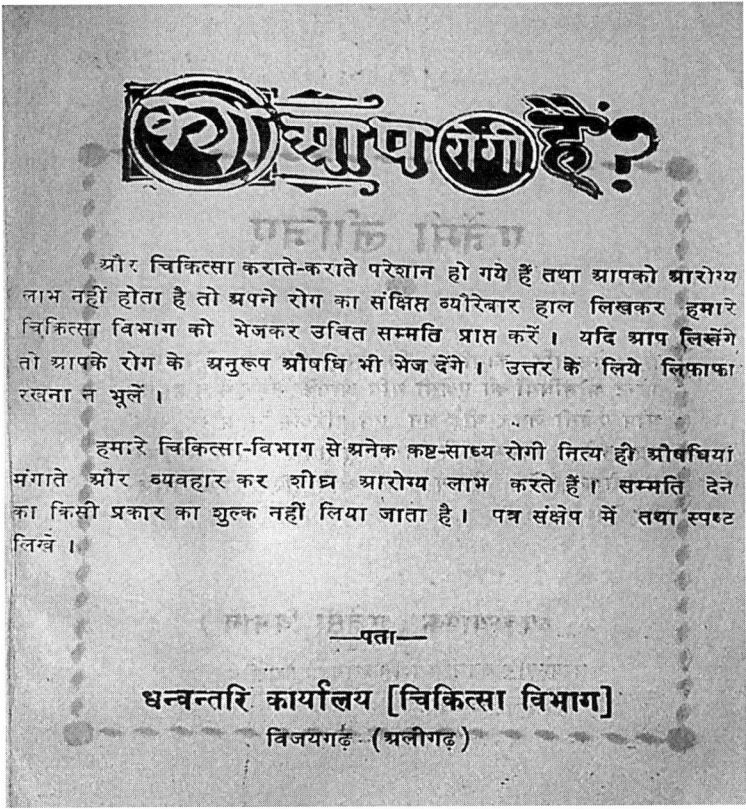

Figure 5.6: Are you ill: An advertisement by Dhanvantari Aushadhalaya, Aligarh, offering free postal assistance to those facing health related problems.[47]

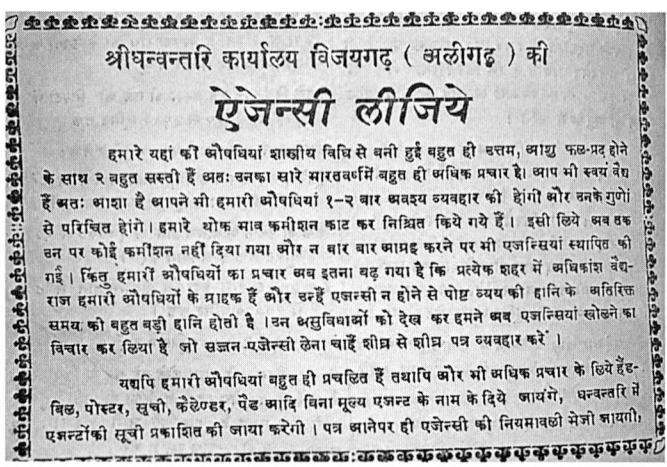

Figure 5.7(a): An advertisement by Dhanvantari Aushadhalaya (Aligarh) for the sale of agency.[48]

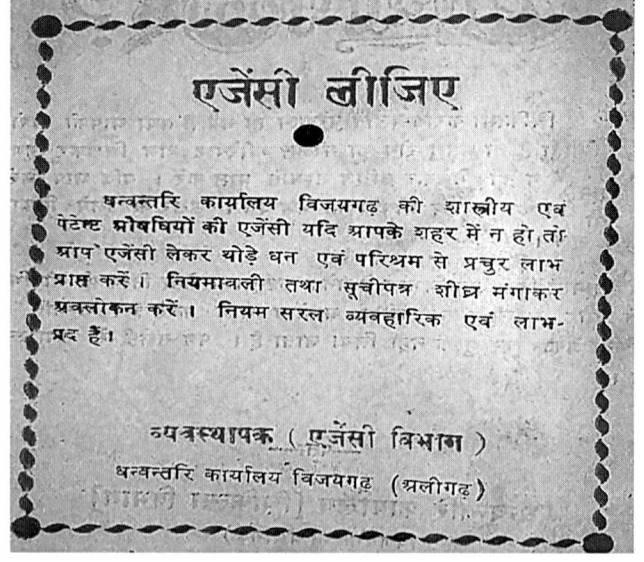

Figure 5.7(b): Another advertisement by Dhanvantari Aushadhalaya (Aligarh) for the sale of agency.[49]

Ayurvedic Mratyunjay Aushadhalaya maintained by Vaid Madhusudan Shastri at his house in Mohalla Nai Basti (Sitapur) on 16 September 1934:[50]

> I found a large crowd of patients both male and female waiting to receive treatment at his [Vaid Madhusudan Shatri's] hands and a large staff of physicians and compounders busy in distributing medicines to them. An examination of his attendance register shows that from 1st January 1934, till yesterday, namely 15th September 1934, 8,355 new patients have been admitted and treated at this Aushadhalaya, excluding 10,890 old patients. The new patients who received treatment and free distribution of medicines this year consists of 4,433 males; 1,728 females and 2,194 children.

Later on, this Aushadhalaya referred to the aforesaid note of the deputy commissioner of Sitapur to substantiate its claim to get into the 'esteemed list' of 'genuine' Ayurvedic pharmacies drafted by the government in 1940.[51]

These Ayurvedic pharmacies revolutionised the market of Ayurvedic drugs, and in turn, that of Ayurveda, in three fundamental respects. First, they ensured a longer shelf-life of the Ayurvedic medicines. Thus, the Ayurvedic drugs could be stored for a longer period, which facilitated their long-distance transportation and sale. Popular Ayurvedic drugs could now be made easily available even in some parts of the countryside. This made the dependence on neighbourhood vaids less stringent. Second, the standardisation of Ayurvedic drugs (along with the growing market of the vernacular Ayurvedic manuals) allowed over-the-counter sale of Ayurvedic drugs. In other words, there was no need for a doctor's prescription for buying any particular medicine. The very fact that these Ayurvedic drugs had supposedly little side-effects further induced this tendency of self-medication.[52] Moreover, it was no longer required to visit the Ayurvedic practitioner frequently merely to get the renewed dose of medicines. Now, one could buy them from the neighbourhood shop on the basis of erstwhile consultation with the vaid. Finally, the Ayurvedic pharmacies ensured mass production of the Ayurvedic drugs. This was essential to fight back the influence of the imported Western medicines which had flooded the Indian drug market. Mass production was also helpful in keeping the prices of the Ayurvedic drugs low and in stabilising this industry.

Besides the Ayurvedic pharmacies, Ayurvedic stores also played an important role in increasing the sale of Ayurvedic drugs. In fact, it were these Ayurvedic stores that had direct contact with the consumers. While one could order medicines from the Ayurvedic pharmacies as well through pre-paid postal schemes offered by them, it could not replace the direct consumer–shopkeeper relationship which was prevalent in the Indian market. Keeping in mind the typical shopping habit of the Indian consumer where purchase-on-credit (popularly known as '*udhari*') was a preferred practice (alongside direct interaction with the producer), small retailers of the towns and the countryside were crucial in widening the supply chain of the Ayurvedic drugs. That is why big Ayurvedic pharmacies often offered several incentives to the small retailers. As Madhuri Sharma puts it, '[S]mall shopkeepers in the surrounding *mofussil* and the rural market towns were promised a generous commission to sell products.'[53]

The speciality of these small shopkeepers was that most of them sold both Western as well as Ayurvedic medicines. And since they shared a direct socio-commercial relationship with the customer, they could convince them to try a particular Ayurvedic drug in place of Western medicine. This was a far more effective way than the newspaper advertisements to induce the customer for using the Ayurvedic drugs. Thus, modes of pre-capitalist communication and marketing techniques continued to have a significant role in a colonial society and economy, thereby overcoming various limitations like that of illiteracy.

Furthermore, many a times, these small medical stores hired a vaid or a doctor, providing him space—that is, a clinic—to carry on his practice. Also, these stores often had contacts with the famous vaids and doctors of the locality and offered them some commission in lieu of prescribing some exclusive medicines. This seemingly 'unfair' business practice proved to be helpful in increasing the sale of a particular medicine produced by an Ayurvedic pharmacy. *Arogya Niketan*, a Bengali novel written by Tarashankar Bandyopadhyaya, explicitly captures this commercial linkage between the medical store and the local vaids and doctors. In this novel, a medical store, named as B.K. Medical Store, used to pay some commission to the protagonist of the novel Jeevan Babu, who was an Ayurvedic practitioner, for prescribing the medicine available only with that store.[54]

ADVERTISING AYURVEDA

The growing acceptance of iconology in history writing (especially in the field of socio-cultural history) has thrown open a new range of historiographical materials such as advertisements to reconstruct the past. Emphasising the significance of advertisements as historiographical source, Peter Burke states: 'The images used in advertising may help historians of the future to reconstruct lost elements of the twentieth century material culture.'[55] According to Burke, the study of advertisement is crucial as they consciously attempt to manipulate the views of the consumers, a process which largely remains unconscious to their mind. However, there is one very major limitation with the historiographical use of advertisements as it often carries the danger of exaggerated interpretation. It is very difficult to assess the real impact of the advertisements on the consumers. To say that the sale of a particular product rose because of the advertisement (and not because of the inherent qualities of that product) carries the risk of exaggerating the impact of advertisements on the human mind. After all, if the advertisements can turn 'users' into 'consumers',[56] then the fraud and deceit prevalent in the market may turn 'consumers' into 'smart consumers' as well. So, it is very speculative to assess the real impact of advertisements on the consumers' minds. However, one can surely say that advertisements do play some role in inducing consumers to try a particular product.

The late nineteenth and early twentieth century Indian market witnessed a plethora of medical advertisements. According to Douglas Haynes, these medical advertisements were 'perhaps the chief form of commercial appeal in Indian newspapers during the late nineteenth century; they remained ubiquitous into the twentieth century and were critical to the incomes of vernacular newspapers, at least until claims they made were regulated in the Drugs and Magic Remedies (Objectionable Advertisements) Act of 1954'.[57] Initially, it were the European medical firms which used the manipulative techniques of advertisements and they almost monopolised the advertising space in English dailies and journals so far as the medical advertisements were concerned. Later on, they started making inroads even into Hindi journals and newspapers. Interestingly, they worked through codes of local culture and targeted mostly the middle-class sensibilities. Some of them were not even hesitant while using Hindu religious symbols and deities to promote their product. For example, one of the advertisements of Woodward's Gripe Water (1930s) used the iconography of *Bal Krishna* (an ideal 'Hindu' child) to touch the sensibilities of the 'Hindu' mother and the family.[58] Similarly, many of them exhibited racial and gender biases in their content. 'Fair babies', 'masculine men' and 'beautiful women' were often portrayed in the medical advertisements of the European firms.[59]

'Indigenous' medical practitioners and pharmacies were quick to learn these manipulative advertising techniques and in some sense they even mastered these techniques better than their European counterparts. The additional avenues available to these 'indigenous' firms made them powerful competitors, at least in the field of medical advertisements. Unlike the European pharmaceutical companies, the Ayurvedic pharmacies, besides using local cultural codes, also invoked nationalist feeling to increase their sale. 'Swadeshi' was definitely a powerful concept at the disposal of these Ayurvedic pharmacies to convince the consumers for using the drugs manufactured by them. The idea of 'National Medicine', which the European firms were invoking back home,[60] was used by the Ayurvedic pharmacies in India. In this regard, one of the advertisements by Ayurvedokt Aushadhalaya (Allahabad) referred to the dominant nationalist idea of the 'Drain of Wealth' to convince the consumer not to use 'English' medicine. The advertisement stated that every year as much as 12 crores of rupees moved out of India in the form of purchase of 'English' medicine, which constituted a major form of drain.[61]

Further, as argued earlier, besides arousing nationalist feeling, the Ayurvedic pharmacies effectively used the social codes and networks to increase their clientele. For example, often the advertisements of Ayurvedic drugs carried testimonials by prominent personalities or some men of authority to authenticate the usefulness of the product. One such advertisement by Mahashakti Aushadhalaya of Benares contained testimonials by renowned literary figures including Premchand (see Figure 5.8).

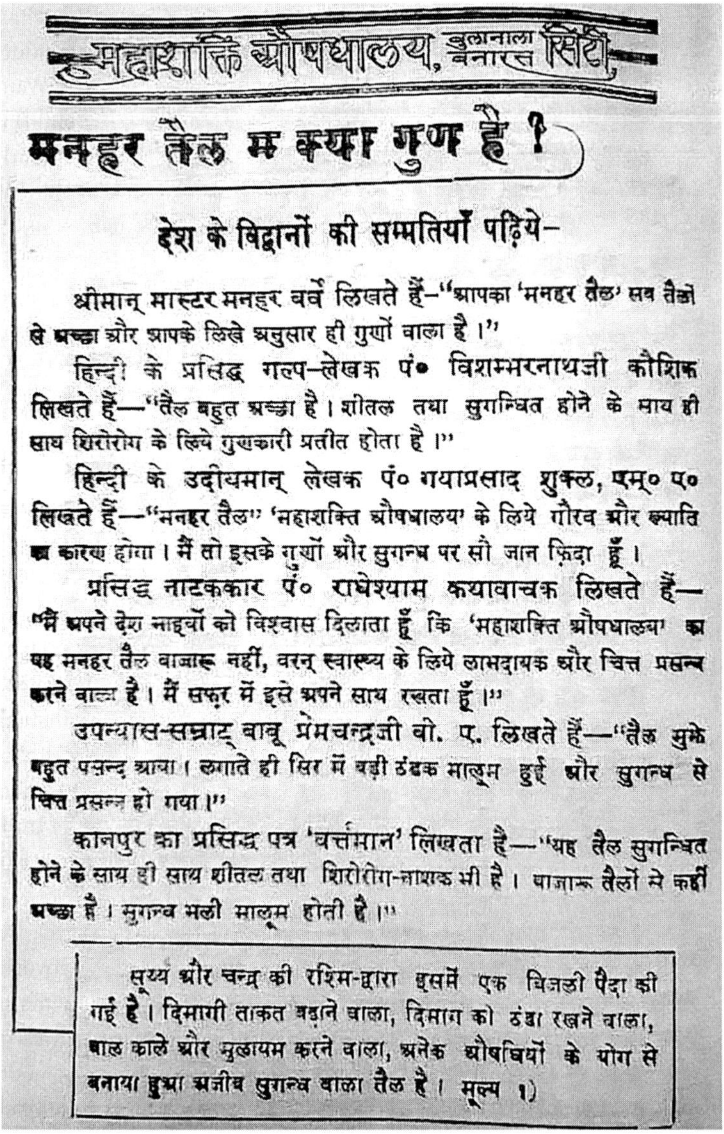

महाशक्ति औषधालय, बुलानाला बनारस सिटी

मनहर तैल में क्या गुण है ?

देश के विद्वानों की सम्मतियाँ पढ़िये—

श्रीमान् मास्टर मनहर बर्वे लिखते हैं—"आपका 'मनहर तैल' सब तैलों से अच्छा और आपके लिखे अनुसार ही गुणों वाला है।"

हिन्दी के प्रसिद्ध गल्प-लेखक पं० विशम्भरनाथजी कौशिक लिखते हैं—"तैल बहुत अच्छा है। शीतल तथा सुगन्धित होने के साथ ही साथ शिरोरोग के लिये गुणकारी प्रतीत होता है।"

हिन्दी के उदीयमान् लेखक पं० गयाप्रसाद शुक्ल, एम्० ए० लिखते हैं—"मनहर तैल" 'महाशक्ति औषधालय' के लिये गौरव और ख्याति का कारण होगा। मैं तो इसके गुणों और सुगन्ध पर सौ जान फ़िदा हूँ।

प्रसिद्ध नाटककार पं० राधेश्याम कथावाचक लिखते हैं—"मैं अपने देश भाइयों को विश्वास दिलाता हूँ कि 'महाशक्ति औषधालय' का यह मनहर तैल बाजारू नहीं, वरन् स्वास्थ्य के लिये लाभदायक और चित्त प्रसन्न करने वाला है। मैं सफ़र में इसे अपने साथ रखता हूँ।"

उपन्यास-सम्राट् बाबू प्रेमचन्द्रजी बी. ए. लिखते हैं—"तैल मुझे बहुत पसन्द आया। लगाते ही सिर में बड़ी ठंढक मालूम हुई और सुगन्ध से चित्त प्रसन्न हो गया।"

कानपुर का प्रसिद्ध पत्र 'वर्त्तमान' लिखता है—"यह तैल सुगन्धित होने के साथ ही साथ शीतल तथा शिरोरोग-नाशक भी है। बाजारू तैलों से कहीं अच्छा है। सुगन्ध भली मालूम होती है।"

सूर्य्य और चन्द्र की रश्मि-द्वारा इसमें एक बिजली पैदा की गई है। दिमागी ताकत बढ़ाने वाला, दिमाग को ठंढा रखने वाला, बाल काले और मुलायम करने वाला, अनेक औषधियों के योग से बनाया हुआ अजीब सुगन्ध वाला तैल है। मूल्य १)

Figure 5.8: *Manhar Tel*: An advertisement by Mahashakti Aushadhalaya (Benares) containing testimonials of prominent personalities, including Premchand.[62]

Similarly, another advertisement by Babu Laxminarayan Kabiraj of Cuttack carried testimonials of a headmaster and a police inspector (both men of authority) to support its claim.[63] Furthermore, authority/recommendations of renowned landlords/petty chieftains (zamindars) of the locality were also used in some of the Ayurvedic advertisements to convince the common public regarding the effectiveness of the concerned drug. For instance, one of the advertisements by Dhanvantari Aushadhalaya used the testimonials of Chaudhari Rambhajan Singh Zamindar and Chaudhari Nayan Singh Zamindar in order to increase the sale of its medicines.[64]

These testimonials were effective in winning over the faith of the consumer as the medical market was full of 'falsified' claims. In fact, if we look closely at some of the medical advertisements of the time, it clearly provides some insight into the prevalence of widespread fraud and trickery in the medical market. That is why the advertisements of a particular Ayurvedic drug often contained words such as '*asli*' (original), '*ek matra*' (one and only), '*sachcha*' (real), '*varshon se ajmayee hui*' (time-tested) and '*nakli maal se savdhan*' (beware of fake items) to convince the consumer. Some of them even offered 'money back' schemes in case of non-relief. In fact, the world of advertised drugs was always seen with suspicion by the consumers and the Ayurvedic pharmacies were very well aware of this fact; hence, they resorted to several techniques to convince the consumers regarding their authenticity.

The following advertisement clearly illustrates the sceptical attitude of the consumer towards the advertised drugs:

> *Jo log anek baar vigyapani aushadhi manga kar thaga chuke hain aur aisi aushadhiyon se vishwas kho chuke hain, nahi samajhte unse kin shabdon mein hum aushadhi mangane ka anurodh karein, tab unse itna hi kahne ka sahas karte hain ki jahan anek baar thaga chuke, tahan ek baar aur bhi himmat kar hamari pariksha kar dekhiye.*[65]

(It is very difficult to convince those who have been deceived several times by placing orders for some advertised drugs or the other, and have lost their faith in such drugs; however, we can only request such people to try our medicines at least once.)

In such a situation, testimonials of some prominent personalities or some men of authority assuring the utility of any medicine had a serious significance.

Another very important aspect of the Ayurvedic advertisements was that they often resorted to 'negative publicity' of Western drugs, condemning them for the alleged mixture of animal fat and other such tabooed materials, such as alcohol. '*Vishuddhata*' (ultra-purity) was the key characteristic feature which the Ayurvedic pharmacies claimed for the medicines they produced. Occasionally, the notion of '*vishuddha*' Ayurvedic medicines acquired profound social underpinnings as well. For instance, the advertisement of Ayurvedokt Aushadhalaya (Allahabad) has already been cited in Chapter 4 wherein it claimed that all kinds of medicines prepared by the aforesaid pharmacy were made either by Brahmins or other superior castes, and instead of ordinary water they used nectar like water of the Ganges.[66] Thus, in this particular advertisement, the Ayurvedic pharmacy claimed to have distanced itself from the alleged 'polluting' appearance of the lower castes/untouchables, thereby emphasising on 'ultra-purity' of the drug manufactured by them.

However, the very fact that the Ayurvedic advertisements were deeply rooted in the nationalist and socio-cultural discourse of the subcontinent does not mean that they failed to take into account the rapid changes in visual culture initiated in the colonial context. The advertisement of *Amrit Dhara* and *Piyush Ratnakar* clearly reflected the incorporation of new cultural tropes which assumed serious significance in colonial India like the attraction towards the 'fair skin' and the idea of 'ameliorating the world from its sufferings' (extension of 'White Man's Burden'). The early twentieth century advertisement of *Amrit Dhara* portrays a fairy which appears like a Greek goddess and nowhere resembles its Indian counterpart, that is, a *pari*, pouring nectar in the mouth of an animated globe.[67] Similarly, G.A. Mishra Ayurvedic Pharmacy of Jhansi came up with the advertisement of an innovative 'Ayurvedic Injection' which explicitly traversed the boundaries of Ayurveda and Western medicine and combined both the systems into one (see Figure 5.9).[68]

Further, in order to woo the consumers, a considerable portion of the advertised Ayurvedic drugs was covered by all-encompassing drugs

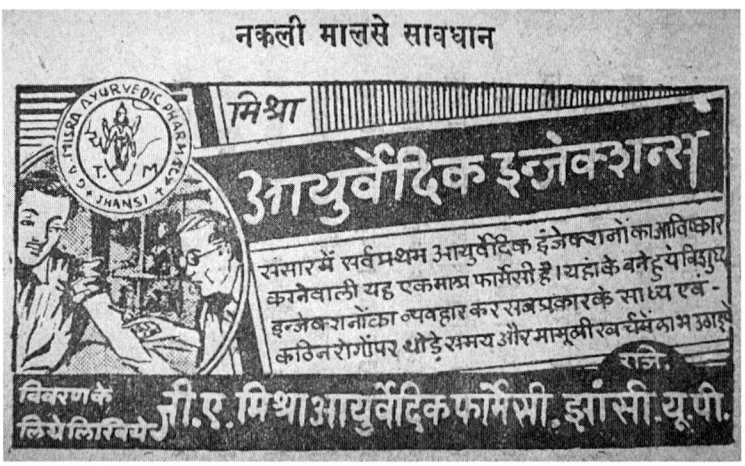

Figure 5.9: An advertisement of Ayurvedic injection by G.A. Mishra Ayurvedic Pharmacy, Jhansi.[69]

or panacea (popularly known as *Ramban Aushadhi*), claiming to cure all the diseases in one stroke, like the arrow of Rama which was powerful enough to sweep away all the evils. Most of the Ayurvedic pharmacies came up with such 'Ramban Aushadhis' [for an illustration, see Figure 5.10(a) and Figure 5.10(b)]. Advertisements of these medicines often made exaggerated and unrealistic claims, but probably they matched the popular mood of the early twentieth century Indian society, which was desperate for overnight miraculous cures in each and every sphere. The language used in the advertisements of these Ramban Aushadhis was really powerful and effective to attract the disappointed minds and hearts. In fact, one can easily feel the real attractive power of the advertisements while looking either at the advertisements of the panacea or at those of the aphrodisiacs.

Incidentally, awards were also instituted for the discovery of Ramban Aushadhis. One such advertisement of award appeared in the *Vaidya Sammelan Patrika* for the discovery of Ramban Aushadhi related to the treatment of snake-bite. It was instituted by the Goodh-chikitsa Mandal, Poonah (an association devoted to the discovery of hidden 'treasures' of Ayurveda). It made a call to the vaids throughout the country to showcase

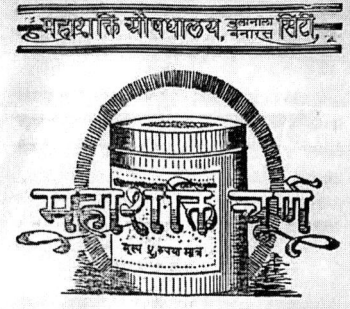
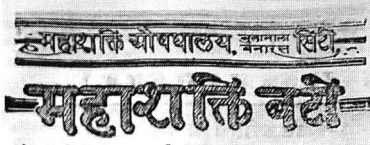

Figure 5.10(a): Some of the advertisements of panacea (*Mahashakti Churna* and *Mahashakti Vati*) by Mahashakti Aushadhalaya, Benares.[70]

their medicines for the effective treatment of snake-bite which could be subsequently certified as panacea for the same.[71]

Like panacea, aphrodisiacs also covered a huge proportion of the Ayurvedic advertisements, so much so that the author of *Raag Darbari*, commenting on the nature of extant medical advertisements, sarcastically claimed that there existed only three 'real' health issues in the country (as appeared from the medical advertisements): dermatophytosis ('*daad*'), hydrocele ('*and-vriddhi*') and impotency ('*namardi*').[72] Promotion of drugs like *Napunsak Vati*, *Kamdev Churna*, *Kamotpadak Vati*, *Madanmanjari*, *Taqat Bahar Goliyan*, *Mahashakti Modak*, *Veeryasindhu* and *Kamdipak Tila* was quite common in the early twentieth century world of print. One can find advertisements of such drugs either in leading Hindi journals of the time like *Abhyudaya*, *Madhuri*, *Vartman* and *Maryada*, or at the back of

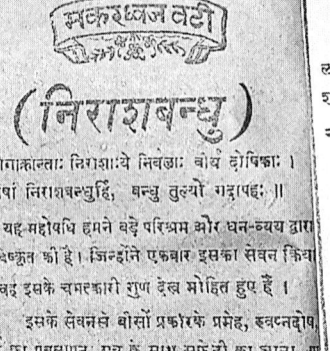

Figure 5.10(b): *Makardhwaj Vati*: A panacea made by the Dhanvantari Aushadhalaya, Aligarh[73]

Ayurvedic books and health tracts [for an illustration, see Figure 5.11(a) and Figure 5.11(b)]. According to Haynes, the popularity of advertised aphrodisiacs was in part due to the fact that the male consumers who used them could avoid admitting 'shameful' sexual problems to medical specialists, such as erectile dysfunction and, more commonly, 'thinness' in semen.[74] Moreover, these advertisements simultaneously addressed prevailing middle-class anxieties about 'lost masculinities' that had become entrenched in the context of colonialism.[75] It is noticeable that the colonial discourses on India from very early on were 'gendered', as the colonised society was feminised and its 'effeminate' character, as opposed to 'colonial masculinity', was held as a justification for its loss of independence.[76] In such a context, aphrodisiacs promised to restore the vigour of the colonised society, particularly that of middle class, often through pseudo-scientific claims.

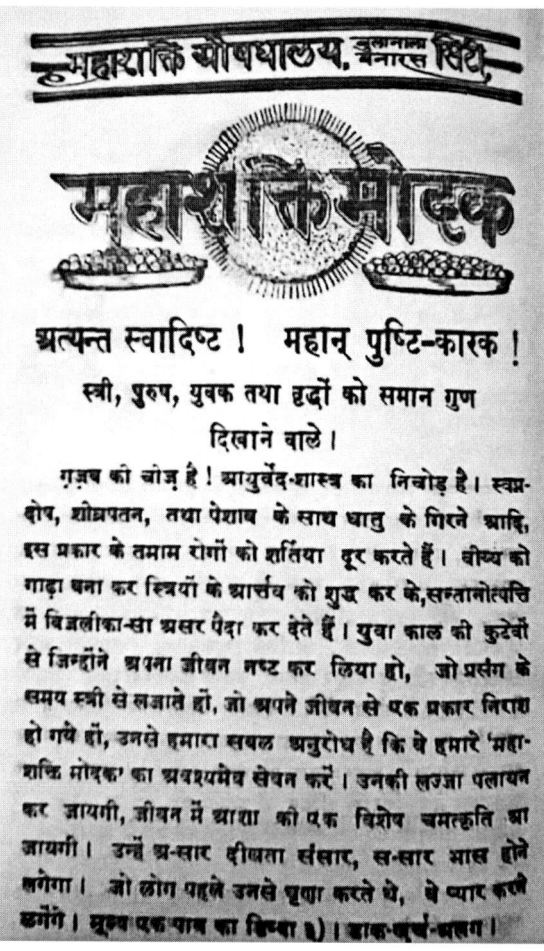

Figure 5.11(a): *Mahashakti Modak*: An advertisement of an aphrodisiac.[77]

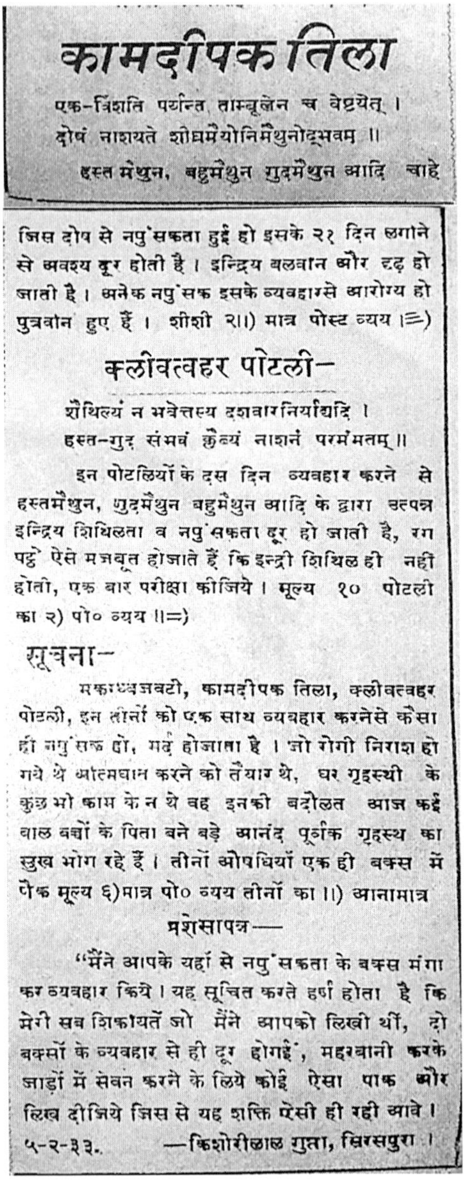

Figure 5.11(b): *Kamdipak Tila*: An advertisement of an aphrodisiac.[78]

Nevertheless, the rampant advertisement of these aphrodisiacs was constantly challenging the discourse over brahmacharya, which was so prominent in the early twentieth century Ayurvedic discourse. While brahmacharya stressed on containment and restraining sexual desires, the aphrodisiacs celebrated sex.[79] In fact, novel ways were offered by Ayurvedic tracts to induce sexual excitement such as through *Vajikaran Gulabjamun* (sweets having aphrodisiac property).[80] Incidentally, expertise (mostly self-proclaimed) over curing sexual impotency or nourishment of semen ('*virya-pushti*') was the reason behind the popularity of many vaids.[81]

However, one should not always take the sale and promotion of aphrodisiacs and the idea of celibacy as antithetical to each other. While it is true that the discourse over brahmacharya was condemning bodily pleasure, something upon which the market of aphrodisiacs was based, Hindu society nowhere celebrated impotency. In fact, impotency was looked down upon and impotent men were heavily despised and mocked at since sexual virility of a man was part and parcel of the overall gendered thought process of society. If one was sexually impotent or unfit, he was deemed to be incapable of performing his usual functions of being a 'man'. In fact, to an extent the discourse over brahmacharya and the sale of aphrodisiacs to cure impotency complimented each other. The whole idea behind brahmacharya was to preserve the sexual power (or, in turn, semen) so that it could be utilised for other 'useful' purposes, that is, in the service of the nation and community. Stored semen was supposed to generate power within the body. On the other hand, if one was sexually impotent, brahmacharya and its associated powers had no meaning for him. So, one could become a brahmachari only after being sexually virile, something which the aphrodisiacs promised. In other words, the discourse over brahmacharya and the sale and promotion of aphrodisiacs were both challenging as well as complimenting each other. Hence, most of the Ayurvedic pharmacies of the early twentieth century came up with such Ayurvedic medicines increasing sexual virility and curing impotency.

Last, but not the least, as argued earlier, compared to their European counterparts, the Ayurvedic practitioners and pharmacies in some sense excelled the art of advertisements. Some of the Ayurvedic practitioners not just advertised the magazines and books published by the printing press owned by them or the medicines prepared by the pharmacies established by them, but they also used the world of advertisements to advertise about themselves and their skills. A classic example in this regard was Yashoda Devi. She brilliantly exploited the world of advertisements to reach her clientele. Advertisements related to her pharmacy and books and magazines published by her often carried some description of Yashoda Devi and her Ayurvedic skills and achievements in the field of female health. Sometimes these descriptions even dominated the main item of the advertisement. For example, one of the advertisements of *Stri Chikitsak* (a monthly magazine published by Yashoda Devi) carried a detailed description of Yashoda Devi, and one can get to know more about Yashoda Devi from this advertisement than the magazine and its contents (see Figure 5.12).

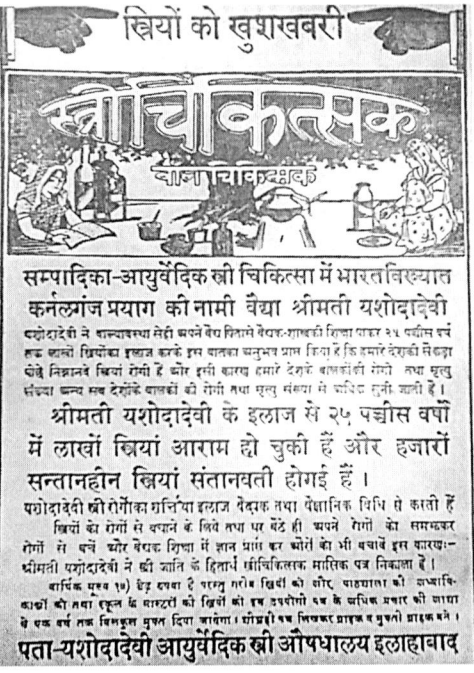

Figure 5.12: Advertisement of *Stri Chikitsak* (a monthly magazine published by Yashoda Devi).[82]

CONCLUDING REMARKS

The market does not work merely within an economic straightjacket; rather, socio-political discourses significantly shape and are, in turn, shaped by the market forces. The preceding discussion on the Ayurvedic print and drug market clearly demonstrates how this interactive relationship shaped the market forces and the socio-political discourses in colonial India. The late colonial Ayurvedic movement launched by the 'new' vaids attested this phenomenon. As argued in the very beginning, the 'new' vaids particularly focussed on those aspects of the medical market which were spared by the monopolistic tendencies unleashed by Western medicine, such as rural healthcare, production of tonics and vitalisers, vernacular health manuals, all-encompassing drugs or panacea, and aphrodisiacs.

This was the reason which made the Ayurvedic pharmacies put greater emphasis on the production of tonics and vitalisers, including panacea and aphrodisiacs, than the drugs meant for specific diseases. Partly, it was the outcome of extant Ayurvedic philosophy which believed not so much in immediate relief of a particular disease but in improving the bodily resistance. In Ayurveda, 'the improvement of *kshetra* (body of the patient) was far more important than the microbe and its destruction'.[83] However, alongside this, there was an economic logic as well. The Ayurvedic pharmacies knew that it was very difficult to penetrate the market of certain allopathic drugs such as quinine which offered quick relief and was very popular with the masses. So, they focussed more on the untapped areas of the medical market instead of directly confronting the market of Western drugs. It demonstrates impressive business sense of the Ayurvedic pharmacies.

Thus, the basic urge was to look for a market and consumers of its own. The various Ayurvedic advertisements that we have discussed also exemplify this attempt by the Ayurvedic practitioners to create 'consumers' out of the 'users' and to carve out a niche for themselves in the medical market. Similar was the objective behind the publication of numerous short, handy, easy-to-consult and affordable Ayurvedic pamphlets, booklets and tracts. Incidentally, this trend has distinct continuities up to the present times if one explores Ayurvedic pharmaceutical companies like Zandu, Dabur and Himalaya and their modus operandi today. These pharmaceutical companies are still engaged in the above-mentioned pursuit of creating the Ayurvedic consumer and the market of its own.[84] In fact, in due course of time, these Ayurvedic pharmaceutical companies through massive proliferation of over-the-counter brands and production of pre-packed traditional Ayurvedic formulas coupled with aggressive marketing strategy have virtually sidelined the vaids in their role as the diagnostician, therapist and the prescriber.[85]

NOTES

1. Brahmanand Gupta, 'Indigenous Medicine in Nineteenth and Twentieth Century Bengal', in Leslie, *Asian Medical Systems*, 368–82; Panikkar, *Culture, Hegemony, Ideology*, 145–75.
2. For example, see Kumar, 'The Indian Drug Industry', 356–85; Maarten Bode, 'Indian Indigenous Pharmaceuticals: Tradition, Modernity and Nature', in Ernst, *Plural Medicine*, 184–203; Madhuri Sharma, 'Creating a Consumer: Exploring Medical Advertisements in Colonial India', in *The Social History of Health and Medicine in Colonial India*, eds Biswamoy Pati and Mark Harrison (London and New York: Routledge, 2009), 213–28.
3. Quoted by Mohan Lal Kothari at the third conference of Madhyabhartiya Vaidya Sammelan held at Nagaud; Mohan Lal Kothari, *Proceedings of Madhyabhartiya Vaidya Sammelan, Nagaud* (Shandilya Kuti, Kashi: Ayurveda Press, 1936).
4. Arnold, *The New Cambridge History of India III.5*, 176.
5. Ulrike Stark, *An Empire of Books: The Naval Kishore Press and the Diffusion of the Printed Word in Colonial India* (Ranikhet: Permanent Black, 2008), 406. Noticeable is the sheer number of Ayurvedic texts published in Hindi/Hindustani.
6. Stark, *An Empire of Books*, 409. It should be noted that the second half of nineteenth century saw an entire movement to develop a 'standard' version of Hindi language, undermining its regional variations and fluidity. This 'standardisation' of Hindi language was often synonymous with incorporation of several Sanskrit terms within its fold and preference given to *Khari boli* over the other variants of the same language such as *Braj*. Print culture played an important role in this entire process which was not devoid of caste, class and community-oriented biases. Incidentally, the United Provinces was the major centre of the aforesaid process of 'standardisation' of Hindi language. For detail on this theme, see Alok Rai, *Hindi Nationalism* (New Delhi: Orient Longman, 2001).

7. Stark, *An Empire of Books*, 410.
8. Ibid.
9. Shrivastava, *Vaidya Priya*.
10. For an extensive list of these vernacular Ayurvedic journals, see Appendix 5.
11. For some recent interventions in this direction, see Stark, *An Empire of Books*. Stark has explored the marketing strategies and networks of the Naval Kishore Press of Lucknow in quite some detail (Stark, *An Empire of Books*, 194–205).
12. Stark, *An Empire of Books*, 198.
13. Chatur Sen Shastri, *Brahmacharya Sadhan* (Lucknow: Ganga Granthagar, 1928).
14. Yashoda Devi, *Dehati Chikitsa* (Allahabad, n.d.).
15. '*Apna ilaj aap hi kijiye*' (treat yourself on your own) or '*kisi doctor ke paas jane ki zaroorat nahi*' (no need to consult a doctor) were some of the popular taglines written in bold letters in the advertisements regarding Ayurvedic texts of the late nineteenth and early twentieth century. See the introductory page of Devi, *Dehati Chikitsa*.
16. *Magh Mela*—A holy fair held at *Sangam* in Allahabad around January–February of every year.
17. Devi, *Dampati Arogyata Jeevanshastra*, 6–7.
18. Ibid., 5.
19. If we look at the vernacular literary market of the United Provinces in the late nineteenth and early twentieth century, then it was full of seemingly 'erotic', 'obscene' and 'semi-pornographic' stuff. In spite of various legal and social regulations, the publication and sale of such literature were very high. Common people were least interested in classical Indian texts and the bestsellers of the time were often sleazy literature on forbidden erotic themes. For detail on this, see Gupta, 'Dirty Hindi Literature'.
20. *Vaidya Sammelan Patrika* 1, nos 3–4, March–April 1936.
21. Yashoda Devi, *Dehati Chikitsa* (Allahabad, n.d.). The language of the advertisement makes every attempt to woo Yashoda Devi's female readership. This advertisement clearly embodies the statements like 'complex issues have been explained in such an easy language that even "foolish" women can understand it quite comfortably' or economic incentives such as 'one gets benefits of a thousand bucks after spending a little money'.
22. Pierre Bourdieu, *The Field of Cultural Production: Essays on Art and Literature*; ed. & intro. by Randal Johnson (Cambridge: Polity Press, 1993).
23. Sisir Kumar Das, *Western Impact—Indian Response: 1800–1910* (New Delhi: Sahitya Akademi, 1991).
24. Bourdieu, *The Field of Cultural Production*, 37–43.

25. Criticising traditional literary history, Hohendahl argues: 'The publicly grounded institution of literature is subject to indirect pressures exerted by political and economic issues on the public sphere. Traditional literary history, which is oriented towards authors, works, or genres, cannot contribute much to the institutional character of literature and thus can comprehend diachronic processes only as isolated series of events.' See Peter Uwe Hohendahl, *Building a National Literature: The Case of Germany, 1830-1870*, trans. Renate Baron Franciscono (Ithaca, NY: Cornell University Press, 1989), 45.
26. Orsini, *The Hindi Public Sphere*.
27. For example, see Chatterjee, *The Nation and Its Fragments*, 4–6; Bayly, *Empire and Information*; Stein Tonnesson and Hans Antlov, eds, *Asian Forms of the Nation* (London: Curzon, 1996).
28. Madhulika Banerjee, 'Ayurvedic Pharmaceuticals: Contesting Economic Hegemony', in *Contesting Colonial Authority: Medicine and Indigenous Responses in Nineteenth and Twentieth Century India*, ed. Poonam Bala (Lanham: Lexington Books, 2012), 35.
29. Banerjee, 'Ayurvedic Pharmaceuticals', 36–37.
30. See Amiya K. Bagchi, *Private Investment in India, 1900–39* (Cambridge: Cambridge University Press, 1972); Sarkar, *Modern India*, 171–72.
31. Kumar, 'The Indian Drug Industry', 382.
32. Ibid., 375.
33. For detailed description of the trajectory of industrialisation and capital investment in the preparation of Ayurvedic medicine and consequent shifts, see Madhulika Banerjee, *Power, Knowledge, Medicine: Ayurvedic Pharmaceuticals at Home and in the World* (Hyderabad: Orient Blackswan, 2009).
34. 'Presidential Address of Pandit Yadavji Vikramji Acharya', in Singh, *Nikhil Bharatvarshiya Ayurveda Mahamandal ka Rajat Jayanti Granth*, 1: 278–91.
35. 'Presidential Address of Pandit Yadavji Vikramji Acharya', 287–88.
36. *Dhanvantari* 9, nos 3–4, August–September 1933. An interesting connection has been drawn between medicine (*aushadhi*) and weapon (*astra*), stating that both should always be up to the mark.
37. Nandini Bhattacharya, 'Between the Bazaar and the Bench: Making of the Drugs Trade in Colonial India, ca. 1900–1930', *Bulletin of History of Medicine* 90, no. 1, 2016, 61–91.
38. Compiled by the author.
39. Also compiled by the author.
40. Singh, *Nikhil Bharatvarshiya Ayurveda Mahamandal ka Rajat Jayanti Granth*, 1: 559.

41. Deepak Kumar, 'Medical Encounters in British India, 1820-1920', *Economic & Political Weekly* 32, no. 4, 1997, 169. Incidentally, Swadeshi movement and the First World War seem to have provided a congenial ground for the growth of Arya Vaidyasala as attested by the rising sales of P.S. Varier's medicines.
42. Kumar, 'Medical Encounters in British India', 169.
43. It should be kept in mind that with the growth of the Indian national movement, the concept of *'swadeshi'* had acquired tremendous economic potential which was exploited by Indian entrepreneurs across the trade.
44. Kumar, 'The Indian Drug Industry', 374.
45. Sharma, *Indigenous and Western Medicine*, 111.
46. For more discussion on this aspect, see the sub-section 'Advertising Ayurveda' of this chapter.
47. Back cover of the Ayurvedic tract by Pandit Ramprasad Mishra 'Rajvaidya', *Kuchimartantram* (Aligarh: Dhanvantari Press, first published in 1925; fourth edition, 1965).
48. *Dhanvantari* 10, no. 3, August 1934, 320.
49. Back cover of the Ayurvedic tract by 'Rajvaidya', *Kuchimartantram*.
50. 'Inspection Notes of R.B.B. Ghanshyam Dass, Deputy Commissioner, Sitapur on 16.09.1934', F. No. 226, Box No. 83, Medical Department, 1938, UPSA.
51. Ibid.
52. Commenting on this tendency of self-medication in contemporary India, Maarten Bode estimates that around 80–90 per cent of Ayurvedic and Unani pharmaceuticals are sold directly (without prescription) to consumers by retailers such as chemists, small grocers as well as supermarkets and beauty parlours (Bode, 'Indian Indigenous Pharmaceuticals', 185–86).
53. Sharma, *Indigenous and Western Medicine*, 111.
54. Tarashankar Bandyopadhyaya, *Arogya Niketan*, 4th edn (Delhi: Rajpal & Sons, 1967), 30.
55. Peter Burke, *Eyewitnessing: The Uses of Images as Historical Evidence* (London: Reaktion Books, 2001), 94.
56. I am borrowing this phraseology of turning 'users' into 'consumers' from Sharma, *Indigenous and Western Medicine*, 120.
57. Douglas E. Haynes, 'Advertising and the History of South Asia, 1880–1950', *History Compass* 30, no. 8, 2015, 364.
58. For the advertisement of Woodward's Gripe Water, see Erwin Neumayer and Christine Schelberger, *Popular Indian Art: Raja Ravi Verma and the Printed Gods of India* (New Delhi: Oxford University Press, 2003), 96.
59. For details on this theme, see Sharma, *Indigenous and Western Medicine*, 123–28.

60. For an interesting example of European firms invoking the idea of 'National Medicine' back home, see one of the advertisements of Beecham's Pills (1920s) which combined the picture of Union Jack along with its product (see Sharma, *Indigenous and Western Medicine*, 147).
61. For the advertisement by Ayurvedokt Aushadhalaya (Allahabad), see page 16 of the pamphlet entitled 'Bharat ki Unnati ka Vaidyak Pratham Anga Hai', in Sharma, *Arogya Darpan*, Vol. 3. Although it is difficult to testify the factual correctness of the given data, the point is that it did invoke and made use of a dominant narrative of the age of economic nationalism in order to convince the consumers to buy its products.
62. Pravasi Lal Verma, ed., *Arogya Mandir* (Benares: Mahashakti Sahitya Mandir, 1927).
63. Biswamoy Pati, *Situating Social History*, 18.
64. *Dhanvantari (Chikitsa Anubhava Ank)* 10, no. 3, August 1934, 23–25.
65. Jagannath Prasad Shukla, *Ayurveda ka Mahatva* (Prayag, 1937), 31. It should be noted that Jagannath Prasad Shukla was the manager of Sudhanidhi Aushadhalaya, Allahabad.
66. For the advertisement, see page 16 of the pamphlet entitled 'Bharat ki Unnati ka Vaidyak Pratham Anga Hai', in Sharma, *Arogya Darpan*, Vol. 3.
67. For the visuals of the advertisement of *Amrit Dhara* and related discussion, see Sharma, 'Creating a Consumer', 220–21.
68. Incidentally, the Ayurvedic practitioners defended the use of these apparent 'Western' therapeutic/diagnostic technologies by arguing that these were clearly described even in the Vedas and other classical Indian texts but by the span of time these had been lost for want of research. For an interesting insight on how injection, stethoscope and other such things were adopted by the Ayurvedic practitioners of the United Provinces, see Madhuri Sharma, 'Knowing Health and Medicine: A Case Study of Benares, *c*. 1900–1950', in *Medical Encounters in British India*, eds Deepak Kumar and Raj Sekhar Basu (Delhi: Oxford University Press, 2013), 170.
69. *Sudhanidhi* 40, no. 10, 16 May 1949. The capstone reads '*nakli maal se savdhan*', that is, 'beware of fake items', which hints at the prevalent fraud and trickery in the medical market.
70. Verma, *Arogya Mandir*. The claims made and the language used in these advertisements are noteworthy.
71. *Vaidya Sammelan Patrika* 1, no. 10, October 1931, 237–39.
72. Shrilal Shukla, *Raag Darbari* (New Delhi: Rajkamal Paperbacks, 2013), 61.
73. *Dhanvantari (Chikitsa Anubhava Ank)* 10, no. 3, August 1934, 24–25.
74. Haynes, 'Advertising and the History of South Asia', 365.

75. Jeremy Schneider, 'Reimagining Traditional Medicine: Tracing the Emergence of Commodified Ayurveda in the Interwar Period' (MSc. thesis in Economic and Social History, Oxford University, 2008), 38–48 (cited in Haynes, 'Advertising and the History of South Asia', 365).
76. For details on such gendered colonial discourses, see Sinha, *Colonial Masculinity*.
77. Verma, *Arogya Mandir*.
78. *Dhanvantari (Chikitsa Anubhava Ank)* 10, no. 3, August 1934, 25.
79. For a profound sociological and iconographical analysis of the advertisements of aphrodisiacs, see Gupta, *Sexuality, Obscenity, Community* (section on 'Brahmacharya, Kaliyug and the Advertisement of Aphrodisiacs'), 66–83; Sharma, *Indigenous and Western Medicine* (section on 'Invading Private Space: Aphrodisiacs and Contraceptives'), 133–36.
80. 'Rajvaidya', *Kuchimartantram*, 42–43.
81. For instance, the real popularity of Vaidya ji—one of the chief characters of the satirical novel *Raag Darbari*—was owing to his pills nourishing semen (see Shukla, *Raag Darbari*, 33, 288, 308).
82. Yashoda Devi, *Dehati Chikitsa* (Allahabad, n.d.).
83. *Dhanvantari* 4, no. 3, 18 February 1925, 133–35; cited in Kumar, 'Medical Encounters in British India', 169.
84. For an interesting insight on this, see Bode, 'Indian Indigenous Pharmaceuticals', 184–203.
85. For a detailed discussion on this relatively recent phenomenon of vanishing of the vaids and hakims with the profusion of branded products, particularly since the last decade of the twentieth century, see Bode, *Taking Traditional Knowledge to the Market*, 59–73.

6

Ayurveda at the Crossroads of Independence

c. 1946–50

So far we have looked at various aspects of the Ayurvedic discourse and the Ayurvedic revivalist movement in colonial India. It would be equally interesting to look at the developments which followed immediately after independence. This is largely because the colonial context, which was hitherto one of the major factors in shaping the characteristic features of the Ayurvedic revivalist movement, was no longer present in a direct manifest form. In the absence of this colonial context, the Ayurvedic movement had to face new kinds of challenges which were internal and relatively subtle vis-à-vis evident colonial onslaught. Besides, such a discussion is equally significant in tracing the postcolonial government attitude towards Ayurveda and other 'indigenous' healing practices which had a lasting imprint on the future development of Ayurveda in independent India.

For quite some time, historians and political theorists deemed independence as a decisive break in Indian history. However, very soon, colonial continuities in postcolonial era became evident across the world, including the Indian subcontinent. As Ashis Nandy argued, '[W]estern colonialism brought with it, not merely economic exploitation and political oppression, but also the unrelenting thrust of a 'civilising' mission based on a worldview which believed in the absolute superiority of the human over the non-human, of the masculine over the feminine, of the historical over the ahistorical, and of the modern over the traditional.'[1] This colonial triumph of the 'modern' over the 'traditional' in the field of 'indigenous' medicine was articulated through postcolonial administrative leanings towards Western medicine while drafting broader health policies for the subject citizens. The nationalist articulation of anti-colonial sentiments in the field of medicine could seldom mitigate the pragmatic contingencies of the newly independent nation modelled on modern framework. Medicine had already become an integral tool of governance for modern nation-states exhibiting a spontaneous and deeply rooted convergence between the requirements of political ideology and those of medical technology.[2] The choice of healing system by the post-independence Indian nation-state depended very much upon this new found virtue of medicine in modern ways of governance.[3] It becomes quite evident when one closely analyses the contemporaneous reports/recommendations of health surveys and subsequent response of the government.

Three reports which become particularly crucial for the purpose of present study are the *Report of the Health Survey and Development Committee*, 1946; *Report of the Committee on Indigenous Systems of Medicine*, 1948; and *Report and Recommendations of the United Provinces Ayurvedic and Unani Systems Reorganisation Committee*, 1949. The present chapter scrutinises each of these reports and consequent response of the related officials extensively to situate the envisaged role of Ayurveda in the biopoiitics[4] of independent India, particularly that of the United Provinces. While doing so, it looks for colonial continuities and disjunctures, if any, of the official attitude towards 'indigenous' medicine in the era of experimental planning. Incidentally, as argued by Rachel Berger, this was the period which witnessed a scramble to lay claim to an authoritative knowledge of Ayurveda and subsequent formulation of policy determining the place of Ayurvedic medicine and practitioners in the larger biopolitics of the state by a plurality of stakeholders, ranging from federal politicians to state bureaucrats to educational instructors to lay authors.[5]

LOCATING AYURVEDA/'INDIGENOUS' MEDICINE IN BHORE AND CHOPRA COMMITTEE REPORTS

With independence in sight, attempts were made both by the officials as well as political groups and voluntary organisations to prepare a roadmap of the public health policy for an imagined postcolonial future.[6] In this regard, it was as early as 1938 that the Indian National Congress set up the National Planning Committee under the chairmanship of Jawaharlal Nehru to prepare an 'all-embracing Plan' for future development of India with health being one of the primary foci. The Health sub-committee headed by Col. S. S. Sokhey was one of the 29 sub-committees of the National Planning Committee. However, the Health sub-committee adopted an ambivalent position towards 'indigenous' medicine.[7] Incidentally, all the members of the Health sub-committee were trained in Western medicine and there was no representative of 'indigenous' medicine as such.[8] As a corollary, Western medicine came to acquire central position in the report of the sub-committee, reducing 'indigenous' systems of healing at their best as an auxiliary to Western medicine. In fact, in its report, the Health sub-committee categorically stated that the issue of 'indigenous' medicine needed to be 'properly solved, otherwise, it [was] likely to *impede terribly the development of scientific medicine in the country*'.[9] The report of the Health sub-committee further argued that likewise many other countries, the pharmacopoeia of 'indigenous' systems of medicine in India had not been 'adequately revised' for centuries and that with the development of the scientific methods of assessing pharmacological and therapeutic value of drugs, most of the 'indigenous' remedies were found to be of 'no value'.[10] Thus, 'indigenous' medicine received little prestige at the hands of the Health sub-committee constituted by the Indian National Congress in its pioneering attempt to plan on the national basis.

Nevertheless, the first extensive official health survey at pan-Indian level outlining the future biopolitics of the Indian nation was the *Report of the Health Survey and Development Committee*, 1946 (popularly known as the Bhore Committee Report).[11] While it acknowledged the conspicuous presence and reach of 'indigenous' systems of healing in India in glaring terms,[12] the *Report* expressed its inability to assess the real value of these systems.[13] That is why the *Report* deliberately remained silent over the place of 'indigenous' systems of medicine in the organised state medical relief in the country. However, emphasising on preventive medicine/health care as the central attribute of future medical organisation, it raised doubts over the validity of 'indigenous' systems of medicine in such a schema as these systems were focused more on improving the long-term bodily resistance than immediate prevention and relief of a particular disease.

Incidentally, such emphasis on preventive aspect of health care, in many ways, forced the Ayurvedic practitioners to shift their focus from 'curative' to 'preventive' aspect of medicine in post-independence India to fit in the biopolitics of the time.[14]

Furthermore, the Bhore Committee Report expressed serious doubts over the element of scientificity and dynamism of 'indigenous' systems of medicine. According to the *Report*, no system of medical treatment which was static in conception and practice and did not keep pace with the discoveries and researches of scientific workers the world over could hope to give the best available ministration to those who sought its aid.[15] In this regard, the *Report* pointed out the absence of some of the vital aspects of modern medicine such as obstetrics, gynaecology, advanced surgery and some other specialties in 'indigenous' systems of medicine.[16] Here the *Report* went on to argue in favour of doing away with the categories like 'Western' and 'Eastern' and talked about a corpus of scientific knowledge and practice belonging to the whole world and to which every country had made its contribution.[17] It further argued that it would be unfair and unjust to deny anyone the benefit of the scientific system and of the daily growing volume of research and achievement in the wide world of science merely because some other method of treatment (that is, 'indigenous' systems of medicine) was claimed to be cheaper.[18] Thus, the cost-effectiveness of 'indigenous' medicine, which was often posed by its proponents to carve out a favourable position vis-à-vis Western medicine, was undermined as imparting benefits of the latest development in science to its citizens was seen as the moral obligation of an independent nation to ensure a healthy future.

Interestingly, the Bhore Committee Report referred to the universal trend of de-recognising 'indigenous' systems of medicine world over. It was argued that in China and Japan, a moratorium extending to a definite period of years had been declared after which the practice of the 'indigenous' systems in those countries would not be recognised. Similar was the case with the Soviet Union where 'indigenous' systems of medical treatment had already been de-recognised. Nonetheless, the Bhore Committee Report expressed its inability to suggest any such measure in the Indian context and left it entirely on the discretion of the provincial governments to decide what part, if any, should be played by 'indigenous' systems in the organisation of public health and medical relief.[19] Here, the Bhore Committee Report endorsed the recommendations of Dr Butt, Dr Narayan Rao and Dr Vishwa Nath who emphasised the continuation of registration of 'indigenous' practitioners through examinations as envisaged by the Bombay Medical Practitioners Act, 1938, as a step in the right direction. It was argued that 'indigenous' practitioners trained and registered under the requirement of the above Act, or similar legislation,[20] could be freely utilised for promoting public health and medical relief in India.[21] It clearly reflects the continued hegemony of institutionally trained 'new' vaids over the 'hereditary' practitioners of 'indigenous' medicine in independent India.

The next landmark report related to the development and future of 'indigenous' systems of medicine in independent India was the *Report of the Committee on Indigenous Systems of Medicine*, 1948, authored under the supervision of Ram Nath Chopra[22] (thereby deriving its popular moniker, the Chopra Report). In fact, the Bhore Committee Report with its aim to strive for a bold plan with tight budgets in the field of health sector remained mostly undertoned while discussing 'indigenous' systems of healing and deliberately cordoned it off for further discussion. Consequently, it created an immediate reaction among those who wished 'indigenous' systems of medicine to have a place in India's future health administration. The Chopra Report was an outcome of this reaction.[23] Simultaneously, the time and context, that is, that of postcolonial nationalist reconstruction of a newly independent nation, in which the aforesaid report was produced also had huge imprints on its various recommendations.

The most crucial recommendation of the Chopra Report was to create a 'unified system (of healing) for the country'.[24] The very phrase itself reflects the most celebrated nationalist agenda of unification, thereby prioritising the broader interest of the nation over factional differences. In fact, the Chopra Report through its emphasis on synthesising a unified system of healing tried to overcome the differences which prevailed among the practitioners of various healing systems along the lines of 'tradition' and 'modernity' on the one hand[25] and 'communal' identity(-ies) on the other.[26] This goal was clearly stated by Ram Nath Chopra in the introduction of the *Report*:

> We wish to emphasise here that the Committee do not believe in the multiplicity of systems of medicine. Science is universal and medical science is no exception. The so-called 'Systems' merely represent different aspects of and approaches to medical science as practiced during different ages and in different parts of the world. Anything of value emerging from these should be utilised for the benefit of humanity as a whole without any reservation and integrated in the form of a unified system for the country.[27]

Thus, the Chopra Committee tried to temporarily resolve the long-standing contradictions and clash of ideologies and status which mark the socio-political history of health and medicine throughout the late colonial period.

Incidentally, in its enthusiasm to prepare the ground for synthesis of a unified system of healing, the Chopra Committee went on to trace the origin of all healing systems of the world from Ayurveda. Identifying the Vedic origin of Ayurveda in India, the Chopra Report described its spread to Egypt, Greece, Rome and Arabia in due course of time, thereby influencing Greek medicine, which, in turn, was the precursor of both the Unani Tibb and Western medicine.[28] Thus, a natural logic was derived that since all other healing systems of the world contain Ayurvedic influences in some form or other, synthesis of a unified system was fairly possible. In other words, even while arguing in favour of a unified system, the nationalist pride was vividly secured by exalting Ayurveda and its inconspicuous history of influence on other systems. However, the government was quick to recognise the futility of such arguments for a unified system of healing. In its final decision after consideration of the aforesaid recommendation of the Chopra Committee, the government of India reached the following conclusion:

> Integration of different systems of medicine on the lines contemplated by the Chopra Committee is impracticable, as the theories and principles of modern medicine are very different from the theories and principles enunciated by Ayurveda and Unani. The evolution of an integrated system will be possible only after the methods of modern scientific research have been applied to the principles and practice of Ayurveda and Unani and it has been ascertained what is of proven merit and value in these systems.[29]

Interestingly, the postcolonial government of India was more interested in continuing modern scientific medicine (or the so-called Western medicine) to serve as the basis for the development of national health services in the country.[30] This very fact fundamentally blurs the prevailing notions of colonial and postcolonial differences and forces us to rethink the existing historical categories in this regard. As argued earlier, the nationalist articulation of anti-colonial sentiments in the field of medicine could not mitigate the pragmatic contingencies of the newly independent nation. The postcolonial Indian nation-state, likewise its predecessor, required the services of Western medicine to rule over the 'body' of its citizens. In fact, for the state, choice of healing system was not solely dependent on 'individual healthcare'; rather the very functioning of modern state system required an efficient device of 'social medicine'. 'Indigenous' systems of healing in their contemporaneous forms could hardly fit into this statist frame.

In tandem with the aforesaid pragmatic necessity of modern state, the Chopra Committee recommended necessary training of six months in public health and other essential subjects to the registered practitioners of 'indigenous' medicine. It comprised of training in topics ranging from first aid to minor surgery to basic obstetrics to elementary bacteriology and preventive medicine.[31] In due course of time, this evolved into Ayurvedic leaning towards *Swasthavratta* which included several topics of biopolitical concerns.[32] It was an effort to make 'indigenous' healing systems fit enough to carry the responsibility of maintaining large-scale public health eschewing their individual-centric perspective.

Yet another important recommendation of the Chopra Committee was related to the curricula of 'indigenous' systems of medicine. The Committee argued that a board of experts should be set up for editing and publishing 'old classics' and the 'right kind' of text-books of the integrated type.[33] This recommendation clearly reflects the long-standing demand of the All India Vaidya Sammelan regarding uniform curricula and training of vaids.[34] At the same time, it also hints towards an attempt to create an 'authentic' text and discourse thereby purging regional variations that had been exhibited by the Ayurvedic treatises across the subcontinent.

Nevertheless, more than the recommendations it is the introductory remarks of the Chopra Committee Report regarding Ayurveda which catch attention for the purpose of the present study. The *Report*, while it deemed Ayurveda as being 'native to the soil' in strict sense of the term (thereby spontaneously denuding Unani of any such status), considered Siddha as part of Ayurveda only. Thus, in the eyes of the Chopra Committee, Ayurveda appeared as the true claimant of an overarching Indian healing system. Further, deliberating on its origin, the Committee emphatically argued that 'its beginning, as of any other thing which deals with man, lie deep in unrecorded history; but the traditional date is around 3000 years ago'. Moreover, it divided the history of Ayurveda into four distinct periods: (i) the Vedic period; (ii) the period of original research and classical authors; (iii) the period of compilation and also of *tantra*s and Siddhas (chemist physicians); and (iv) the period of stagnation and recompilation (coterminous with the medieval and colonial periods, respectively).[35]

All these notions regarding origin and evolution of Ayurveda were in perfect symmetry with the late colonial Ayurvedic discourse which exhibited similar perceptions. In other words, the proponents of Ayurveda successfully managed to ensure their predominance over other 'indigenous' healing systems in independent India, at least in the official discourse. This dominance appeared more blatantly in the provincial health planning and administration of the United Provinces wherein the word 'Ayurveda' came to be used as a generic term for all 'indigenous'/Indian systems of healing, including Unani. In fact, the very naming of the post 'deputy director (Ayurveda), medical and health services'—an official responsible for development of 'indigenous' systems of healing throughout the province—hints at the extent to which Unani was sidelined as a system having marginal importance and Ayurveda being the 'real representative' of 'indigenous'/Indian systems of medicine in the official discourse of the post-independence United Provinces.

REORGANISING AYURVEDA AND UNANI IN THE UNITED PROVINCES

The aforesaid reports and recommendations by the two committees headed by Joseph William Bhore and Ram Nath Chopra respectively were mostly suggestive in nature. Public health and sanitation being a state subject, the provinces had the final authority over the fate of 'indigenous' healing systems. In this regard, the report which showed glimpses of the future role of 'indigenous' healing systems in the health administration of the

United Provinces was the *Report and Recommendations of the United Provinces Ayurvedic and Unani Systems Reorganisation Committee*, 1949. However, before examining its major recommendations and subsequent stand of the state government, let us first examine the contentious issue of extension of registration for the practitioners of 'indigenous' medicine—a demand that appeared immediately after independence. This issue is particularly significant largely because it opened up a Pandora's box of designating 'qualified' and 'unqualified' practitioners (or, to be more precise, 'vaids/hakims' on the one hand and 'quacks' on the other) in the field of 'indigenous' medicine. This, in turn, brought forth extant social predilections vis-à-vis various aspects of folk healing and associated subaltern healers.

The recent scholarship on subaltern therapeutics has pointed out that Ayurveda and Unani—in their more erudite, textually grounded forms— have been, and still are, largely inaccessible for the mass of the people.[36] This created space for thriving of a number of subaltern healers in the countryside imparting folk medicine mixing popular Ayurvedic/Unani remedies with those of naturopathy and Western medicine eclectically. It made the terrain of South Asian 'indigenous' medical culture intriguingly complex. In Chapter 3 of the present study we have already looked at the conscious efforts on the part of the All India Vaidya Sammelan to purge these subaltern healers from within its fold, condemning their 'pretentious' medical wisdom. It matched perfectly with the colonial stigmatisation of these folk healers active in the rural hinterland as 'quacks'. Thus, during the colonial period, subaltern therapeutics that was eclectic and unsystematised faced the brunt of both the hegemonic colonial medical notions as well as the revived and regenerated Ayurvedic system of healing.

However, the independence of India from colonial yoke generated a lot of enthusiasm and hopes among different sections of the practitioners of 'indigenous' medicine, including subaltern healers. In this regard, many members of the Board of Indian Medicine[37] of the United Provinces believed that independence would lead to freedom from the hegemony of Western medicine and Ayurveda would be the primary healing system of independent India. Related to this belief, a considerable number of the Board members were also in favour of the extension of the authority of the Board and bringing many more 'indigenous' practitioners within the purview of the Board. They were, in fact, arguing emphatically to bring many folk healers claiming Ayurvedic/Unani authority, such as *Kohals*,[38] *Jarrahs*[39] and dais[40], within the category of 'registered' practitioners through the extension of registration to them.[41]

The Board members believed that registering these folk healers as 'Ayurvedic practitioners', although of lower ranks,[42] would enable the Board to exercise some control over their practice which, in turn, would be in the broader interest of the public health. It was pointed out that non-registration of these 'Ayurvedic practitioners' who had been practising only on sectional lines like eye, ear, nose, throat, bones, dentistry and child birth would ultimately kill all Ayurvedic knowledge and practice of ancient surgery in howsoever crude form it existed. In contrast, registration would raise the standard of these medical practitioners and would tone their skills.[43]

The aforesaid intention of the Board members was reciprocated with equal enthusiasm by the folk healers. For instance, Anjuman-i-Jarrahan, the association of the Jarrahs located at Muzaffarnagar, had been sending continuous petitions since 1941 to bring the Jarrahs within the fold of registration. Consequently, in a meeting held in December 1947, the Board of Indian Medicine made an arrangement for the registration even of dais, Kohals, Jarrahs, etc., on an experimental basis, at a relatively lower registration fee,[44] despite the fact that there was no such provision of registration of these folk healers in the United Provinces Indian Medicine Act, 1939.

However, as soon as the government came to know about the aforesaid arrangements of registration of the folk healers by the Board of Indian Medicine, it created a lot of furore. In a letter dated 1 January 1950, the secretary, Medical 'B' Department, United Provinces, asked for a full report from the chairman, Board of Indian Medicine, regarding such arrangements and the logical basis of it, and meanwhile suspended any further registration of the folk healers until further orders. The matter was subsequently raised in the legislative council in the meeting held on 12 October 1950. Subsequent to this, the government directed the Board of Indian Medicine to stop any such registration of the folk healers immediately.[45]

Nonetheless, the Board and the associations of Kohals and Jarrahs (such as Kohal Netra Vaidya Sabha, Kanpur, and Anjuman-i-Jarrahan,

Muzaffarnagar) kept pushing for the registration of folk healers and revoke the government's decision on this matter. Numerous petitions, memorandums and letters were sent. Consequently, the entire matter was once again referred to the deputy director (Ayurveda), medical and health services [DDMHS(A)] by the government. Incidentally, D. A. Kulkarni, deputy director (Ayurveda), came vehemently against any such arrangement of registering the folk healers like Kohals and Jarrahs. He believed that it would be like legalising 'quackery'. He called a meeting with the delegates of Kohal Netra Vaidya Sabha, Kanpur, on 4 May 1953 in his office and was alarmed by the responses of the delegates. Kulkarni, on the basis of this brief interaction, pointed out the following facts to the government:[46]

- There was no college or institution which used to give any theoretical or practical training in this art of eye treatment.[47]
- The Kohals hardly had any knowledge of 'modern' anatomy, physiology and pathology of eye disease.[48]
- The Kohals lacked the 'exact' and 'standard' knowledge of Ayurvedic and Unani Tibb and had no 'scientific' knowledge of any of these systems.[49]
- The Kohals mostly learn their art through apprenticeship and received no standardised training to become an expert.[50]

In the light of the above facts, in his letter to the secretary, Medical 'B' Department, United Provinces (dated 9 May 1953) Kulkarni categorically stated that 'these *Kohals* and *Netra Vaidya*s could not be considered as Ayurvedic practitioners and should not be registered as vaids and hakims by the Board of Indian Medicine, U.P.'. Subsequently, this assessment of Kulkarni was accepted by the government, restricting the entry of these folk healers in the state-recognised system of Ayurveda.[51] Thus, the movement that had begun in the 'colonial' era in the late nineteenth and early twentieth century to purge Ayurveda of its low-caste folk healing influences reached its logical culmination in 'independent' India, receiving an official seal.

At the same time, it marked the victory of 'one Ayurveda' over 'many ayurvedas'.[52] The Orientalist/nationalist construct of Ayurveda eventually superseded, at least in the official discourse, many subaltern healing traditions that were handed down to it historically over generations. However, it should not be seen as the end of the story for the subaltern healers. As Helen Lambert argues, despite modernity's narrative of progress and routine construal of folk medicine as a dying and rapidly disappearing practice, the empirical evidence suggests its continued presence.[53] These folk healers, in due course of time, resorted to various strategies through which they sought to maintain integrity of their practice in rapidly changing times, thereby surviving on their own terms.[54] In fact, the very flexibility and non-canonical nature of subaltern therapeutics, which deems it misfit to be recognised by the state, allows it to thrive outside the statist health infrastructure traceable across diverse subaltern and even elite domains.[55]

Coming back to the *Report and Recommendations of the United Provinces Ayurvedic and Unani Systems Reorganisation Committee,* 1949, as argued earlier, it was this report and subsequent reaction of the government over its various provisions/propositions which provided a glimpse into the future place of 'indigenous' healing systems, including Ayurveda, in the health administration of the province. To begin with, one of the key recommendations of the Reorganisation Committee was to train the practitioners of 'indigenous' systems of healing in public health and social medicine. In fact, both the Reorganisation Committee and the government believed that:

> [S]ocial medicine, public health and environmental hygiene should receive greater recognition than curative medicine, both by the public and the Medical Colleges. The success of a physician should be judged by the improvement in the general health level of the people and lowering of incidence of diseases in the area in which he serves. More stress should, therefore, be given in the syllabus of studies for medical course specially that of the Indian systems of medicine on the study of the subject of social medicine, public health and environmental hygiene with special emphasis on conduct in daily life – *Dina Charya, Ratri Charya, Ritu Charya, Aahar* and *Vihar,* so that the new physicians turned out by Ayurvedic Colleges may be able to guide the people in their respective areas in reforming their habits on healthy lines and improving sanitation of their locality.[56]

Thus, the attempt was to make Ayurveda and Unani systems more 'pragmatic', both from the viewpoint of health of an individual as well as biopolitics. In this regard, the revised syllabus, as recommended by the Reorganisation Committee, clearly shows its emphases on the preparation of 'general practitioner' of Ayurveda with less stress on specialisation at the graduate level; 'practical training' of vaids and hakims; inclusion of 'useful modern methods and ideas' of Allopathic treatment in the curriculum designed for vaids and hakims; and eventually the training of vaids and hakims in preventive and social medicine and environmental hygiene.[57]

Here the Committee criticised the school of thought which advocated that there should be no mixing of Ayurveda/Unani with modern science or medicine and only '*shuddh*' (pure) Ayurveda and Tibb, as contained in the classical Sanskrit/Arabic/Persian texts, should be taught. Contrastingly, the Committee believed that 'Ayurveda if confined only to the few ancient texts which have come down to us in a thrice redacted form and if divorced from the advances made in modern times in the domain of medical and other sciences, will never be able to attain the position of the *Great National System of Medicine*. Also, the products of the so-called *Shuddh* Ayurvedic course will not be efficient and competent medical practitioners capable of replacing with success the Allopathic practitioners turned out by the modern Allopathic Colleges will never be produced.'[58] That is why the Committee included things like modern physics, chemistry, biology, bacteriology, parasitology and physiology along with the study of classical texts in the proposed curricula for the Ayurvedic/Unani course.

At the same time, the Reorganisation Committee also agreed with the Bhore and Chopra committees' recommendation that the teaching of preventive and social medicine should permeate the whole course, for the aim of future medical practitioners should be primarily to root out causes that lead to disease (that is, preventive) and only secondarily to cure disease (that is, curative). Reflection of this can be found in the inclusion of a paper on Swasthavratta in the proposed curriculum which broadly dealt with public health and hygiene. It clearly shows the attempt to make Ayurveda as influential a tool of biopolitics as modern medicine was in the hands of the state. Perfectly in tune with this larger objective, the detailed syllabus of the paper on Swasthavratta[59] included topics like designing and building of dwelling places, collection and handling of vital statistics of birth and death, study of the impact of climate and profession on personal health, preservation of health during fairs and festivals, epidemiology and prevention of common communicable diseases, water supply, waste management and rural healthcare. All these were vital aspects associated with biopolitics. The attempt was to train the Ayurvedic practitioners to handle public health and body in such a manner that it allows the smooth functioning of the economy and maintenance of law and order by ensuring a healthy 'subject'.

The government was also keenly interested in the aforesaid biopolitical aspect of the training of Ayurvedic and Unani students. That is why, in March 1951, when D. A. Kulkarni recommended that the district medical officer of health or any other local officer of the public health department should be attached to every affiliated college of the Board of Indian Medicine as a part-time professor in public health and social medicine for imparting adequate training of right standard in the modern aspect of this subject, the government readily approved it. Subsequently, on 4 May 1953, the governor approved, on an experimental basis, the utilisation of the services of district/municipal medical officer of health for giving a maximum number of 20 lectures and 10 practical demonstrations to the students of the four Ayurvedic and Unani colleges[60] on the modern aspect of social medicine and public health.[61] In fact, the syllabus designed for these lectures by the public health officers further expanded and streamlined the erstwhile syllabus on Swasthavratta and included several other topics of biopolitical concerns more clearly and categorically (for the detailed syllabus of these lectures, see Appendix 6).

Thus, the above discussion substantially reveals the attempts for the absorption of Ayurveda/Unani in the biopolitics of the post-independence United Provinces (now, Uttar Pradesh). For this purpose, many a time, even the fundamental concepts and focus of these systems were compromised and even altered to fit in the larger system of state-run health administration. For instance, while the Ayurvedic philosophy, as delineated in classical texts, believed not so much in immediate relief of a particular disease and rather focused on improving bodily resistance through long-term measures, it was now supposed to bring immediate relief, thereby bringing the situation under control as soon as possible. This was largely because prolonged illness on a broader scale could threaten the law and order. Similarly, while Ayurvedic philosophy believed in personalised and specific remedy for every individual based on rigorous observation of habits and lifestyle of the individual, the biopolitical concerns forced it to consider 'public on the whole' as its basic unit for future research and prescription. These were the tendencies that had already appeared within the Ayurvedic movement itself towards the end of the colonial rule to fit in the 'future' health administration of an independent nation. However, it came in a much more visible form in the post-independence period.

The new-found interest and stress on Swasthavratta and the readiness to learn the skill of managing public health and preventive medicine was the clear-cut manifestation of both the aspiration as well as desperation of the Ayurvedic practitioners to be absorbed in the state system of health administration. However, their path was not so easy. One of the recommendations of the Reorganisation Committee was that the Ayurvedists trained in public health measures of environmental hygiene should be given charge of, say, 20 municipalities out of the present number of 86 and 10 districts out of 49 districts for the purpose of health relief to start with, so that they might be able to demonstrate practically the usefulness of the Ayurvedic teachings on Swasthavratta.[62] When this recommendation reached the health ministry of the province for consideration, S. P. Pande (secretary, ministry of health, United Provinces) sought the opinions of the deputy director (Ayurveda) and director of medical health and services (DMHS). Now, the difference of opinions could be seen between deputy director (Ayurveda) and DMHS over this issue. While D. A. Kulkarni, deputy director (Ayurveda), favoured the idea and proposed that the entire public health work at least of one district and of one municipality should be placed under the charge of suitable qualified Ayurvedists on an experimental basis,[63] A. P. Bajpayee, DMHS, considered it an unnecessary experiment playing with human life. Bajpayee, in fact, raised serious doubts over the potential of Ayurvedic practitioners in handling matters of public health. He stated:

> I do not understand as to what is meant by 'Ayurvedist trained in public health measures of environmental hygiene,' as this training is largely dependent on an overall modern scientific conception of bacteriology, biochemistry and hygiene, which was not at all developed when the practice of Ayurveda was in vogue. Smattering of a few principles of public health without any proper background does not make for public health training. I cannot, therefore, see how men not trained in theory and practice of the latest scientific medicine

can be put in charge of health measures covering areas of 20 municipalities and 10 districts consisting of millions of people, and how the State can accept the responsibility of entrusting the lives of so many people to the charge of imperfectly trained workers.[64]

In the wake of this conflict of opinions between deputy director (Ayurveda) and DMHS, S. P. Pande resorted to a careful policy and advised the health minister to wait for the decision of the Government of India on the recommendations of the Chopra Committee over the future of Ayurveda.[65]

Another occasion when the attempts of the Ayurvedic practitioners to make an inroad into the existing health infrastructure of the province got frustrated came around the same time. One crucial recommendation of the Reorganisation Committee was that 'separate wards in each district hospital should be allotted for treatment on the lines of Indian system, and that these wards should be put in the charge of competent physicians of the Indian systems who should be controlled directly by the Deputy Director (Ayurveda) and not by the Civil Surgeon except in matters of local administration'. The Committee also proposed that 'an Ayurvedic section in the out-door department of these hospitals should also be started immediately'.[66] Once again S. P. Pande (secretary, ministry of health, United Provinces) directed D. A. Kulkarni [deputy director (Ayurveda)] to discuss this recommendation with A. P. Bajpayee (DMHS, United Provinces) and put up, if possible, an agreed plan for improving the health conditions in the rural areas of the province on 'Ayurvedic' lines.[67] At the same time, Pande also advised that while doing so, it should be kept in mind that the province was passing through an acute financial crisis and whatever scheme was submitted to the government had to be workable on practical lines.[68]

Replying to this, D. A. Kulkarni wholeheartedly supported the scheme with a little change. He expected the vaids and hakims who were to be in-charge of the proposed separate wards to work under the administrative control of the civil surgeons only and not under the direct control of the deputy director (Ayurveda).[69] Detailed discussions took place between D. A. Kulkarni, officials of the DMHS and also director of punchayati raj, United Provinces, over this scheme. While at this time deputy director (Ayurveda) and DMHS showed some agreement in support of the aforesaid scheme, most of the recommendations were rejected by the ministry itself, on 11 December 1951, owing to the financial crunch and to avoid 'confusion in the minds of patients' which was supposed to be generated by creation of separate wards.[70] Frustrated with this, Kulkarni made another desperate attempt to clear the doubts of the secretary to the government, medical department, United Provinces, in his letter addressed to him on 25 January 1952. However, the secretary in his response to it paid no heed to his plea and stuck with his earlier orders.[71]

Several other recommendations of the Reorganisation Committee were either thoroughly rejected or postponed by the government stating that 'time is not yet ripe'.[72] Thus, Ayurveda's journey to make inroads into the biopolitics of the province was full of obstacles. Officials in general were not very interested in assigning this role to Ayurveda despite the recommendations and attempts of the Ayurvedic and Unani Systems Reorganisation Committee and its appraisal by the deputy director (Ayurveda). Western medicine continued to be the basic tool for bioploitical concerns of the state and hence the government seemed to be least interested in promoting 'indigenous' systems of medicine on the ground. Official discourse of promotion and development of 'indigenous' systems of medicine, as was/is the case with many other official discourses, remained only on paper.

An interesting digression here would be to discuss a unique recommendation of the Reorganisation Committee and subsequent reaction of the government over this recommendation. The Reorganisation Committee made a suggestion to establish a 'Leper Asylum' in the province, imparting treatment exclusively on the lines of Indian systems of medicine. While making this recommendation, the Committee argued that 'it is our firm conviction that the Indian systems of medicine contain several very good and effective medicines for the treatment of leprosy and other skin diseases...In the course of the medical census of Benares and Meerut towns we came across a number of vaids and hakims *who claim to have successfully cured* a number of leprosy cases'.[73] In this regard, S. P. Pande (secretary, ministry of health, United Provinces) recommended a proposal to the health minister on 3 June 1949 to immediately provincialise the Aman Sabha Leper Asylum of Bahraich district owing to financial problems faced by this asylum and turn it into the Leper Asylum to be run on purely

'Ayurvedic' lines as envisaged by the Reorganisation Committee. According to Pande, such a step seemed 'extremely desirable' keeping in mind 'the declared policy of the government to place Ayurveda on a sound footing'.[74]

Interestingly enough, unlike the several other cases mentioned above where the prior opinions of both the deputy director (Ayurveda) and the DMHS were sought, Pande did not refer this matter for consideration of the deputy director (Ayurveda) before sending his aforesaid proposal to the health minister. It was only when the consented proposal reached the deputy director (Ayurveda) to chalk out the plans for establishing such a 'Leper Asylum' running exclusively on Ayurvedic lines that it was revealed by the deputy director (Ayurveda) that there was no vaid or hakim in the department who could run such an asylum efficiently. Consequently, the plan to establish an Ayurvedic Leper Asylum had to be abandoned midway for the time being.[75]

This classic instance of exemplary carelessness and haste of the medical secretary S. P. Pande to realise 'the declared policy of the government' shows the attitude of the state and its officials towards the leprosy-affected and other marginal groups (such as the 'insane') requiring serious medical attention. In fact, these groups were hardly a matter of serious concern for the government and could be subjected to experimental schemes without any substantial discussion and deliberation. The concerns related to 'proper scientific knowledge', 'authenticity of claims', 'precious human life', etc., hardly appeared in their case. This attitude was in some way inherited by the postcolonial government from its colonial predecessor[76] which made the poor and people at the margins as 'guinea pigs', making another case for seriously reconsidering these binaries of 'colonial' and 'postcolonial' in the field of health administration.

Coming back to the anomaly between 'the declared policy' of the government to put Ayurveda on a sound footing and the ground reality, in 1950–51, D. A. Kulkarni proposed to establish 100 additional state Ayurvedic and Unani dispensaries to promote 'indigenous' systems of healing. He argued that at present there were 372 state Ayurvedic and Unani dispensaries in the rural areas of the province and 70 more were being established during the current year (that is, 1949–50), raising the total number of such dispensaries to 442. Kulkarni believed that since these dispensaries continued to do good work at comparatively less expense and were popular with the rural public, there was need to open such 100 additional dispensaries in the ensuing year.[77]

Now, while the provincial government accepted the need for the establishment of more such dispensaries as 'an established fact', in view of financial stringency and doubt in the receipt of subsidy for such dispensaries from the Government of India, it was proposed to establish only 50 such dispensaries during the year 1950–51. Not only this, as the prospect of absence of subsidy for such dispensaries from the Centre in future years became more evident, a sudden question that floated amongst the official circle of the province was how feasible it was to establish such new dispensaries in the years to come. Of course, it was not possible to abolish already established dispensaries, but the top officials grew more and more reluctant about opening new dispensaries which had been there since 1947–48.[78] Thus, gradually, both the Centre and the state government were becoming unenthusiastic to establish such government-funded Ayurvedic and Unani dispensaries and their commitment to the cause of promoting 'indigenous' systems of healing remained confined only to paper and some ritualistic deliberations.

At a different terrain, the communalisation of healing systems, which had already begun in the first half of the twentieth century, reached new heights in post-independence era. We have already discussed how communal ideas gripped the Ayurvedic movement primarily under the aegis of the All India Vaidya Sammelan, subsequent to which communities came to be identified as preferring a particular healing system.[79] Further, it has also been delineated (particularly in Chapter 1) how this entire phenomenon of communalisation of healing systems was in sharp contrast with the efforts of someone like Ajmal Khan who contemplated 'indigenous' healing practices as representatives of pluralistic culture of India. Incidentally, at the height of communal hatred and mistrust in the 1940s, Ahmed Husain, a hakim from Madras, in his letter to Muhammad Ali Jinnah lamented that 'Hakim Ajmal Khan Sahib in the prime of his effort of reviving Unani medicine *lost himself by turning a nationalist in good faith of the Gandhian type* and shunned the progress of Unani'.[80] Husain further argued that while Ayurveda found a place in the 'national life of the Hindus', Unani failed to progress due to neglect of the Muslims. Hence, he urged Jinnah to include revival and encouragement of the Unani medicine in the reconstruction programme of the Muslim League.[81]

Not only Ayurveda and Unani came to be identified with separate communal identities, but in fact, there is evidence which illustrates that the institutions devoted to the learning of these systems often became potential breeding ground for communal forces. In this regard, a confidential report of S. C. Kapoor shows that the Rishikul Ayurvedic College, Haridwar, turned into an important site of the activities of the Rashtriya Swayamsevak Sangh (RSS) in the 1940s. In fact, the RSS used this College to mobilise youths towards its ideology and cause. The confidential report of S. C. Kapoor reveals that many of the staff and students of this College were active members of the RSS. It facilitated the organisation of a big rally of RSS by Basant Rao (provincial organiser of the RSS) on 19 January 1948 in Haridwar, in which the Ayurvedic college became the main rendezvous of the RSS workers. In this rally and other meetings, a Hindi booklet entitled *Hindustan va Pakistan me Youdh Hoga* ('War is Inevitable between Hindustan and Pakistan') written by Swami Vishuddhananda Saraswati was circulated widely. Consequently, on 5 February 1948, the police arrested some of the students and staff of the College for their prominent part in the RSS activities for spreading communal hatred.[82]

However, following the ban on the RSS after the assassination of Mahatma Gandhi, the College authorities made an attempt to dissociate themselves and the institution from the RSS and its activities. In fact, even a ban was imposed on its students from participating in RSS-run gymnasiums. Subsequently, the College authorities in their various statements attempted to prove their participation in nationalist activities and their disassociation with the RSS.[83]

CONCLUDING REMARKS

Thus, on the whole, the disappearance of the colonial context did not make the quest of Ayurveda to enter the state-sponsored public health system easier. Rather it became more complex and frustrating at times. It shows how continuously changing political and social contexts were the key factors in shaping the fate of Ayurveda in India. It was in a peculiar socio-political context that the Ayurvedic revivalist movement had emerged and gained momentum in late colonial times, challenging the hegemony of Western medicine. In other words, the Ayurvedic challenge to the hegemony of Western medicine was more political and social than medical. Hence, the change of context (that is, political independence from foreign rule) severely affected the future of Ayurvedic revivalist movement.

As the aforesaid examples show, the attitude of the postcolonial government officials, planners and decision-making authroities, particularly those of the United Provinces, was unexpectedly not better than their colonial counterparts when it came to promote Ayurveda and other 'indigenous' systems of medicine. Once independence was achieved, Western medicine appeared to them as a more 'pragmatic' and 'scientific' healing system, both from the perspective of an individual and the state, as compared to 'indigenous' medicine. In fact, a controversy which came up in 1950 over the use of the terms 'medical officer' and 'doctor' for vaids and hakims in-charge of the state Ayurvedic and Unani dispensaries clearly shows the continuation of colonial attitude towards 'indigenous' systems of healing and associated practitioners. In 1950, a petition was given by Shri Prakash Pandey, in-charge of the state indigenous dispensary, Lucknow, urging the health minister to allow the use of the term 'medical officer' for the in-charge of state indigenous dispensaries 'as they do the equal work as the in-charge of government hospitals imparting Allopathic treatment'.[84] According to him, not allowing the vaids and hakims to use this term maintains the colonial difference of status among the practitioners of 'indigenous' and Western medicine.

However, the provincial government felt that there was no reason vaids and hakims should be so keen for these titles and failed to see the status associated with these terms. Both the medical secretary and the deputy director (Ayurveda) believed that the practitioners of 'indigenous' system should be proud in using the terms like *kaviraj*/vaid/hakim only and should have a separate identity of their own. Use of terms like 'medical officer' and 'doctors' by the practitioners of 'indigenous' medicine, it was pointed out, would increase confusion and was unnecessary.[85] Here the government failed to take cognizance of the fact that the term 'medical officer' (very much like the term 'civil surgeon' of colonial times) was primarily a term of status than a mere title belonging to a practitioner trained in a particular system. Nonetheless, this petition and subsequent response of the government exhibit the discrimination that the practitioners of 'indigenous' healing systems continued to face in independent India.

NOTES

1. Ashis Nandy, 'A Post-colonial View of the East and the West,' *Alternatives: Global, Local, Political* 8, no. 1, January 1982, 25.
2. Foucault, *The Birth of the Clinic*, 38–39.
3. In fact, ironically enough, as argued by Indudharan Menon, in post-independence India, Western medicine made its dominant presence felt even more blatantly than it did during the colonial period, which eventually forced the standardised version of Ayurveda to become more and more compliant with biomedicinal principles. See Indudharan Menon, *Hereditary Physicians of Kerala: Traditional Medicine and Ayurveda in Modern India* (Oxon and New York: Routledge, 2019).
4. In the context of the present work, I am using the term 'biopolitics' in Foucauldian sense which denotes the use of medical knowledge and health infrastructure as a 'control apparatus' used by the state to exercise its authority over the subject population. For details on Foucauldian notion of 'biopolitics', see Michel Foucault, *Society Must be Defended: Lectures at the College de France, 1975–76* (New York: Picador, 2003), 239–64; and Michel Foucault, *The Birth of Biopolitics: Lectures at the College de France, 1978–79* (New York: Picador, 2010).
5. Berger, *Ayurveda Made Modern*, 157.
6. It was the cumulative result of these attempts that at the moment of independence, as Sunil Amrith points out, the value of public health was well established in Indian political culture; however, it was a deeply contested value. See Sunil Amrith, 'Political Culture of Health in India: A Historical Perspective', *Economic & Political Weekly* 42, no. 2, 13–19 January, 2007, 117.
7. For details on the report of the Health sub-committee and its attitude towards 'indigenous' medicine, see Shubhneet Kaushik, 'Planning for a Healthy Nation: Report of the Health Sub-Committee of National Planning Committee', in *Redefining India*, ed. Rahul Kumar Mohanta (Delhi: Kumud Publications, 2019), 116–27.
8. Kaushik, 'Planning for a Healthy Nation', 117.
9. K. T. Shah, *National Health: Report of the Sub-Committee of National Planning Series* (Bombay: Vora & Co. Publishers Ltd., 1948), 45 (emphasis added).
10. Shah, *National Health*, 50.

11. Set up in 1943 by the Government of India under the chairmanship of Sir Joseph William Bhore, an Indian civil servant born in Nasik (Bombay Presidency), the aforesaid committee dealt extensively with the issue of primary health care in post-War India with its two-pronged strategy of a short-term measure and a long-term programme. The *Report* firmly entrenched health as an important component of state planning and politics. Accepted by the government of newly independent India in 1952, the proposals of the *Report*, although not implemented immediately, continued to have guiding influence over subsequent health surveys and planning in India.
12. Commenting on the merits and popularity of indigenous healing systems, the Bhore Committee Report in its short section on 'Indigenous Systems of Medicine' (Chapter XXIII) stated: 'We realise the hold that these systems exercise not merely over the illiterate masses but over considerable sections of the intelligentsia. We have also to recognise that treatment by practitioners of these systems is said to be cheap, and it is claimed that the empirical knowledge, that has been accumulated over centuries has resulted in a fund of experience of the properties and medicinal use of minerals, herbs and plants which is of some value.' Furthermore, acknowledging the patriotic value associated with these 'indigenous' healing systems, the *Report* argued that 'the undoubted part that these systems have played in the long distant past in influencing the development of medicine and surgery in other countries of the world has naturally engendered a feeling of patriotic pride in the place they will always occupy in any world history of the rise and development of medicine'. According to the *Report*, this feeling has not been without its effect on the value which is attached by some of the practice of these systems. See 'Chapter XXIII: Indigenous Systems of Medicine', in *Report of the Health Survey and Development Committee* (New Delhi: Government of India Press, 1946), 2: 455.
13. 'Chapter XXIII: Indigenous Systems of Medicine', 455. According to the authors of the *Report*, they were 'unfortunately not in a position to assess the real value of these ['indigenous'] systems of medical treatment as practiced today' due to the lack of time and opportunities at their disposal which was a pre-requisite to conduct any investigation into such matter.
14. For a detailed discussion on this shift, see the following discussion on the *Report and Recommendations of the United Provinces Ayurvedic and Unani Systems Reorganisation Committee*, 1949.
15. 'Chapter XXIII: Indigenous Systems of Medicine', 455.
16. Ibid.
17. This idea of doing away with categories like 'Western' and 'Eastern' systems of medicine was taken quite seriously by the subsequent *Report of the Committee*

on Indigenous Systems of Medicine, 1948 (popularly known as the Chopra Committee Report). It emphasised the universal applicability of useful medical knowledge regardless of systemic affiliations.
18. 'Chapter XXIII: Indigenous Systems of Medicine', 456.
19. Ibid.
20. As, for instance, the United Provinces Indian Medicine Act, 1939.
21. 'Chapter XXIV: Regulation of the Professions Responsible for Health Services to the Community', in *Report of the Health Survey and Development Committee*, 2: 461.
22. Born in Punjab in 1882, Ram Nath Chopra is particularly remembered for his path-breaking contributions in Indian pharmacology. Trained by Dr Walter E. Dixon, who was appointed as the first professor of pharmacology in the University of Cambridge, Ram Nath Chopra himself pioneered pharmacological teaching and research in India. In fact, following in the footsteps of his teacher (that is, Dr Dixon), Chopra was the first professor of pharmacology at the Calcutta School of Tropical Medicine which he joined in 1921, and later became its director. Chopra was particularly interested in 'indigenous' drugs and related medical systems, promotion of which became his long-term goal. His famous text *Indigenous Drugs of India* (1933) along with his engagement in ethnopharmacological activity, which resulted into several publications on the Indian materia medica, testifies the aforesaid commitment of Chopra. For further details on life and work of Ram Nath Chopra, see Harkishan Singh, 'Ram Nath Chopra (1882-1971) - A Visionary in Pharmaceutical Science', *Indian Journal of History of Science* 43, no. 2, 2008, 231–64.
23. Dagmar Wujastyk, 'The Evolution of Indian Government Policy on Ayurveda in the Twentieth Century', in Wujastyk and Smith, *Modern and Global Ayurveda*, 63. Interestingly, Wujastyk goes on to argue that non-inclusion of Ram Nath Chopra in the Bhore Committee despite his professional eminence in the early 1940s and prominent and substantial statements on health reform is tempting enough to conjecture that Chopra's interest in 'indigenous' medicine disqualified him in Bhore's eyes.
24. See 'Introduction', in *Report of the Committee on Indigenous Systems of Medicine, Vol. I: Recommendations* (New Delhi: Ministry of Health, Government of India, 1948), 1–8.
25. Differences along this line were basically between the practitioners of 'indigenous' systems of healing and Western medicine.
26. The most pertinent example of differences on this line was that between Ayurveda and Unani which had been linked with 'Hindu' and 'Muslim' identities respectively by this time.

27. 'Introduction', *Report of the Committee on Indigenous Systems*. Similar ideas were re-uttered by Ram Nath Chopra in his presidential address at the thirty-fifth Indian Science Congress held in January 1948 at Patna. For the complete lecture delivered by Ram Nath Chopra on this occasion, see Col. Sir Ram Nath Chopra, 'Rationalisation of Medicine in India: Presidential Address', *Everyman's Science* 43, no. 1, April–May 2008, 5–22.
28. 'Introduction', *Report of the Committee on Indigenous Systems*.
29. Cited in the *Report of Udupa K.N. Committee on Ayurveda Research Evaluation* (Delhi: The Times of India Press, 1958), 5.
30. *Report of Udupa K.N. Committee*, 5.
31. 'The Organisation of Rural Medical Relief', in *Report of the Committee on Indigenous Systems*, 114–26.
32. For a detailed discussion on *Swasthavratta*, see the next section on reorganisation of Ayurveda and Unani in the United Provinces.
33. 'Education and Medical Institutions', in *Report of the Committee on Indigenous Systems*, 95–113.
34. For a discussion on this theme, see Chapter 3 of the present work.
35. 'Introduction', *Report of the Committee on Indigenous Systems*.
36. David Hardiman and Projit Bihari Mukharji, eds, *Medical Marginality in South Asia: Situating Subaltern Therapeutics* (London and New York: Routledge, 2012), 1.
37. It was a statutory body entrusted with the task of keeping record of all the registered medical practitioners of 'indigenous' medicine in the province and time-to-time framing rules to ensure proper conduct and standard on the part of these practitioners in performance of their duties.
38. *Kohal* is the term used for folk eye-surgeons who supposedly derive their knowledge from Ayurveda. They mostly used to treat cataracts in the rural countryside. Etymologically, Kohal means '*kajal*', a common eye cosmetic used in most of north India.
39. *Jarrah* is the term used for the orthopaedists who supposedly derive their knowledge from the Unani system of healing. Active in the rural countryside, they are primarily the bone setters, adjusting joint dislocations, and physiotherapists. They mostly use non-surgical means to treat fractures, dislocation, sports injuries and set the bone without applying any plaster. They use the art of treating orthopaedic problems with bare hands and supplementing it with regular essential oil massages and specially prepared Unani medicinal pastes.
40. Dais are basically midwives. While there was a provision for registering those midwives having some sort of elementary training in modern childcare,

'indigenous' countryside dais were mostly outside the purview of registration. Even in case of registered trained midwives and assistant midwives, caste and class predilections continued to linger on their status. This became quite visible when an amendment was proposed, in 1943, in the constitution of the United Provinces Nurses and Midwives Council which used to carry the registration of midwives, assistant midwives and nurses, and kept supervision on their training and activities. The proposed amendment along with several other recommendations argued in favour of inclusion of one registered assistant midwife (to be elected by the registered assistant midwives) among the elected members of the United Provinces Nurses and Midwives Council. However, Dr D. P. Bali, deputy inspector general of civil hospitals (women), United Provinces, in a letter to the secretary, medical department, United Provinces (dated 30 November 1943) advocated that 'as no educational qualification is laid down for the assistant midwives before they take up midwifery training, majority of the assistant midwives are *illiterate*. The standard of their training in midwifery is very elementary and the duration of training is very short. In fact, *they are no better than ordinary indigenous Dais*. So to have a person of this *very low standard* with practically no education and without ability to understand the legislation and follow the proceedings of meetings, would be, in my opinion, *an insult* to a body like Nurses and Midwives Council where *an educated an enlightened member can be a very great asset*. The assistant midwives should, therefore, have no seat in the Council.' Subsequently, the Bill was further amended and provisioned for inclusion of two representatives from the registered midwives and assistant midwives to be elected jointly by them. Thus, the provision was diluted under the class attack launched against 'illiterate' assistant midwives. See 'Bill to Amend the U.P. Midwives and Assistant Midwives and Health Visitors Registration Act of 1934', F. No. 301, Box No. 1, 1943, Medical 'B' Department, UPSA (emphasis added).

41. See 'Registration of Kohals and Midwives by the Board of Indian Medicine, Lucknow', F. No. 1541, Box No. 58, 1949, Medical 'B' Department, UPSA.
42. It is interesting to note that the Board members were arguing in favour of extension of registration to the folk healers but with hierarchical gradations.
43. See the 'Letter from the Chairman, Board of Indian Medicine, Uttar Pradesh to the Secretary to Government, Medical 'B' Department, Uttar Pradesh', dated 17 January 1950 in 'Registration of Kohals and Midwives', UPSA.
44. Registration fee for dais was set at Rs 1 and for Kohals, Jarrahs, etc., at Rs 5. 'Registration of Kohals and Midwives', UPSA.
45. 'Registration of Kohals and Midwives', UPSA.
46. Ibid.

47. Incidentally, Kulkarni refused to pay any heed to the delegates who insisted that the government should take steps for establishing a college for reviving this art.
48. It was ironical that the upholders of 'ancient' knowledge were derogated on the basis of absence of 'modern' knowledge. It shows the hegemonic potential of 'modernity' itself wherein 'ancient' 'traditional' knowledge also had to conform to the modern standards. In fact, as argued by Biswamoy Pati and Mark Harrison in their recent work on society, medicine and politics in colonial India, while it seems paradoxical, 'tradition' was often put to the service of modernity, normalising and legitimising new values and formations. Revitalisation of 'traditional' systems of healing in India was nowhere an aberration to this phenomenon (Pati and Harrison, *Society, Medicine and Politics*, 8).
49. Kulkarni actually reached this conclusion when the delegates were asked about the number of eye diseases according to Ayurveda and Unani Tibb. The chairman of the Kohal Netra Vaidya Sabha replied that there were about 115 of them according to Ayurveda and 70 according to Tibb, although as Kulkarni pointed out, as a matter of fact the number of eye diseases, according to Ayurveda, was 77 only. Also, according to Kulkarni, none of the members could name even a few of the eye diseases on Ayurvedic lines. Neither could tell about any medicines used for eye diseases according to Ayurveda except the 'Ark of Triphala'. This, however, clearly shows that textual authority was prioritised and even hegemonised over practical aspects of healing by the deputy director (Ayurveda). 'Registration of Kohals and Midwives', UPSA.
50. In fact, the delegates stated that generally a training of one year under an expert was enough to enable a person to start his practice, which was actually more than the training of mere three months in eye diseases imparted by the Jhansi University which the Kohals doubted and considered insufficient. 'Registration of Kohals and Midwives', UPSA.
51. 'Registration of Kohals and Midwives', UPSA.
52. For a summary of this distinction between 'one Ayurveda' and 'many ayurvedas', see Banerjee, *Power, Knowledge, Medicine*, 21. According to Banerjee, despite the fact that Ayurveda is not an oral tradition as its fundamental principles are guided by some elementary texts, that is, *Charaka*, *Sushruta* and *Vagbhata* samhitas, it is not canonical like other textual traditions. It permitted generously many practices not mentioned in the elementary texts so long as the basic parameters of analysis remain the same. In other words, as per Banerjee, Ayurveda is based upon a textual tradition which is open-ended: closed at one end by its epistemology, but open at the

other to learning from empirical situations. Nevertheless, by mid-twentieth century, this open-endedness of Ayurvedic tradition was eventually sealed thereby making it 'one' 'homogenous' system.

53. Helen Lambert, 'Wrestling with Tradition: Towards a Subaltern Therapeutics of Bonesetting and Vessel Treatment in North India', in Hardiman and Mukharji, *Medical Marginality in South Asia*, 109–25.
54. For a recent intervention on these survival strategies of folk healers, see Gauri Raje, 'The Modernising Bhagat', in Hardiman and Mukharji, *Medical Marginality in South Asia*, 152–70.
55. Here it is worth noticing that worldwide the statutory support to 'modern' medicine pushed all other systems or practices of healing and their practitioners outside the purview of legality, thereby criminalising them at once. Nevertheless, outlawing or criminalisation of non-official healing practices fails to eliminate its practitioners completely. There always existed 'gray zones' of medicine displaying complex performative healing practices. For detail on such 'gray zones' of medicine, especially in the Latin American context, see Diego Armus and Pablo F. Gómez, eds, *The Gray Zones of Medicine: Healers and History in Latin America* (Pittsburgh: University of Pittsburgh Press, 2021).
56. 'Recommendations of the United Provinces Ayurvedic and Unani Systems Reorganisation Committee—Training in Public Health and Social Medicine', F. No. 19 RC, Box No. 31, 1949, Medical 'B' Department, UPSA.
57. 'Recommendations of the United Provinces Ayurvedic and Unani Systems Reorganisation Committee—Basic Qualifications, Curriculum and Pre-admission Test', F. No. 13 RC, Box No. 114, 1949, Medical 'B' Department, UPSA.
58. Ibid.; emphasis added.
59. It was designed and proposed by the Expert Committee headed by D. A. Kulkarni, deputy director (Ayurveda), in consultation with the Education Committee of the Board of Indian Medicine, Uttar Pradesh, on 11 July 1951.
60. These four colleges were Rishikul Ayurvedic College, Haridwar; Lalit Hari Ayurvedic College, Pilibhit; Bundelkhand Ayurvedic College, Jhansi; and Unani Medical College, Allahabad.
61. See 'Recommendations of the United Provinces Ayurvedic and Unani Systems Reorganisation Committee—Training in Public Health and Social Medicine', F. No. 19 RC, Box No. 31, 1949, Medical 'B' Department, UPSA.
62. 'Recommendations of the United Provinces Ayurvedic and Unani Systems Reorganisation Committee', F. No. 22 RC, Box No. 110, 1949, Medical 'B' Department, UPSA.

63. The district and municipality suggested by Kulkarni for this experimental purpose were the newly created district of Tehri-Garhwal and municipality of Rishikesh (see the letter of D. A. Kulkarni to S. P. Pande dated 19 December 1949 in Ibid.).
64. See the letter of A. P. Bajpayee to S. P. Pande dated 4 January 1950 in Ibid.
65. 'Recommendations of the United Provinces Ayurvedic and Unani Systems Reorganisation Committee', F. No. 22 RC, Box No. 110, 1949, Medical 'B' Department, UPSA.
66. 'Recommendations of the United Provinces Ayurvedic and Unani Systems Reorganisation Committee', F. No. 34 RC, Box No. 111, 1949, Medical 'B' Department, UPSA.
67. Here it is interesting to note the way 'Indian systems' (the term used in the aforesaid recommendation of the Committee) became synonymous with 'Ayurveda' in the official health discourse of the province by this time.
68. See the letter by S. P. Pande to D. A. Kulkarni dated 17 November 1949 in 'Recommendations of the United Provinces Ayurvedic and Unani Systems Reorganisation Committee', F. No. 34 RC, Box No. 111, 1949, Medical 'B' Department, UPSA.
69. See the letter by D. A. Kulkarni to S. P. Pande dated 1 June 1950 in Ibid.
70. See the letter by K. P. Srivastava (assistant secretary to the government, medical department, Uttar Pradesh) to D. A. Kulkarni dated 11 December 1951 in Ibid.
71. Ibid.
72. For example, the recommendation to bring the scale and pay of the Ayurvedic graduates in government service at par with the graduates in Western medicine; recommendation to give facilities and authority to vaids and hakims graduated from chartered university or possessing a diploma or degree granted by the Board of Indian Medicine to conduct minor surgical cases, etc., faced equal aversion on the part of the government. (See 'Recommendations of the United Provinces Ayurvedic and Unani Systems Reorganisation Committee', F. No. 35 RC, Box No. 114, 1949, Medical 'B' Department, UPSA.)
73. 'Recommendations of the United Provinces Ayurvedic and Unani Systems Reorganisation Committee', F. No. 9 RC, Box No. 114, 1949, Medical 'B' Department, UPSA (emphasis added).
74. Ibid.
75. Ibid.
76. The colonial public health policy, in fact, often poised to remove or control the movement of these marginalised sections of sufferers, that is, lepers and insanes into jails/asylums. Incidentally, this colonial desire to incarcerate

lepers and insanes received support of the upper-caste middle-class Indian elite as well. For this culpable nexus between upper-caste middle-class Indian elite and colonial rule in invisibilising lepers and insanes, see Biswamoy Pati and Chandi P. Nanda, 'The Leprosy Patient and Society: Colonial Orissa, 1870–1940s', in Pati and Harrison, *The Social History of Health and Medicine*, 113–28; and Biswamoy Pati, 'Confining 'Lunatics': The Cuttack Asylum, c. 1864–1906', in Pati and Harrison, *Society, Medicine and Politics*, 196–231.

77. 'Establishment of Additional 50 State Ayurvedic and Unani Dispensaries during 1950–51', F. No. 1437, Box No. 58, 1949, Medical 'B' Department, UPSA.

78. It was in sharp contrast with the enthusiasm that one can see during the phase of provincial Congress ministries in the late 1930s when the United Provinces government under the leadership of Govind Ballabh Pant decided to open several subsidised aushadhalayas and dawakhanas with whatever meager fund it had at its disposal (as delineated in Chapter 2 of the present work).

79. See Chapter 4 of the present work.

80. 'Letter from Ahmed Husain to Muhammad Ali Jinnah (dated August 28, 1944)', in *Quaid-e-Azam Mohammad Ali Jinnah Papers*, Volume 11 (Islamabad: National Archives of Pakistan, 2005), available at http://thepartitionofindia.blogspot.in/2012/07/unani-medicine.html (accessed on 16 July 2019).

81. Highlighting this complaining attitude of the Unani practitioners, particularly in post-independence era, Neshat Quaiser argues that a communally charged post-partition situation produced palpable medical communalism with its everyday manifestations. This postcolonial medical communalism went on to construct a 'complaining' Unani-Muslim subject for whom Ayurveda and the post-partition Indian state emerged as the immediate principal adversarial 'others' in place of Western medicine. For details on this subject, see Neshat Quaiser, 'Tension, Placation, Complaint: Unani and Post-Colonial Medical Communalism,' in *Medical Pluralism in Contemporary India*, eds V. Sujatha and Leena Abraham (Hyderabad: Orient BlackSwan, 2012), 130–62.

82. 'R.S.S. Activities at Rishikul Ayurvedic College, Haridwar', F. No. 1088, Box No. 03, 1948, Medical 'C' Department, UPSA. In fact, Govind Ballabh Pant was particularly alarmed by the news of disappearance of a large quantity of sulphur and other chemicals from the Rishikul Ayurvedic College as it could be used by the RSS in perpetrating widespread violence. However, the confidential report of S. C. Kapoor considered this news of disappearance of chemicals as mere rumour.

83. See the letter from sabhapati, Rishikul Ayurvedic College, to the deputy secretary, health department, United Provinces Government (dated 18 May 1948) in Ibid.

84. 'Use of the Terms—Medical Officer and Doctor for Vaids and Hakims In-charge of State Indigenous Dispensaries, U.P., F. No. 1388, Box No. 44, 1950, Medical 'B' Department, UPSA.
85. Ibid. It should be noted that almost a similar controversy had appeared in 1933. At that time, the Board of Indian Medicine (United Provinces) insisted on the use of term 'Licentiate' (likewise the practitioners of Western medicine) for vaids and hakims who had passed out of the institutions recognised by the Board and had received formal training on 'modern' lines to distinguish them from other (that is, hereditary/non–institutionally trained) vaids and hakims. The Board believed that such 'high-sounding' title of being 'Licentiate' was essential to raise the reputation of those vaids and hakims who had passed out of these institutions. To this proposal, the secretary, medical department, United Provinces, responded harshly by saying that use of such terms by 'indigenous' medical practitioners might bear confusion and mislead the public with the practitioners of Western medicine. Consequently, he suggested the use of old Sanskrit and Persian terms such as 'Ayurveda Visharad' and 'Tabib-i-Alim' for those passing out of Ayurvedic/Unani schools and 'Ayurveda Acharya' and 'Hakim-i-Fazil' for those passing out of Ayurveda/Unani colleges (see 'Board of Indian Medicine', F. No. 131, Box No. 59, 1933, Medical Department, UPSA). Compare the line of arguments given in this case with the one that took place in 1950.

Conclusion

Addressing the fourteenth annual general meeting of the Countess of Dufferin's Fund that took place in the Town Hall on 3 March 1899, the then Viceroy of India Lord Curzon talked about the three 'boons' which the British had brought to India as 'gifts' in their hands—religion, law and science.[1] According to Curzon, while some doubts might be 'legitimately' entertained about some of these 'gifts', no two opinions could be there about the benefits of Western science, particularly medicine. Curzon further went on to claim that

> [T]here may be *prejudices*, and there may be *scruples arising from long custom*, or from *ignorance*, or from other causes, but doubts there cannot possibly be; and I say this, if we had come back to you (the Indians) from the West with our medicine in our hand, and with that alone, we should have been justified in our return.[2]

In fact, invoking Rudyard Kipling, Curzon found in Western medicine an accomplishment in fulfilling the 'White man's burden'.[3] Curzon further declared that Western medicine was 'no mere collection of pragmatical or experimental rules', it was 'built on the rock-bed of pure, irrefutable science', and it was 'a boon which is offered to all, rich and poor, Hindu and Mohammedan, woman and man'.[4] Moreover, according to Curzon, Western medicine lifted the veil of purdah 'without irreverence' and it was so far the only dissolvent which broke down the barriers of caste 'without sacrilege'.[5]

None of the above claims made by Curzon actually stand firm in the wake of the recent works on the history of health and medicine in colonial India. While historians like David Arnold, Mark Harrison and many others have clearly brought out the imperialist motives of Western medicine in India, scholars like Biswamoy Pati, Charu Gupta, Kavita Sivaramakrishnan, Madhuri Sharma and Rachel Berger have seriously undermined the role of Western medicine in overcoming caste, class and gender-related boundaries. In fact, adoption of many of the modern medical tools and technologies such as stethoscopes and thermometers by Ayurvedic practitioners,[6] as shown by Madhuri Sharma, allowed to maintain the purdah norms as they could be used to access women's bodies and to make an accurate diagnosis without touching them physically.[7] Similarly, these tools and technologies allowed in many ways to maintain the caste and class norms as well.

Things were not very different in the case of 'indigenous' medicine as well. As the present work shows, the late colonial Ayurvedic discourse and movement were equally fraught with social and political content as well as intent. Nationalism and anti-colonial independence movement were key factors grooming and shaping the Ayurvedic discourse during the period under discussion. This overall political context was significant for the movement to revive Ayurveda as the champion of 'indigenous' medicine, often claiming the status of 'national healing system' of India. However, as it has been delineated, in its pursuit of creating a distinct 'indigenous' identity different from that of 'colonial' Western medicine, Ayurveda, in fact, imbibed many of the characteristic features of Western medicine itself such as institutionalisation, pharmaceuticalisation, standardisation and professionalisation. Such ambiguity perhaps is the distinctive trait of any revivalist movement. Nevertheless, what makes the Ayurvedic revivalist movement more interesting is that while Ayurvedic practitioners incorporated many of the traits of Western medicine, they almost failed to inculcate its most important feature—spirit of enquiry/experiment. In the absence of such spirit, the Ayurvedic practitioners remained focused on blind adoption of what may be called 'ancient received wisdom' in modern times. It was precisely this lack of spirit of enquiry which made even Mahatma Gandhi hesitant to fully endorse this 'swadeshi' healing system (that is, Ayurveda) in the field of medicine.[8] In fact, in many ways, Ayurvedic practitioners were trying to create their hegemony in the field of medicine without substance. They focused themselves on discourse, organisation, mobilisation, etc., to revive Ayurveda as 'indigenous' medicine, but very few of them actually worked in the direction of advancing new research in Ayurveda.

This was the reason why Ayurveda apparently ended on a losing side in independent India as the disappearance of the colonial context after 15 August 1947 stripped Ayurvedic revivalist movement of its most influential mobilising tool, that is, the all-pervasive anti-colonial struggle. This shift in political context and its impact on the Ayurvedic revivalist movement comes out explicitly if one reads Chapter 2 and Chapter 6 of the present book side-by-side. In fact, in many ways, the Ayurvedic practitioners till today blame the lack of state patronage as the most important reason behind the present condition of Ayurveda and other 'indigenous' healing systems instead of looking inwards and realising the hollowness of their efforts which has been aspiring for 'hegemony without substance'.[9]

The present work emphatically delineates the social dimension and content of the late colonial Ayurvedic discourse as well. Simultaneously, the economic context in which the Ayurvedic revivalist movement unfolded has been discussed with special emphasis on the Ayurvedic print and drug market. All this clearly establishes the connections between the emerging discourses on the Ayurveda, the 'nation' and various aspects of society (that is, caste, class, community and gender) in the late colonial period.

Incidentally, as illustrated in chapters 3 and 4, the social culture exhibited by the Ayurvedic discourse of the period under discussion was highly casteist, communal, and class- and gender-biased. There was constant attempt to blame the 'Others', that is, lower castes/classes, Muslims, women, etc., for spreading various diseases resulting into the degenerating health of the 'Hindu' male. Thus, the content and reference point of study for the Ayurvedic practitioners of the time was not simply a biological human body; rather it was quite often a 'Hindu' 'male' body. In other words, the Ayurvedic publicists were actively involved not just in the 'reconstruction of a tradition' but also in reconstructing the society and the 'nation' as a whole along specific lines.

Actually, like colonialism used the 'scientific' discourses to meet its own requirements, similarly the proponents of 'indigenous science' also used the 'scientific' discourses to recast the 'indigenous' society, tradition and culture and linked them with the historical process of making of a nation. Thus, the 'rational' and 'objective' scientific discourses, be they colonial or 'indigenous', were equally 'prejudiced' and 'subjective' in their content, and one needs to approach these 'scientific' discourses critically. Interestingly, the tendencies summarised above linger on till today. Ayurveda as a 'true' representative of 'indigenous' healing system of India holds the fascination of many contemporary political representatives, governments, social groups and non-governmental organisations (NGOs). Attempts are being made to push the history of Ayurveda as old as possible;[10] efforts are going on to establish the superior scientificity of this particular healing system without laboratory evidences;[11] and endeavours are being made to establish its 'hegemony without substance' by creating mere discourse. Simultaneously, the typical tendencies exhibited by the Ayurvedic drug market in colonial period such as extra emphasis on vitalisers, tonics, panacea, aphrodisiacs, negative publicity of allopathic drugs, adulteration and deceit in the name of 'time-tested' Ayurveda have reached new heights in contemporary times. Roadside make-shift stalls/tents claiming 'ancient' Ayurvedic authority; advertisements of medicines invoking the 'secrets' of Ayurveda to increase male potency and sexual vigour; and promotion of utterly non-Ayurvedic drugs in the name of Ayurveda have become quite a common sight in present times.

NOTES

1. *Speeches by Lord Curzon of Kedleston, Vol. I* (Calcutta: Office of the Superintendent of Government Printing, 1900), 54–60.
2. *Speeches by Lord Curzon*, 57 (emphasis added).
3. Curzon here quoted the famous poem of Rudyard Kipling where he wrote:

    'Take up the white man's burden,
    The savage wars of peace,
    Fill full the mouth of famine,
    And bid the sickness cease.'
    (*Speeches by Lord Curzon of Kedleston, Vol. I*, 57).

4. *Speeches by Lord Curzon*, 57.
5. Ibid.
6. It is worth noticing that the embrace of a range of mundane modern technologies in the late nineteenth and early twentieth century changed the entire outlook of the Ayurvedic practitioners towards body and

healing. For a recent intervention on this theme, see Mukharji, *Doctoring Traditions*. Deriving inspiration from David Arnold's fascinating work on the revolutionary potential of everyday technologies in shaping 'new ideas of time, space, of body, self, and other' (David Arnold, *Everyday Technology: Machines and the Making of India's Modernity* [Chicago and London: University of Chicago Press, 2013]), Mukharji delineates the therapeutic changes that the Ayurvedic healing system underwent owing to the introduction and assimilation of small technologies such as pocket watches, thermometers, stethoscopes, microscopes, injections and even glass phials. Moreover, as argued by Mukharji, adoption of these small technologies was not necessarily a product of hegemonic influences of Western medicine; rather these were conscious adoptions on the part of the Ayurvedic practitioners to improve their system which, in turn, became the catalysts for further change. In fact, as delineated by Mukharji, the Ayurvedic practitioners who were involved in deploying these modern technologies which, in turn, led to a fundamental shift in their approach towards the human body, nowhere saw them as 'alien' or 'new' to Ayurveda. Rather these small-scale technologies often acquired new genealogies or 'histories' in Ayurvedic discourse, thereby making them integral to Ayurveda from 'time immemorial'. For instance, Mukharji shows how the clinical uptake of a relatively new practice of diagnosing the pulse using pocket watches by Ayurvedic practitioners was sanctified by invoking the concept of *nadipariksha* as the iconic and exemplary instance of Kobiraji knowledge.

7. Here Madhuri Sharma gives an interesting reference of Dr Raghubir Sahaya Bhargav, doctor of homeopathic medicines, who, while explicating the usefulness of stethoscope, argued: 'Major benefit of the stethoscope...those women who wanted to get their chest examined hold the one end of the tool which should be kept on the patient and doctor *behind the curtain* can put both leads of the tool into his ear and can hear the rhythm' (see Sharma, *Indigenous and Western Medicine*, 51).

8. 'Speech at Opening of Tibbi College, Delhi, February 13, 1921', *CWMG*, 22: 342.

9. Tripathi, interview, 17 April 2014. During the interview, Vaid Guru Prasad Tripathi lamented the fact that the present Indian state has no interest in promoting Ayurveda which is the 'original' healing system of this land. Getting nostalgic, this nonagenarian Ayurvedic practitioner took the names of some of the politicians of his youth who were great admirers and supporters of Ayurveda such as Madan Mohan Malviya, Dr Sampoornanand, Raghunath Vinayak Dhulekar, Kanhaiya Lal Munshi, Govind Ballabh Pant, Purushottam

Das Tandon, Lal Bahadur Shastri and Morarji Desai. Interesting to note here is the absence of the name of Jawaharlal Nehru.

10. For instance, see the response of the AYUSH Department to the question, 'What is the origin of Ayurveda?' (cited in the 'Introduction' of the present work).

11. An interesting example of such efforts is the recent controversy over *putrajeevak beej*—an Ayurvedic product by Baba Ramdev's Divya Pharmacy that promises a male child. Similarly, Baba Ramdev also claims to treat HIV-AIDS and cancer through yoga and Ayurvedic products.

See *Financial Express*, 'Ramdev Baba Drug 'Putrajeevak Beej' Promises Male Child'. 1 May 2015, available at https://www.financialexpress.com/industry/controversy-hits-ramdev-drug-promising-birth-of-male-child-hits-modis-beti-bachao-campaign/68323/ (accessed on 22 July 2019); Randeep Ramesh, 'TV Swami Offers a Cure for All Ills', *The Guardian*, 14 June 2008, available at https://www.theguardian.com/world/2008/jun/14/india.television (accessed on 20 July 2023).

Appendices
Appendix 1

Rules Related to the Admission of Patients to the European Civil Hospital, Allahabad (June 1920)[1]

General

1. The European Civil Hospital is a government institution intended for:
   Class (I)—European and Anglo-Indian patients, who are poor and destitute, or have only limited means and are unable to afford adequate medical attendance and nursing at their own homes during a serious illness.
   Class (II)—European and Anglo-Indian servants of the government in all civil departments.
   Class (III)—Wives and families of European and Anglo-Indian civil officers.
   Class (IV)—All Europeans and Anglo-Indians not included in the above.
2. Indians cannot be admitted.

Appendix 2

Principal Features of Scheme for Establishing Subsidised Dispensaries of 'Indigenous' Medicine in the United Provinces, 1938[2]

1. Subsidised dispensaries (of 'indigenous' medicine) were to be set up and subsidised practitioners (vaids and hakims) settled under this scheme only in those areas where facilities for medical aid under the allopathic or the 'indigenous' systems (Ayurveda and Unani) were inadequate or non-existent.
2. Such dispensaries and/or private practitioners were to be controlled by statutory bodies like District Boards, Town Area and Notified Area Committees, suitable registered bodies like managing committee of charitable endowments and even by philanthropic individuals. The controlling authority was supposed to provide the necessary buildings for the location of the dispensary and for the residence (whether on payment or free of rent) of the vaid or the hakim. The buildings could either belong to or be rented by the controlling authority.
3. Aushadhalayas or Dawakhanas were to be established under this plan only in the larger villages where suitable buildings were available (such institutions were to be under the charge of only registered vaids and hakims). Where a full fledged dispensary was not needed or where other suitable building for the purpose was not available, a qualified vaid or hakim willing to settle down might be subsidised; the qualifications held being such as were recognised adequate by the United Provinces Board of Indian Medicine.
4. The cost of maintaining an Aushadhalaya or a Dawakhana was estimated at Rs 600 per annum, viz.:

Medicines — Rs 150
Vaid or hakim at Rs 25 per month — Rs 300
Compounder and general servant at Rs 10 per month for both — Rs 120
Miscellaneous — Rs 30

Total — Rs 600

5. It was proposed that for subsidised vaids and hakims, the rate of subsidy will be Rs. 360 per annum for a Class 'A' vaid/hakim and Rs. 240 per annum for a Class 'B' vaid/hakim. In addition to the subsidy such a practitioner would get Rs. 180 and Rs. 120 per annum respectively on account of the cost of medicines for free distribution. One-fourth of such subsidy under both categories was to be payable by or through the controlling authority.
6. Dispensaries or vaids or hakims working under this scheme were open to regular inspection by members and officers of the Board of Indian Medicine, United Provinces; the gazetted district staff; the member of the United Provinces Legislature (both Houses) and other authorised persons residing in the district.
7. Proper accounts of income and expenditure of the dispensaries and reports on the working of such dispensaries and the subsidised medical practitioners were to be submitted to the Chairman of the Board of Indian Medicine, United Provinces, Lucknow by June 1, of every year.
8. An application for a grant-in-aid under this scheme could be made at anytime by the District Boards or interested bodies or individuals through the Chairman of the Board of Indian Medicine, United Provinces.
9. The government reserved for itself the right to withdraw the subsidy anytime on account of failure to carry out the main object of this scheme or to render accounts punctually and correctly, or for misuse of funds, or of any other defect.
10. The allotment available for this scheme during the current year (1938–39) was set at Rs. 37,500.

Appendix 3

District-wise List of 'Genuine' Ayurvedic and Unani Pharmacies Drawn by the Board of Indian Medicine, United Provinces[3]

S. No.	Name of District	Ayurvedic Pharmacy	Unani Pharmacy
1.	Saharanpur	i. Rishikul Ayurvedic College Pharmacy, Haridwar ii. Gurukul Kangri Pharmacy, Haridwar iii. Kumaun Ayurvedic Pharmacy, Kankhal	–
2.	Dehradun	–	–
3.	Muzaffarnagar	–	–
4.	Meerut	–	Shifai Dawakhana, Karim Ali Street
5.	Bulandshahr	–	–
6.	Agra	Bhartiya Dawakhana, Rawatpara	(selling both Ayurvedic and Unani medicines)
7.	Muttra (that is, Mathura)	i. Gurukul Pharmacy, Brindaban ii. Sukh Sancharak Company	–
8.	Mainpuri	–	–
9.	Etah	–	–
10.	Aligarh	–	–
11.	Jhansi	Bundelkhand Ayurvedic College Pharmacy	–

S. No.	Name of District	Ayurvedic Pharmacy	Unani Pharmacy
12.	Jalaun	–	–
13.	Hamirpur	–	–
14.	Banda	–	–
15.	Allahabad	Sewa Samiti Pharmacy	Unani Dawakhana
16.	Cawnpore	i. Chand Aushadhalaya ii. Ayurvedic College and Pharmacy Works, Nayaganj	–
17.	Fatehpur	–	–
18.	Farrukhabad	–	–
19.	Etawah	–	–
20.	Bareilly	–	–
21.	Bijnor	–	–
22.	Badaun	–	Dawakhana Ashrarul Shafa
23.	Moradabad	–	–
24.	Shahjahanpur	Saraswati Aushadhalaya	–
25.	Pilibhit	i. Lalit Hari Ayurvedic College Pharmacy ii. Dinbandhu Aushadhalaya	–
26.	Garhwal	–	–
27.	Almora	–	–
28.	Nainital	–	–
29.	Mirzapur	–	–
30.	Jaunpur	–	–
31.	Ghazipur	–	–
32.	Ballia	i. Pratap Datavya Aushadhalaya, Kutchery Road ii. Shri Maheshwari Aushadhalaya	–
33.	Gorakhpur	–	–
34.	Basti	–	–

S. No.	Name of District	Ayurvedic Pharmacy	Unani Pharmacy
35.	Azamgarh	–	–
36.	Benares	i. Ayurvedic Pharmacy, BHU ii. Ayurvedic Pharmacy, Kashi Rasayanshala, Gyanvapi	–
37.	Unnao	Swatantra Aushadhalaya, Sadr Bazar	–
38.	Sitapur	Ayurvedic Pharmacy, Jail Road	–
39.	Hardoi	–	–
40.	Kheri	–	–
41.	Rae Bareli	–	–
42.	Lucknow	i. Mool Chand Rastogi Trust Aushadhalaya ii. Swatantra Aushadhalaya iii. Ayurveda Bhaskar Aushadhalaya	i. Unani Takmil-uttila Pharmacy ii. Desi Dawakhana, Cantonment Road iii. Indian Dawakhana, Gwyne Road
43.	Fyzabad	–	–
44.	Gonda	–	–
45.	Sultanpur	–	–
46.	Pratabgarh	–	–
47.	Barabanki	–	–
48.	Bahraich	i. Mishra Bandhu Aushadhalaya ii. M.C. Sharma Vaidya & Sons	–

Appendix 4

Suggestions Made by Mool Chand Rastogi Trust Aushadhalaya[4]

1. Compiling of a common pharmacopoeia for the use of rural dispensaries be proposed with the specifications of the names of medicines as well as the name of books containing their preparations so as to avoid the confusion as medicines of similar names were prescribed by authors of various books, for the same as well as different diseases; and were, according to them, prepared in different manner.
2. Patent medicines of any of the approved firms should be rarely used in the government dispensaries as patenting of medicine gave undue advantage to some pharmacies.
3. The government should devise some machinery for checking the genuineness of the medicine supplied.
4. If the rates quoted by any firm were abnormally low, the District Medical Officer of Health before accepting such a tender should either call for samples of medicines by the firm concerned or ask the firm to assign reasons for such cheap rates. Also, when the medicines were actually supplied, they should be periodically tested to ensure that cheaper medicines were not substituted.

Appendix 5

List of Ayurvedic Journals being Published from Different Parts of the United Provinces[5]

S. No.	Ayurvedic Journal	Place	Starting Year	Editor/Proprietor
1.	Sudhanidhi	Prayag	1909	Jagannath Prasad Shukla
2.	Vanausadhi Prakash	Meerut	1913	Baburam Sharma
3.	Vaidya Sammelan Patrika (later renamed as Ayurveda Mahasammelan Patrika)	Prayag	1914	Mouthpiece journal of All India Vaidya Sammelan
4.	Chikitsak	Kanpur	1917	Kishori Dutt Shastri
5.	Vaidya	Moradabad	1917	Shankar Lal Gupt
6.	Ayurveda Pracharak	Kashi	1921	Shandilya Dwivedi
7.	Stri Chikitsak	Allahabad	1922	Yashoda Devi
8.	Illaj	Allahabad	1923	Girivar Sahay Saxena
9.	Anubhoot Yogmala	Etawah	1923	Visheshwar Dayalu
10.	Rakesh	Etawah	–	Rupendra Nath Shastri
11.	Arogya Sindhu	Etawah	–	Pandit Lakshmi Narayan
12.	Dhanvantari	Aligarh	1923	Devisharan Garg
13.	Ayurveda Keshari	Kanpur	1925	Rameshwar Mishra
14.	Swasthya Bandhu	Aligarh	1925	Ramchandra Sharma
15.	Ayurveda Samachar	Aligarh	1926	Bankelal Gupt
16.	Pranacharya	Kanpur	1928	Ram Narayan Shastri

S. No.	Ayurvedic Journal	Place	Starting Year	Editor/Proprietor
17.	Ratnakar	Etawah	1930	Vaidyaraj Chhote Lal Jain
18.	Vanausadhi Darpan	Haridwar	1934	Mangal Dutt Shukla
19.	Vanausadhi	Kashi	1934	Kedarnath Sharma
20.	Jeevan Shakti	Haridwar	1935	Shilajit Depot
21.	Swasthya	Mathura	1936	Jagannath Das
22.	Parivar Bandhu	Agra	1939	–
23.	Gharelu Chikitsa	Prayag	1940	Mahendranath Pandey
24.	Ayurveda Keshari	Lucknow	1940	Shivaram Dwivedi
25.	Ayurveda College Patrika	Benares	1942	Banaras Hindu University
26.	Vaidyaraj	Meerut	–	Pandit Narayan Dutt
27.	Banaspati Vigyan	Kanpur	–	–
28.	Grih Chikitsa	Mathura	–	–
29.	Ban Lakshmi	Aligarh	–	–
30.	Haridwar Samachar	Haridwar	–	Pandit Shiv Chandra

Appendix 6

Syllabus of the Paper on *Swasthavratta*[6]

Social and Preventive Medicine Syllabus

In the teaching of this subject stress should be laid on fundamental and basic principles of the Science and art of Social and Preventive medicine. Details are to be avoided as they are not required of a 'Basic Medical Man'. Throughout the whole period of study the attention of the student should be directed by the teachers of various branches of indigenous medicine to the importance of its preventive aspect. Emphasis should be laid more on practical training and inculcation of a preventive outlook rather than on didactic lectures. Social aspect of medicine together with its special importance in the administration of a welfare state should receive due attention. The students are to be trained with the purpose of providing qualified personnel trained in the art and science of promotion, preservation and restoration of health of all and to relieve human suffering, but not for providing so-called practitioners engaged in commercialised medicine. This new outlook in the teaching of medicine is required to be given utmost importance.

1. HEALTH – Definition and conception of health, Promotion of preservation of health as fundamental human right, Effect of heredity and environment on health, Inherited traits, Healthy environment.
2. PERSONAL HYGIENE – Cleanliness, clothing, sleep, rest, exercise, recreations, healthy habits, care of health in tropics, health consciousness.
3. VENTILATION, AIR CONDITIONING AND LIGHTING – Fresh air, vitiated air, air temperature, humidity and movement; Dust and

smoke; Natural and artificial ventilation; Comfort zones and air conditioning; Overcrowding, Tropical climate and its effect on health; Natural purification of air; Examination of ventilation condition; Air-borne diseases.

4. DWELLING AND WORK PLACES – Dwelling site, aspect, damp-proofing and rat-proofing; Residential houses, workshops, schools, hospitals, cinemas, hostels and restaurants, slaughter-houses, dairies, markets.
5. WATER SUPPLY – Sources, impurities, purification; Public water supplies; Physical, chemical and bacteriological characters of good water; Water-borne diseases.
6. FOOD AND NUTRITION – Food requirements, common food products; Inspection of food stuffs, adulteration, food storage, food deficiencies and nutritional disorders; Balanced diet; Nutritional survey; Food-borne diseases.
7. WASTES – Collection, removal and disposal of refuse, sullage and sewage, conservancy and water carriage systems; Utilisation of wastes, composting, sullage and sewage farms; Disposal of dead bodies.
8. CAMP AND RURAL SANITATION – Fairs, camps, medical and sanitary arrangements; Rural sanitation; Diseases due to insanitation.
9. PREVENTIVE MEDICINE – (a) Infection, resistance and immunity; Reservoirs of infection, Modes of transmission of infection and Portals of discharge and entry of infection; Cross infection collection and dispatch of samples to laboratories.

    (b) General principles of prevention and control of communicable diseases; Notification, recognition, segregation and isolation, quarantine, treatment of carriers, placarding, disinfection, disinfestations, immunisation, treatment of cases, specific chemotherapy; General, environmental and traffic sanitation, railways, trains, buses and other conveyances.

    (c) Epidemiology and prevention of common communicable disease of tropics with special reference to plague, cholera, small pox, malaria, kala-azar, filariasis, diphtheria, tuberculosis, typhus, rabies, leprosy, venereal diseases, helminthic infections, enteric fever and dysenteries; Animal disease transferable to man; Insect-borne diseases; Insect control (fly, mosquito, louse, fleas, ticks and sand fly).

10. VITAL STATISTICS – Population, registration, birth, death and other morbidity and mortality rates; Collection, compilation and tabulation of statistical data, common statistical errors.
11. PUBLIC HEALTH ORGANISATIONS – (a) Medical and Public Health Organisation in Centre and Uttar Pradesh, World Health Organisation
    NON-OFFICIAL ORGANISATIONS:
    (b) Maternity and Child Welfare.
    (c) School Health Work.
    (d) Industrial Health organisation, Occupational hazards, health safety and welfare of workers.
    (e) Health education.
    (f) Medical and Public Health Institutions and their administration, clinics, dispensaries, hospitals, sanatoria, health units.
    (g) Important Public Health Regulations.
    (h) Health Insurance and other welfare or social security measures.

Appendix 7

Lord Dhanvantari[7]
(Idol at the Lord Dhanvantari Temple, All India Ayurvedic Congress, Punjabi Bagh, New Delhi, 19 January 2015)

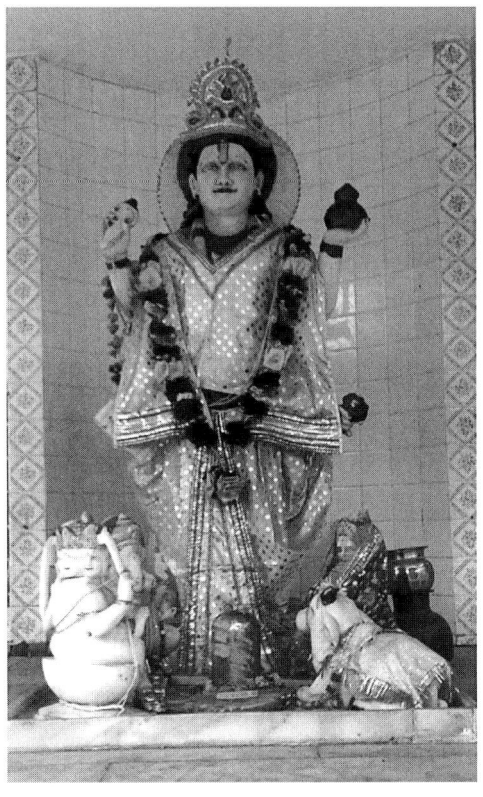

Appendix 8

Vaid Guru Prasad Tripathi[8]
(Lucknow, 14 April 2014)

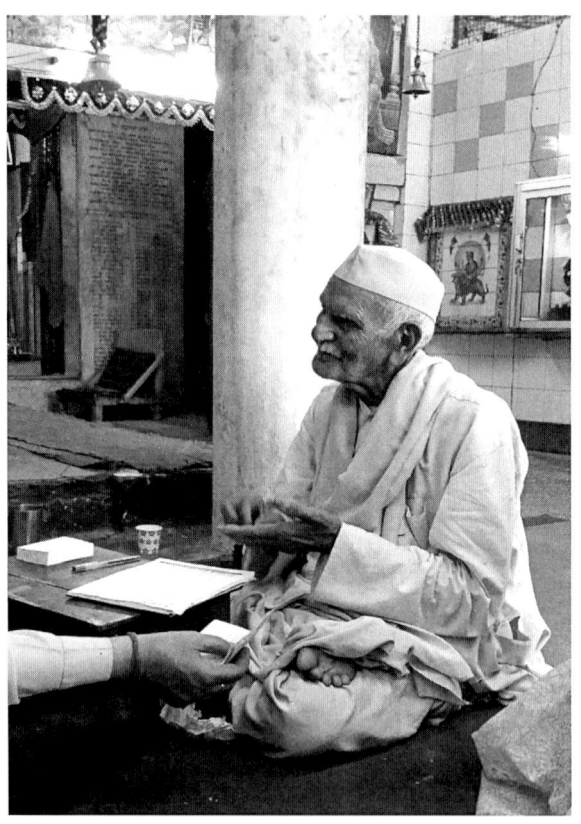

NOTES

1. 'Rules for the Admission of Patients to the European Hospital, Allahabad', F. No. 65, Box No. 31, 1919, Medical Department, UPSA.
2. 'Payment of Grants for Subsidised 'Dawakhanas' and 'Aushadhalayas' during 1939–40', F. No. 155, Box No. 82, 1938, Medical Department, UPSA.
3. 'List of Approved Ayurvedic and Unani Pharmacies in U.P.', F. No. 226, Box No. 83, 1938, Medical Department, UPSA.
4. 'List of Approved Ayurvedic and Unani Pharmacies in U.P.', F. No. 226, Box No. 83, 1938, Medical Department, UPSA.
5. Compiled by author.
6. 'Recommendations of the United Provinces Ayurvedic and Unani Systems Reorganisation Committee—Training in Public Health and Social Medicine', F. No. 19 RC, Box No. 31, 1949, Medical 'B' Department, UPSA.
7. Photograph by author.
8. Photograph by author.

Bibliography

PRIMARY SOURCES

Archival Materials

National Archives of India, New Delhi

Education, Health and Land Department, Health Proceedings
Home Department, Medical Proceedings
Home Department, Public Proceedings
Home Department, Sanitary Proceedings

Uttar Pradesh State Archives, Lucknow

Uttar Pradesh Government, Medical Department Proceedings
Uttar Pradesh Government, Sanitation Department Proceedings
Uttar Pradesh Government, Public Health Department Proceedings

Regional Archives, Allahabad

Commissioner's Office Records, Fyzabad
Commissioner's Office (Post-Mutiny Records), Allahabad

Government Reports and Official Publications

Report of the Health Survey and Development Committee. Vols 1 and 2. New Delhi: Government of India Press, 1946.

Report of the Committee on Indigenous Systems of Medicine, Vol. 1: Recommendations. New Delhi: Ministry of Health, Government of India, 1948.

Report and Recommendations of the United Provinces Ayurvedic and Unani Systems Reorganisation Committee. Allahabad: Health Department, Government of United Provinces, 1949.

Report of Udupa K. N. Committee on Ayurveda Research Evaluation. Delhi: The Times of India Press, 1958.
Speeches by Lord Curzon of Kedleston. Vol. 1. Calcutta: Office of the Superintendent of Government Printing, 1900.
The Gazetteer of India: History and Culture. Vol. 2. 6th ed. (first edition published in October 1973). New Delhi: Publications Division, 2003.
The Collected Works of Mahatma Gandhi (different volumes). 3rd revised ed. New Delhi: Publication Division, 2000.
Trivedi, Rekha, ed. *Smriti Ke Prishth: Swatantrata Senaniyon ke Sansmaranon par Aadharit.* Lucknow: UP State Archives, Department of Culture, 1998.

Hindi Tracts

Agarwal, Rishilal. *Manchahi Santan.* Allahabad, 1928.
Bhargava, Ayodhya Prasad. *Santati Shastra.* Benares City, 1923.
Chand, Rai Pooran. *Plague Darpan.* Patna City: Satya Sudhakar Press, 1916.
Devi, Yashoda. *Shishu Raksha Vidhan arthat Balrog Chikitsa.* Allahabad, 1912.
———. *Santan Palan.* Allahabad, 1913.
———. *Ghar ka Vaid.* Allahabad, 1914.
———. *Dampati Arogyata Jeevanshastra.* Allahabad, 1927.
———. *Dehati Chikitsa.* Allahabad, n.d.
Ghanekar, Ayurvedacharya Bhaskar Govind. *Auspargic Rog.* Benares, 1937.
Gupt, Babu Kedarnath. *Swasthya aur Jal Chikitsa.* Allahabad: Chhatra Hitkari Pustakmala, 1933.
Kedia, Baijnath. *Vyang Chitravali.* Calcutta and Benares: Hindi Pustak Academy, 1932.
Lal, Hazari. *Vaidyak Sar.* Benares, 1910.
Pade, Shankar Daji Shastri. *Gorasadi Aushadhi.* Allahabad: Sudhanidhi Granthavali, n.d.
Pandey, Mahendranath. *Hamare Bachche.* Prayag, 1931.
'Rajvaidya', Pandit Ramprasad Mishra. *Kuchimartantram.* 4th ed. (first published in 1925). Aligrah: Dhanvantari Press, 1965.
Sharma, Pandit Ganesh Dutt. *Dadru-Chikitsa.* 1st ed. Benares, 1932.
Sharma, Pandit Jagannath. *Arogya Darpan.* Vol. 3. Prayag, 1898.
———. *Santan Palan.* Benares, 1933.
Sharma, Pannalal. *Yuva-Rakshak.* Agra, 1908.
Shastri, Acharya Chandrashekhar. *Sharir Vigyan.* Delhi, 1937.
Shastri, Chatursen. *Brahmacharya Sadhan.* Lucknow: Ganga Granthagar, 1928.

Shrivastava, Jawahir Singh. *Vaidya Priya*. Lucknow: Naval Kishore Press, 1924.
Shukla, Jagannath Prasad. *Ayurveda ka Mahatva*. Prayag, 1937.
———. *Ayurvedic Patron ka Itihas*. 2nd ed. (first edition published in 1942). Prayag: Sudhanidhi Press, 1953.
Singh, Kaviraj Pratap, ed. *Nikhil Bharatvarshiya Ayurveda Mahamandal ka Rajat Jayanti Granth*. Vols 1 and 2. Benares: Mahashakti Press, 1935 and 1936.
Singh, Suryabali. *Brahmacharya ki Mahima*. Benares, 1931.
Thakur, Keshavkumar. *Grihastha Jeevan*. Prayag, 1932.
Vaidya, Babu Haridas. *Chikitsa Chandrodaya*. Agra, 1935.
Verma, Pravasi Lal, ed. *Arogya Mandir*. Benares: Mahashakti Sahitya Mandir, 1927.
Vyas, A. G. *Su-Santati Shastra*. Mathura, 1929.

Journals/Magazines/Newspapers (Select Issues)

Anubhoot Yogmala (Etawah)
Dhanvantari (Aligarh)
Saraswati (Benares)
Sudhanidhi (Allahabad)
The Gentleman's Magazine
Vaidya Sammelan Patrika (Prayag)

Novels/Stories

Bandyopadhyaya, Tarashankar. *Arogya Niketan*. 4th ed. Delhi: Rajpal & Sons, 1967.
Premchand. *Nirmala*. Benares: Saraswati Press, 1923.
———. *Godan: A Novel of Peasant India*, tr. Jai Ratan and P. Lal. 16th enlarged ed. Bombay: Jaico Publishing House, 2002.
———. 'Doodh ka Daam', in *Naya Mansarovar*, Vol. 8, ed. Kamal Kishore Goenka, 68–78. New Delhi: Sasta Sahitya Mandal Prakashan, 2017.
Renu, Phanishwar Nath. *Maila Anchal*. New Delhi: Rajkamal Paperbacks, 2013.
Shukla, Shrilal. *Raag Darbari*. New Delhi: Rajkamal Paperbacks, 2013.

Interviews

Vaid Guru Prasad Tripathi, Lucknow, India, 17 April 2014.
Ahsan Husain, Lucknow, India, 14 April 2014.

SECONDARY SOURCES

Alavi, Seema. 'Unani Medicine in the Nineteenth Century Public Sphere: Urdu Texts and the Oudh Akhbar'. *Indian Economic and Social History Review* 42, no. 1, 2005, 101–29.

———. *Islam and Healing: Loss and Recovery of an Indo-Muslim Medical Tradition, 1600–1900*. Ranikhet: Permanent Black, 2007.

All India Women's Conference. *All India Women's Conference: Annual Report*. Calcutta, 1934.

Alter, Joseph S. 'Celibacy, Sexuality and the Transformation of Gender into Nationalism in North India'. *The Journal of Asian Studies* 53, no. 1, February 1994, 45–66.

———. 'Somatic Nationalism: Indian Wrestling and Militant Hinduism'. *Modern Asian Studies* 28, no. 3, 1994, 557–88.

———. *Gandhi's Body: Sex, Diet, and the Politics of Nationalism*. Philadelphia: University of Pennsylvania Press, 2000.

Amrith, Sunil. 'Political Culture of Health in India: A Historical Perspective'. *Economic & Political Weekly* 42, no. 2, 2007, 114–21.

Anderson, Walter K., and S. D. Damle. *The Brotherhood in Saffron: The Rashtriya Swayamsevak Sangh and Hindu Revivalism*. Boulder: Westview Press, 1987.

Andrews, Charles F. *Mahatma Gandhi's Ideas*. London: Allen and Unwin, 1929.

Armus, Diego and Pablo F. Gómez, eds. *The Gray Zones of Medicine: Healers and History in Latin America*. Pittsburgh: University of Pittsburgh Press, 2021.

Arnold, David. 'Touching the Body: Perspectives on Indian Plague, 1896–1900'. In *Subaltern Studies V*, ed. Ranajit Guha, 55–90. Delhi: Oxford University Press, 1987.

———. *Imperial Medicine and Indigenous Societies*. Delhi: Oxford University Press, 1989.

———. *Colonising the Body: State Medicine and Epidemic Disease in Nineteenth-Century India*. Berkeley: University of California Press, 1993.

———. *The New Cambridge History of India III.5: Science, Technology and Medicine in Colonial India*. Cambridge: Cambridge University Press, 2000.

———. 'Plurality and Transition: Knowledge Systems in Nineteenth Century India'. Unpublished paper presented at The Princeton History of Science Seminar, October 2003. Available at http://www.princeton.edu/~hos/Workshop%20I%20papers/Arnold%20History%20of%20Science%20paper.htm (accessed on 23 May 2019).

———. *Everyday Technology: Machines and the Making of India's Modernity*. Chicago and London: University of Chicago Press, 2013.

Ashby, Philip H. *Modern Trends in Hinduism*. New York: Columbia University Press, 1974.

Attewell, Guy. *Refiguring Unani Tibb: Plural Healing in Late Colonial India*. Hyderabad: Orient Longman, 2007.

Bagchi, Amiya K. *Private Investment in India, 1900–39*. Cambridge: Cambridge University Press, 1972.

Bala, Poonam. 'State and Indigenous Medicine in Nineteenth and Twentieth Century Bengal: 1800–1947'. PhD diss., Department of Sociology, University of Edinburgh, 1987.

——. 'Medical Revivalism and the National Movement in British India'. *Ancient Science of Life* 10, no. 1, July 1990, 1–5.

——. *Imperialism and Medicine in Bengal: A Socio-Historical Perspective*. New Delhi: Sage Publications, 1991.

——. *Medicine and Medical Policies in India: Social and Historical Perspectives*. Lanham: Lexington Books, 2007.

Ballhatchet, K. *Race, Sex and Class under the Raj*. London: Weidenfeld & Nicholson, 1980.

Banerjee, Madhulika. *Power, Knowledge, Medicine: Ayurvedic Pharmaceuticals at Home and in the World*. Hyderabad: Orient Blackswan, 2009.

——. 'Ayurvedic Pharmaceuticals: Contesting Economic Hegemony'. In Poonam Bala, ed. *Contesting Colonial Authority: Medicine and Indigenous Responses in Nineteenth and Twentieth Century India*, 29–50. Lanham: Lexington Books, 2012.

Bayly, C. A. *Empire and Information: Intelligence Gathering and Social Communication in India, 1780–1870*. Cambridge: Cambridge University Press, 1996.

Berger, Rachel. 'Ayurveda and the Making of the Urban Middle Class in North India, 1900–1945'. In Dagmar Wujastyk and Frederick M. Smith, eds. *Modern and Global Ayurveda: Pluralism and Paradigms*, 101–16. Albany: State University of New York Press, 2008.

——. 'From the Biomoral to the Biopolitical: Ayurveda's Political History'. *South Asian History and Culture* 4, no. 1, 2013, 48–64.

——. 'Between Digestion and Desire: Genealogies of Food in Nationalist North India'. *Modern Asian Studies* 47, no. 5, September 2013, 1622–43.

——. *Ayurveda Made Modern: Political Histories of Indigenous Medicine in North India, 1900–1955*. Hampshire: Palgrave MacMillan, 2013.

Bhattacharya, Nandini. 'Between the Bazaar and the Bench: Making of the Drugs Trade in Colonial India, ca. 1900–1930'. *Bulletin of History of Medicine* 90, no. 1, Spring 2016, 61–91.

Bhattacharya, Sabyasachi. *Financial Foundations of the Raj: Ideas and Interests in the Reconstruction of Indian Public Finance 1858–1872*. Hyderabad: Orient Longman, 2005.

Bhishagratna, Kaviraj Kunjalal, tr. *Sushruta Samhita*. Calcutta: Self-published by the author-cum-translator, 1907.

Billington, M. F. *Woman in India*. First published, 1895, reprint. New Delhi: Amarko Book Agency, 1973.

Bode, Maarten. 'Indian Indigenous Pharmaceuticals: Tradition, Modernity and Nature'. In *Plural Medicine, Tradition and Modernity, 1800–2000*, ed. Waltraud Ernst, 184–203. London: Routledge, 2002.

———. *Taking Traditional Knowledge to the Market: The Modern Image of the Ayurvedic and Unani Industry, 1980–2000*. Hyderabad: Orient Longman, 2008.

Bourdieu, Pierre. *The Field of Cultural Production: Essays on Art and Literature*. Ed. & intro. Randal Johnson. Cambridge: Polity Press, 1993.

Brass, Paul. 'The Politics of Ayurvedic Education: A Case Study of Revivalism and Modernisation in India'. In Susanne Hoeber Rudolph and Lloyd I. Rudolph, eds, *Education and Politics in India: Studies in Organisation, Society, and Policy*, 342–74. Delhi: Oxford University Press, 1972.

Burke, Peter. *Eyewitnessing: The Uses of Images as Historical Evidence*. London: Reaktion Books, 2001.

Caplan, Pat. 'Celibacy as a Solution? Mahatma Gandhi and Brahmacharya'. In Pat Caplan, ed., *The Cultural Construction of Sexuality*, 271–95. London: Routledge, 1987.

Chakravarti, Uma. 'Whatever Happened to the Vedic Dasi? Orientalism, Nationalism and a Script for the Past'. In Sangari and Vaid, *Recasting Women*, 27–87.

Chandra, Bipan. *Communalism in Modern India*. New Delhi: Vikas Publishing House, 1984.

Chandra, Bipan, Mridula Mukherjee, Aditya Mukherjee, Sucheta Mahajan and K. N. Panikkar. *India's Struggle for Independence*. New Delhi: Penguin Books, 1989.

Chatterjee, Partha. *Nationalist and the Colonial World: A Derivative Discourse*. London: Zed Books, 1986.

———. 'Colonialism, Nationalism and Colonised Women: The Contest in India'. *American Ethnologist* 16, no. 4, 1989, 622–33.

———. 'The Nationalist Resolution of the Women's Question'. In Sangari and Vaid, *Recasting Women*, 233–53.

Chatterjee, Partha. *The Nation and Its Fragments: Colonial and Postcolonial Histories*. Princeton: Princeton University Press, 1993.

Chattopadhyaya, Debiprasad, ed. *Studies in the History of Science in India*. Vol 1. New Delhi: Editorial Enterprises, 1982.

Chopra, Col. Sir Ram Nath. 'Rationalisation of Medicine in India: Presidential Address'. *Everyman's Science* 43, no. 1, April–May 2008, 5–22.

Crawford, D. G. *A History of the Indian Medical Service, 1600–1913*. 2 vols. London: W. Thacker & Co., 1913–14.

———. *Roll of the Indian Medical Service, 1615–1930*. London: W. Thacker & Co., 1930.

Das, Sisir Kumar. *Western Impact—Indian Response: 1800–1910*. New Delhi: Sahitya Akademi, 1991.

Datta, P. K. *Carving Blocs: Communal Ideology in Early Twentieth Century Bengal*. Delhi: Oxford University Press, 1999.

Denoon, Donald. *Public Health in Papua New Guinea: Medical Possibility and Social Constraint, 1884–1984*. Cambridge: Cambridge University Press, 1989.

Douglas, Mary. *Purity and Danger: An Analysis of Concepts of Pollution and Taboo*. London: Routledge, 1966.

Dumont, Louis. *Homo Hierarchicus: The Caste System and Its Implications*. Tr. Mark Sanisbury, Louis Dumont and Basia Gulati. Chicago: University of Chicago Press, 1980.

Ernst, Waltraud, ed. *Plural Medicine, Tradition and Modernity, 1800–2000*. London: Routledge, 2002.

Financial Express. 2015. 'Ramdev Baba Drug 'Putrajeevak Beej' Promises Male Child'. 1 May. Available at https://www.financialexpress.com/industry/controversy-hits-ramdev-drug-promising-birth-of-male-child-hits-modis-beti-bachao-campaign/68323/ (accessed on 22 July 2019).

Forbes, Geraldine. 'Managing Midwifery in India'. In *Contesting Colonial Hegemony: State and Society in Africa and India*, eds Dagmar Engels and Shula Marks, 152–72. London: British Academy Press, 1994.

Foucault, Michel. *Madness and Civilisation: A History of Insanity in the Age of Reason*. London: Tavistock, 1961.

———. *The Archaeology of Knowledge*. London: Tavistock, 1969.

———. *The Birth of the Clinic: An Archaeology of Medical Perception*. New York: Pantheon Books, 1973.

———. *Society Must be Defended: Lectures at the College de France, 1975–76*. New York: Picador, 2003.

Foucault, Michel. 'The Crisis of Medicine or the Crisis of Antimedicine?' Tr. Edgar C. Knowlton Jr., William J. King and Clare O'Farrell. *Foucault Studies*, no. 1, December 2004, 5-19. Available at https://rauli.cbs.dk/index.php/foucaultstudies/article/view/562/607 (accessed on 2 July 2019).

———. *The Birth of Biopolitics: Lectures at the College de France, 1978-79*. New York: Picador, 2010.

Freitag, Sandria B. *Collective Action and Community: Public Arenas and the Emergence of Communalism in North India*. Berkeley: University of California Press, 1989.

Gandhi, M. K. *Hind Swaraj*. 17th reprint. Ahmedabad: Navjivan Publishing House, 2005.

———. *A Guide to Health*. Tr. A. Rama Iyer. Madras: S. Ganesan Publisher, 1921.

Ganesan, Uma. 'Medicine and Modernity: The Ayurvedic Revival Movement in India, 1885-1947'. *Studies on Asia* 4, 2001, 108-31.

Ghosh, Anindita. *Power in Print: Popular Publishing and the Politics of Language and Culture in a Colonial Society, 1778-1905*. New Delhi: Oxford University Press, 2006.

Girija, K. P. *Mapping the History of Ayurveda: Culture, Hegemony and the Rhetoric of Diversity*. London and New York: Routledge, 2022.

Guha, Supriya. 'From Dais to Doctors: The Medicalisation of Childbirth in Colonial India'. In *Understanding Women's Health Issues: A Reader*, ed. Lakshmi Lingam, 145-60. New Delhi: Kali for Women, 1998.

Gupt, Atridevji, tr. *Charaka Samhita*. Benares: Bhargava Pustakalaya, 1948.

Gupta, Brahmanand. 'Indigenous Medicine in Nineteenth and Twentieth Century Bengal'. In Charles Leslie, ed. *Asian Medical Systems: A Comparative Study*, 368-82. California: University of California Press, 1977.

Gupta, Charu. 'Dirty Hindi Literature: Contests about Obscenity in Late Colonial North India'. *South Asia Research* 20, no. 2, 2000, 89-118.

———. *Sexuality, Obscenity, Community: Women, Muslims, and the Hindu Public in Colonial India*. Delhi: Permanent Black, 2001.

———. 'Procreation and Pleasure: Writings of a Woman Ayurvedic Practitioner in Colonial North India'. *Studies in History* 21, no. 1, 2005, 17-44.

Hardiman, David. 'Indian Medical Indigeneity: From Nationalist Assertion to the Global Market'. *Social History* 34, no. 3, August 2009, 263-83.

Hardiman, David, and Projit Bihari Mukharji, eds. *Medical Marginality in South Asia: Situating Subaltern Therapeutics*. London and New York: Routledge, 2012.

Harrison, Mark. *Public Health in British India: Anglo-Indian Preventive Medicine, 1859-1914*. Cambridge: Cambridge University Press, 1994.

Haynes, Douglas E. 'Advertising and the History of South Asia, 1880-1950'. *History Compass* 30, no. 8, 2015, 361-74.

Haynes, Douglas E., and Gyan Prakash, eds. *Contesting Power: Resistance and Everyday Social Relations in South Asia*. Berkeley: University of California Press, 1992.

Hobsbawm, Eric. 'Introduction: Inventing Traditions'. In Hobsbawm and Ranger, *The Invention of Tradition*, 1-14.

Hobsbawm, Eric and Terrence Ranger, eds. *The Invention of Tradition*. Cambridge: Cambridge University Press, 1983.

Hohendahl, Peter Uwe. *Building a National Literature: The Case of Germany, 1830-1870*. Tr. Renate Baron Franciscono. Ithaca, NY: Cornell University Press, 1989.

Jaggi, O. P. *Medicine in Medieval India*. Delhi: Atma Ram, 1977.

Jeffery, Roger. 'Recognising India's Doctors: The Institutionalisation of Medical Dependency, 1918-39'. *Modern Asian Studies* 13, no. 2, 1979, 301-26.

Jha, D. N. *Early India: A Concise History*. New Delhi: Manohar Publishers, 2004.

Jha, Prasadilal. 'Achchi Daiyon ki Avashyakta'. *Stri Darpan* 29, no. 3, September 1923.

John, Rosselli. 'The Self-Image of Effeteness: Physical Education and Nationalism in Nineteenth Century Bengal'. *Past and Present* 86, 1980, 121-48.

Jones, Kenneth W. *The New Cambridge History of India Vol. III.1: Socio-Religious Reform Movements in British India*. Cambridge: Cambridge University Press, 1989.

Kaushik, Shubhneet. 'Planning for a Healthy Nation: Report of the Health Sub-Committee of National Planning Committee'. In Rahul Kumar Mohanta, ed., *Redefining India*, 116-27. Delhi: Kumud Publications, 2019.

Kavadi, Shirish N. 'Philanthropy, Medicine, and Health in Colonial India'. In Helaine Selin, ed., *Encyclopaedia of the History of Science, Technology, and Medicine in Non-Western Cultures*. Dordrecht: Springer, 2016.

Kothari, Mohan Lal. *Proceedings of Madhyabhartiya Vaidya Sammelan, Nagaud*. Shandilya Kuti, Kashi: Ayurveda Press, 1936.

Koselleck, Reinhart. *The Practice of Conceptual History*. California: Stanford University Press, 2002.

Kumar, Anil. *Medicine and the Raj: British Medical Policy, 1835-1911*. New Delhi: Sage Publications, 1998.

———. 'The Indian Drug Industry under the Raj, 1860-1920'. In Biswamoy Pati and Mark Harrison, eds. *Health, Medicine and Empire: Perspectives on Colonial India*, 356-85. New Delhi: Orient Longman, 2001.

Kumar, Deepak. 'Medical Encounters in British India, 1820-1920'. *Economic & Political Weekly* 32, no. 4, 25-31 January, 1997, 166-70.

Kumar, Shankar. 'Ancient Indian Medicine in the Work of Charaka, Sushruta and Vagbhata—A Textual and Historical Study'. PhD diss., Department of History, University of Delhi, 2013.

Lambert, Helen. 'Wrestling with Tradition: Towards a Subaltern Therapeutics of Bonesetting and Vessel Treatment in North India'. In David Hardiman and Projit Bihari Mukharji, eds. *Medical Marginality in South Asia: Situating Subaltern Therapeutics*, 109-25. London and New York: Routledge, 2012.

Langford, Jean M. *Fluent Bodies: Ayurvedic Remedies for Postcolonial Imbalance*. Durham: Duke University Press, 2002.

'Letter from Ahmed Husain to Muhammad Ali Jinnah (dated August 28, 1944)'. In *Quaid-e-Azam Mohammad Ali Jinnah Papers*. Vol. 11. Islamabad: National Archives of Pakistan, 2005. Available at http://thepartitionofindia.blogspot.in/2012/07/unani-medicine.html (accessed on 16 July 2019).

Leslie, Charles. 'The Professionalising Ideology of Medical Revivalism'. In Milton Singer, ed., *Modernisation of Occupational Cultures in South Asia*, 691-708. Durham: Duke University Press, 1973.

———. 'The Modernisation of Asian Medical Systems'. In John Poggie and R. Lynch, eds, *Rethinking Modernisation: Anthropological Perspectives*, 377-94. Westport: Greenwood Press, 1974.

———. 'The Ambiguities of Medical Revivalism in Modern India'. In Leslie, *Asian Medical Systems*, 356-67.

———, ed. *Asian Medical Systems: A Comparative Study*. Berkeley: University of California Press, 1976.

Liebeskind, Claudia. 'Arguing Science: Unani Tibb, Hakims and Biomedicine in India, 1900-50'. In Waltraud Ernst, ed., *Plural Medicine, Tradition and Modernity, 1800-2000*, 58-75. London: Routledge, 2002.

Lyotard, Jean Francois. *The Postmodern Condition: A Report on Knowledge*. Tr. Geoffrey Bennington and Brian Massumi. Minneapolis: University of Minnesota Press, 1984.

Macleod, Roy. 'Introduction'. In Roy and Lewis, *Disease, Medicine and Empire*, 1-18.

Macleod, Roy and Milton Lewis, eds. *Disease, Medicine and Empire: Perspectives on Western Medicine and the Experience of European Expansion*. London: Routledge, 1988.

Majumdar, R. C. 'Medicine'. In D. M. Bose, S. N. Sen and B. V. Subbarayappa, eds, *A Concise History of Science in India*, 213-68. New Delhi: Indian National Science Academy, 1971.

Majumdar, Susmita Basu. 'Medical Practitioners and Medical Institutions: Gleanings from Epigraphs'. *Proceedings of the Indian History Congress*, 69th Session, Kannur, 2008, 196–210.

Malhotra, Anshu. *Gender, Caste, and Religious Identities: Restructuring Caste in Colonial Punjab*. New Delhi: Oxford University Press, 2002.

———. 'Of Dais and Midwives: 'Middle Class' Interventions in the Management of Women's Reproductive Health in Colonial Punjab'. In Sarah Hodges, ed., *Reproductive Health in India: History, Politics, Controversies*, 199–226. Delhi: Orient Longman, 2006.

Manderson, Lenore. *Sickness and the State: Health and Illness in Colonial Malaya, 1870–1940*. Cambridge: Cambridge University Press, 1996.

Mani, Lata. 'Contentious Traditions: The Debate on Sati in Colonial India'. *Cultural Critique* 7, 1987, 119–56.

Mayo, Katherine. *Mother India*. New York: Blue Ribbon Books, 1927.

Menon, Indudharan. *Hereditary Physicians of Kerala: Traditional Medicine and Ayurveda in Modern India*. Oxon and New York: Routledge, 2019.

Metcalf, Barabara D. 'Nationalist Muslims in British India: The Case of Hakim Ajmal Khan'. *Modern Asian Studies* 19, no. 1, 1985, 1–28.

Mill, James. *The History of British India*. London: Baldwin, Cradock and Joy, 1817.

Mukharji, Projit Bihari. *Doctoring Traditions: Ayurveda, Small Technologies and Braided Sciences*. Chicago: University of Chicago Press, 2016.

———. *Nationalising the Body: The Medical Market, Print and Daktari Medicine*. London: Anthem Press, 2009.

Mukherjee, Girindranath. *History of Indian Medicine, Vol. 3*. New Delhi: Munshiram Manoharlal Publications Pvt. Ltd., 2003.

Mukherjee, Sujata. 'Ayurvedic Medicine in Colonial Bengal: Challenge and Response'. In Syed Ejaz Hussain and Mohit Saha, eds, *India's Indigenous Medical Systems: A Cross-Disciplinary Approach*, 100–13. New Delhi: Primus, 2015.

Murlidhar, Paliwal, and Byadgi P.S. 'Charaka—The Great Legendary and Visionary of Ayurveda'. *International Journal of Research in Ayurveda and Pharmacy* 2, no. 4, 2011, 1011–15. Available at http://www.ijrap.net/admin/php/uploads/541_pdf.pdf (accessed on 9 July 2019).

Nanda, B. R., ed. *Selected Works of Govind Ballabh Pant*. Different volumes. Delhi: Oxford University Press, various years.

Nandy, Ashis. 'A Post-colonial View of the East and the West'. *Alternatives: Global, Local, Political* 8, no. 1, January 1982, 25–48.

Nehru, Jawaharlal. *The Discovery of India*. New Delhi: Penguin Books, 2004.

Neumayer, Erwin, and Christine Schelberger. *Popular Indian Art: Raja Ravi Verma and the Printed Gods of India*. New Delhi: Oxford University Press, 2003.

Nizami, Zafar Ahmad. *Hakim Ajmal Khan*. New Delhi: Publications Division, 1988.

Oldenburg, Veena. *The Making of Colonial Lucknow: 1856–77*. Princeton: Princeton University Press, 1984.

Orsini, Francesca. *The Hindi Public Sphere, 1920–1940: Language and Literature in the Age of Nationalism*. Oxford: Oxford University Press, 2002.

Oxford Advanced Learner's Dictionary. 6th ed. Oxford: Oxford University Press, 2000.

Panikkar, K. N. 'Indigenous Medicine and Cultural Hegemony: A Study of the Revitalisation Movement in Keralam'. *Studies in History* 8, no. 2, 1992, 283–308.

———. *Culture, Hegemony, Ideology: Intellectuals and Social Consciousness in Colonial India*. New Delhi: Tulika, 1995.

Pati, Biswamoy. 'Siting the Body: Perspectives on Health and Medicine in Colonial Orissa'. *Social Scientist* 26, nos 11–12, 1998, 3–26.

———. *Situating Social History: Orissa (1800–1997)*. New Delhi: Orient Longman, 2001.

———. 'Confining 'Lunatics': The Cuttack Asylum, c. 1864–1906'. In Pati and Harrison, *Society, Medicine and Politics*, 196–231.

Pati, Biswamoy, and Chandi P. Nanda. 'The Leprosy Patient and Society: Colonial Orissa, 1870–1940s'. In Pati and Harrison, *The Social History of Health and Medicine*, 113–28.

Pati, Biswamoy, and Mark Harrison, eds. *Health, Medicine and Empire: Perspectives on Colonial India*. New Delhi: Orient Longman, 2001.

———, eds. *The Social History of Health and Medicine in Colonial India*. London and New York: Routledge, 2009.

———. *Society, Medicine and Politics in Colonial India*. London and New York: Routledge, 2018.

Prakash, Gyan. *Another Reason: Science and Imagination of Modern India*. New Jersey: Princeton University Press, 1999.

Quaiser, Neshat. 'Politics, Culture and Colonialism: Unani's Debate with Doctory'. In Pati and Harrison, *Health, Medicine and Empire*, 317–55.

———. 'Tension, Placation, Complaint: Unani and Post-Colonial Medical Communalism'. In V. Sujatha and Leena Abraham, eds, *Medical Pluralism in Contemporary India*, 130–62. Hyderabad: Orient BlackSwan, 2012.

Rai, Alok. *Hindi Nationalism*. New Delhi: Orient Longman, 2001.

Rai, Saurav Kumar. 'Indianisation of the Indian Medical Service, *c.* 1890s–1930s'. *Proceedings of the Indian History Congress*, 75th Session, New Delhi, 2014, 826–32.

Raina, B. L. *Health Science in Ancient India*. New Delhi: Commonwealth Publishers, 1990.

Raje, Gauri. 'The Modernising Bhagat'. In David Hardiman and Projit Bihari Mukharji, eds. *Medical Marginality in South Asia: Situating Subaltern Therapeutics*, 152-70. London and New York: Routledge, 2012.

Ramesh, Randeep. 'TV Swami Offers a Cure for All Ills'. *The Guardian*, 14 June 2008, available at https://www.theguardian.com/world/2008/jun/14/india.television (accessed on 20 July 2023).

Roy, Pratap Chandra, tr. *The Mahabharata*. Calcutta: Bharata Press, 1884.

Saha, Ranjana. 'Infant Feeding: Child Marriage and 'Immature Maternity' in Colonial Bengal, 1890s–1920s'. *Proceedings of the Indian History Congress*, 75th Session, New Delhi, 2014, 708–15.

Sangari, Kumkum, and Sudesh Vaid, eds. *Recasting Women: Essays in Indian Colonial History*. New Brunswick: Rutgers University Press, 1990.

Saraswati, Gananath Sen. *Lectures of M. M. Gananath Sen Saraswati*. Varanasi: Chowkhambha Sanskrit Series Office, 2002.

Sarkar, Natasha. 'Fleas, Faith and Politics: Anatomy of an Indian Epidemic, 1890–1925'. PhD diss., Department of History, National University of Singapore, 2011.

Sarkar, Sumit. *Modern India: 1885–1947*. Delhi: Macmillan, 1983.

———. *Modern Times: India, 1880s–1950s*. Ranikhet: Permanent Black, 2015.

Sehrawat, Samiksha. *Colonial Medical Care in North India: Gender, State and Society, c. 1840-1920*. New Delhi: Oxford University Press, 2013.

Shah, K. T. *National Health: Report of the Sub-Committee of National Planning Series*. Bombay: Vora & Co. Publishers Ltd., 1948.

Shah, Shalini. 'Representation of Female Sexuality in the Ayurvedic Discourse of the Early Medieval Period'. *Studies in History* 22, no. 1, 2006, 45–58.

Sharma, Madhuri. 'Creating a Consumer: Exploring Medical Advertisements in Colonial India'. In Pati and Harrison, *The Social History of Health and Medicine*, 213–28.

———. *Indigenous and Western Medicine in Colonial India*. Delhi: Foundation Books, 2012.

———. 'Knowing Health and Medicine: A Case Study of Benares, *c.* 1900–1950'. In *Medical Encounters in British India*, eds Deepak Kumar and Raj Sekhar Basu, 160–86. Delhi: Oxford University Press, 2013.

Sharma, P. V. *History of Medicine in India: From Antiquity to 1000 A.D.* New Delhi: Indian National Science Academy, 1992.

Sharma, R. S. *India's Ancient Past*. Delhi: Oxford University Press, 2005.

Shastri, Hari Prasad, tr. *The Ramayana of Valmiki*. Vol. 1. London: Shanti Sadan, 1952.

Shrivastava, A. K., ed. *Akhil Bhartiya Ayurveda Mahasammelan ka Shatabdi Granth*. Delhi: All India Ayurvedic Congress, 2009.

Singh, Harkishan. 'Ram Nath Chopra (1882–1971)—A Visionary in Pharmaceutical Science'. *Indian Journal of History of Science* 43, no. 2, 2008, 231–64.

Sinha, Mrinalini. *Colonial Masculinity: The 'Manly Englishman' and the 'Effeminate Bengali' in the Late Nineteenth Century*. Manchester: Manchester University Press, 1995.

Sivaramakrishnan, Kavita. 'The Use of Past in a Public Campaign: Ayurvedic *Prachar* in the Writings of Bhai Mohan Singh Vaid'. In *Invoking the Past: The Uses of History in South Asia*, ed. Daud Ali, 178–91. New Delhi: Oxford University Press, 1999.

———. *Old Potions, New Bottles: Recasting Indigenous Medicine in Colonial Punjab, 1850–1945*. New Delhi: Orient Longman, 2006.

Snow, C. P. *The Two Cultures and Scientific Revolution*. New York: Cambridge University Press, 1959.

Stark, Ulrike. *An Empire of Books: The Naval Kishore Press and the Diffusion of the Printed Word in Colonial India*. Ranikhet: Permanent Black, 2008.

Tharu, Susie. 'Tracing Savitri's Pedigree: Victorian Racism and the Image of Women in Indo-Anglican Literature'. In Sangari and Vaid, *Recasting Women*, 254–68.

The Imperial Gazetteer of India, Vol. 24, New edition, published under the authority of His Majesty's Secretary of State for India in Council. Oxford: Clarendon Press, 1907–09.

Todorov, Tzvetan. *The Conquest of America: The Question of Other*. New York: Harper Perennial, 1992.

Tonnesson, Stein, and Hans Antlov, eds. *Asian Forms of the Nation*. London: Curzon, 1996.

Tripathi, Brahmanand. *Ashtang Hridayam of Srimad Vagbhata*. Delhi: Chaukhamba Sanskrit Pratisthan, 2014.

Wallerstein, Immanuel. 'The Heritage of Sociology: The Promise of Social Sciences'. *Current Sociology* 47, no. 1, 1999, 1–37.

White, Hayden. *Metahistory: The Historical Imagination in Nineteenth Century Europe*. Baltimore: Johns Hopkins University Press, 1973.

Wujastyk, Dagmar. 'The Evolution of Indian Government Policy on Ayurveda in the Twentieth Century'. In Wujastyk and Smith, *Modern and Global Ayurveda*, 43–76.

Wujastyk, Dagmar, and Frederick M. Smith, eds. *Modern and Global Ayurveda: Pluralism and Paradigms*. New York: State University of New York Press, 2008.

Zimmerman, Francis. *The Jungle and the Aroma of Meats*. Delhi: Motilal Banarsidas, 1999.

Zysk, Kenneth G. *Ascetism and Healing in Ancient India: Medicine in the Buddhist Monastery*. New York and Oxford: Oxford University Press, 1991.

INDEX

Acharya, Yadavji Trikamji, 86, 100n11, 162
adulteration, 163–64, 224, 237
Agra, 27, 31, 75–76, 85, 152, 230, 235
Alexander, 89
Allahabad, 26, 29, 50, 69, 84–85, 93, 115–16, 118, 121, 153, 158, 231, 234
    Ayurvedokt Aushadhalaya, 110, 172, 175
    European Civil Hospital, 31, 227
    Stri Aushadhalaya, 74, 164–65
    Stri Shiksha Pustakalaya, 84–85, 153
    Sudhanidhi Pharmacy, 74, 164
    Sudhanidhi Press, 85, 153
    Unani Dawakhana, 74, 231
    Unani Medical School, 73
All India Ayurvedic and Unani Tibbi Conference, 32–34, 60–61, 79n6, 92, 103n33, 113
All India Muslim League, 32, 60, 209
All India Unani Tibbi Conference, 34
All India Vaidya Sammelan, 9, 16, 33–34, 39, 84–99, 109, 112–14, 116, 118, 162, 196, 198, 208
All India Women's Conference, 133
Anderson, Benedict, 160
Anjuman-i-Jarrahan, 199

Anjuman-i-Tibia, 34
antur ghar, 133–34, 146n106
aphrodisiac, 149, 176–81, 183, 224
Arya Vaidyasala, Kottakal, 42, 165–66
Aryan heritage, 14, 113
Ashvins, 7
Association of Surgeons, 66
Atharvaveda, 7, 10, 12, 14, 107
Aurangzeb, 89, 116
aushadhalayas, 69–73, 228
Ayurvedic and Unani Tibbia College, 32, 61, 63, 74
Ayurvedic anthem, 44–45
Ayurvedic drug market, 6, 16, 137, 149, 151, 161–70, 183, 223–24
    over-the-counter sale, 169
Ayurvedic flag, 44–45
Ayurveda Mahamandal, 103n39
Ayurvedic medical stores, 85, 162, 164, 169–70
Ayurvedic print market, 6, 16, 150–60, 223
Ayurvedic Vidyapith, 93
AYUSH, 12, 20n26, 21n41
Aziz, Abd al, 34

Bahraich, 206, 232
Bajpayee, A.P., 204–05
Banaras Hindu University, 114, 235

Ayurvedic College, xxiii, 42, 73, 126
Ayurvedic Pharmacy, 74, 164–65, 232
Kayachikitsa Department, 20n26
Bandyopadhyaya, Tarashankar, 170
barber, 93, 107, 129, 140n15
Benares, 42, 73–74, 85, 125, 165, 206, 232, 235
Mahashakti Aushadhalya, 74, 172–73, 177
Mahashakti Sahitya Mandir, 85, 153
Bengal Chemicals and Pharmaceutical Works, 162, 165
bhagats, 56n63, 110–11
Bharadvaja, 7–8
Bhore, Joseph William, 194, 212n11
Bhore Committee Report, 134, 147n115, 191–97, 202
Bielby, Elizabeth, 130
Billington, Mary Frances, 131
biopolitics, 78, 191–93, 196, 202–04, 206, 211n4
Board of Indian Medicine, 39, 48–49, 58n77, 72–75, 77–78, 94, 198–200, 203, 228–30
Bogus medical institutions, 36–37
Bombay, 68, 110, 164–65
Legislative Council, 38
Medical Registration Bill, 38
Medical Practitioners Act, 194
Bomford, G., 48
Bose, Subhash Chandra, 67
Bourdieu, Pierre, 159–60
Brahma, Lord, 7
brahmacharya (celibacy), 3, 16, 46, 107, 116, 119, 121–29, 181
brahmanisation, 110, 117

Brahmin, 2, 43, 109–10, 175
breastfeeding, 110, 139n11
Buddhism, 11, 89
Burman, S.K., 166

Calcutta, 42, 112, 114, 164–66
Ashtanga Ayurveda Vidyalaya, 63–64
C.K. Sen & Company, 42, 164
European General Hospital, 31
Central Provinces, 68, 94
Chand, Rai Pooran, 109, 118, 138n6
Charaka, 8, 10–11, 13, 86, 137
Samhita, 5, 7–8, 10–12, 13, 86, 113, 136
Chhangani, Govardhan Sharma, 97
child birth, 130–34, 199
child care, 109, 119–20, 130, 132
child marriage, 125
cholera, 77, 139n6, 237
Chopra, Ram Nath, 194, 197, 213n22
Chopra Committee Report, 191, 194–97, 202, 205
Civil Disobedience Movement, 67–68
civil surgeon, 28–29, 94, 205, 210
civilising mission, 130, 146 n 96
coachman, 127
colonialism, 3, 6, 24, 26, 28, 46, 129, 151, 161–62, 178, 190, 223
commercialisation, 6, 151
communalisation,14, 33, 70, 72, 112–17, 123, 208
conquistadors, 26
constipation, 125, 139n6
consumer, 42, 149, 159, 166, 170–72, 174–75, 178, 183–84
Cowasjee, 111
cow protection, 92, 114–15
Cox, C.L., 30–31

Curzon, Lord, 221

Dabur, 164, 166, 183
dai, 43, 46, 110–11, 127, 129–35, 199, 214n40
dawakhanas, 69–73, 228
delerium tremens, 29
Delhi, 32, 34, 38, 49, 61, 63, 74, 112
   Hindustani Dawakhana, 74
   Madrasa-i-Tibbia, 38
democracy, 9
deputy director (Ayurveda), 197, 200, 204–07, 210
dermatophytosis/ringworm, 107–08, 177
Devi, Yashoda, 84–85, 100n15, 115, 118–21, 125, 127, 142n51, 153, 155–56, 158, 160, 165, 182, 234
dhai, 43, 109, 135
Dhanvantari, Lord, 8, 9, 91, 95–98, 117, 239
Dhanvantari (journal), 84, 98, 99n1, 121, 163, 178, 234
Dhanvantari Aushadhalaya, 164–65, 167–68, 174, 178
Dhanvantari Divas, 9
Dhanvantari Mahotsava, 16, 84, 95–98, 117
dispensaries, 28–30, 47, 49–50, 66, 69–72, 76–77, 84, 151, 207–08, 210, 228–29, 233, 238
divine origin of Ayurveda, 8, 9, 20n25–26, 101n20
Divodasa, 8, 95
Drain of Wealth, 44, 172
Dufferin, Lady Harriet, 130
   Countess of Dufferin's Fund, 130, 132, 221
dying Hindu race, 92, 114

Enlightenment, 35
epidemics, 25–26, 109, 139n6
Epidemic Diseases Act, 26
Etawah, 87, 231, 234–35

Fergusson, J.C., 48
fisherman, 127
folk healers, 41, 73, 93, 198–201
Fyzabad, 28, 232

Galen, 13
Gandhi, Mahatma, 15, 59–60, 62–66, 68, 122, 209, 222
Ganges, 110, 175
gardener, 93, 127
Ghazni, Mahmud, 89
Ghori, Muhammad, 89, 116
Government of India Act, 1935, 59, 67–68
governor-general in council, 28
Gupt, Maithilisharan, 151–52
Guptas, 89
gynaecology, 193

Haffkine, W.M., 139n6
Hanuman, 126
Hardoi, 50, 70, 96, 232
Haridwar, 131, 162, 165, 209, 235
   Gurukul Kangri Pharmacy, 75, 165, 230
   Rishikul Ayurvedic College, 73–74, 77, 209, 230
hereditary vaids, 37–39, 41, 83
Himalaya (mountain), 7, 65, 89
Himalaya (pharmacy), 183
Hindi Sahitya Sammelan, 113
Hindu Mahasabha, 113
Hindu Sabhas, 112
Homeopathy, 36, 156

homosexuality, 116, 124–27, 129
Huns, 89
Husain, Ahmed, 208

ilm, 33
independence, xxiii, xxvii, 17, 46, 65, 126, 179, 190–91, 198, 210, 222
  post–independence, 191, 193, 197, 203–04, 208
Indianisation, 1, 60
Indian Medical Service (IMS), 1, 17n1, 24–25, 28, 48–49, 78n3
Indian National Congress, 1, 15, 32, 59–60, 65, 67–69, 72–73, 76, 113, 192
  ministry, 50, 66–69, 77–78, 78n3, 219n78
Indra, Lord, 7, 89
insane, 207, 218n76
institutionalisation, 4, 9, 16, 32, 35–36, 84, 93, 222
International Congress on Traditional Asian Medicine (ICTAM), 20n25–26
Irving, J., 29

Jain, Prakashvati Devi, 120, 142n52
Jarrahs, 199–200, 214n39
  Anjuman–i–Jarrahan, 199
Jhansi, 165, 216n50, 230
  G.A. Mishra Ayurvedic Pharmacy, 175–76
Jinnah, Muhammad Ali, 208
Julahas, 117

Kanishka, 11
Kanpur, 26, 84, 109, 118, 165, 199–200, 234–35
Kapoor, S.C., 209, 219n82

Kaur, Bibi Mahindra, 134
Khan, Chengiz, 116
Khan, Hakim Abdul Majeed, 61
Khan, Hakim Ajmal, 15, 32–34, 59–62, 65, 92, 208
Kid Mantra, 90, 102n29
Kipling, Rudyard, 221, 224n3
Kirtikar, Ranchhor Das, 88
kobiraj, 5, 174
kohals, 199–200, 214n38
  Kohal Netra Vaidya Sabha, 199–200, 216n49
Kshatriya, 109–10
ksheer-sagar, 8, 95
Kulkarni, D.A., 200, 203–07
Kushana, 11

Lal, Dr Panna, 77
lawyers, 94
Leper Asylum, 206–07
  Aman Sabha Leper Asylum, 206
leprosy, 107, 206–07, 237
Lucknow, xxiii, 31, 34, 60–61, 71, 85, 125, 165, 210, 232, 235, 240
  Ganga Granthagar, 85, 153–54
  Indian Dawakhana, 74
  Lucknow Family of Abd al Aziz, 34
  Mool Chand Rastogi Trust Aushadhalaya, 76–77, 232–33
  National Medical Store, 57n71
  Naval Kishore Press, 85, 152–54
  Unani Medical School, 73

Madras, 68, 165, 208
  Ayurvedic Pharmacy, 63
  Medical Gazette, 47
Mahabharata, 12, 95, 113
malaria, 3, 25, 62, 139n6, 237

Malviya, Madan Mohan, 42, 59, 225n9
Manusmriti, 12
Maratha, 111, 117
masturbation, 124–26
Mathura, 88, 165, 230, 235
Mayo, Katherine, 132
measles, 26
meat, 30, 137, 148n123
medical entrepreneurship, 42
medical gaze, 2, 17n5
medical modernity, 36
medical nationalism, 1
medical registration bill/acts, 38, 61
medical revivalism, xxiv, xxvii, 3, 4, 6, 35
Meerut, 206, 230, 234–35
Mhaskar, K.S., 93
middle class, 43–44, 50, 85, 106–07, 109, 120, 130–35, 138n5, 159, 172, 178–79
midwifery, 16, 39, 44, 46, 107, 111, 121–22, 129–36, 214n40
professionalisation of, 44, 46, 130–34
Mishra, Premvati, 27, 52n17
Montagu-Chelmsford/Montford reforms, 47, 49, 55n55, 71
Moradabad, 121, 231, 234
Mughals, 116
Muhammad, Prophet, 116
Muhammedan Educational Conference, 61
mulk, 34
Muslim vaids, 54n40
Mysore, 45, 86, 90, 111

Narayan, Jayprakash, 68

Nasik, 87–88, 112
nation, xxiv, 2–3, 34, 44, 46, 61, 109, 120, 122–23, 125, 132, 181, 191–94, 196, 204, 223
nation-state, 44, 191, 196
national healing system, 1, 44, 222
National Institute of Sciences of India, 11
National Medical Store, 57n71
national medicine, 15, 46, 57n71, 172
National Planning Committee, 192
nationalisation, 45
native, 1, 25–26, 29–30, 47, 67, 125, 196
nature cure, 65
nautch girls, 126
nectar, 8, 95, 105n58, 110, 115, 137, 175
Nehru, Brijlal, 64
Nehru, Jawaharlal, 11, 67–68, 192, 226n9
'new' vaids, xxiii–xxiv, 4, 9, 36–39, 41–43, 73, 83–84, 87, 93, 106, 136, 149, 151–52, 162, 183, 194
night-fall/wet dreams, 125–26
North Western Provinces and Oudh, 26, 29
N.N. Sen & Company, 42, 164

obstetrics, 193, 196
Orientalist, 11, 200
Orissa, 43, 68

Pade, Shankar Daji Shastri, 102n26, 112, 115
panacea/*Ramban Aushadhi*, 93, 149, 176–78, 183, 224
Pande, S.P., 204–07

Panini, 10
Panna, Maharani of, 130
Pant, Govind Ballabh, 15, 59–60, 65–68, 219n82
parliamentarianism, 9
Patanjali, 10
Patel, Vallabhbhai, 62, 68
Patiala, 36, 45
Patna, 90, 94
patriarchy, 2, 118, 134, 142n51
Pax Britannica, 90, 101n22
Pitamah, Bhishma, 126
plague, 3, 25, 77, 109, 139n6, 237
    anti–plague movement, xxvi, 2, 26
    plague riot, 26
postal guidance/assistance, 43, 166–67
postcolonial, 190–91, 194–96, 207, 210
potters, 110–11, 140n15
Prajapati, 7
Prasad, Rajendra, 68
Pratap, Maharana, 116
Premchand, 111–12, 135–36, 172–73
princes, 45, 132, 151, 159
print (public) culture, 85–87, 151, 153–54, 159–60
professionalisation, 4, 9, 35–36, 222
    of midwifery, 44, 46, 130–34
prostitute, 124–26
public health, 31, 48–49, 59, 70, 76–77, 91, 131, 152, 191, 194, 196–97, 199, 201–04, 209, 238
pulse, 5, 63, 67, 118, 120,
Punarvasu, Atreya, 8
Punjab, 129, 134
purdah, 3, 27, 118, 121, 221–22

qaum, 33–34
quacks, 198

quackery, 9, 31, 200
quinine, 62, 183

Raebareli, xxiii
Ramayana, 12, 95, 113
Rashtriya Swayamsevak Sangh, 113, 123, 209
Ray, P.C., 42, 166
Renaissance, 35
'Renu', Phanishwar Nath, 47
Report and Recommendations of the United Provinces Ayurvedic and Unani Systems Reorganisation Committee, 1949, xxvii, 17, 191, 198–207
rhinoplasty, 110–11
Rigveda, 11
Risley, H.H., 138n5

sale of agency, 166, 168
Sanatan Dharma Mahaparishad, 104n50, 112
Sankaran, 65
Saraswati, Swami Vishuddhananda, 209
sati, 130
scientificity, 9, 36, 97, 193, 224
Scythians, 89
semen, 124, 137, 178, 181
    preservation of, 125–26, 137
Sen, Gananath, 64, 86, 90, 100n13, 113, 116
Shah, S.P., 69
Sharma, Jagannath, 84–85, 117, 126
Sharma, Pandit Thakur Dutt, 91
Shastri, Chandrashekhar, 114, 141n32
Shastri, Chatursen, 127
Shastri, Kishori Dutt, 84, 131, 165, 234

Shastri, Madhusudan, 169
Shatpatha Brahmana, 11
Shivaji, 116
Shudra, 109–10
Shukla, Jagannath Prasad, 9, 33, 84, 88, 90, 94, 96, 102n26, 112, 160, 165, 234
Siddha, 32, 197
Singh, Kunwar Saryu Prasad Narayan, 94, 101n22, 104n41
Singh, Maharaja Ranjit, 116
Singh, Raghava Prasad Narayan, 140n21
Singhabhum, 2
Sinhji, Bhagvat, 45
Sitala, 2
Sitapur, 75, 167, 169, 232
smallpox, 2, 26, 51n10, 237
snake-bite, 43, 56n63, 110–11, 176–77
social medicine, 196, 201–03
Sokhey, Col. S.S., 192
Srinivasmurthy, G., 87
Staatsmedizin, 27
standardisation, 4, 9, 36, 41–42, 86, 89, 93–94, 161–64, 169, 222
stethoscope, 5, 222, 225 n 27
Stridharma Sikshak, 118–19
subaltern therapeutics, 198, 201
subaltern vaids/healers, 93, 94, 198, 201
Sultan, Tipu, 54n40, 111
Sushruta, 8, 10, 13, 86, 114, 137, 148n123
 Samhita, 7–8, 10–12, 86, 95, 110–11, 113, 136–37, 153
sutika griha, 133–34, 146n106
swadeshi, 2, 62, 166, 172, 222
 movement 187n41

swaraj, 160
swarajists, 68
Swasthavratta, 196, 202–04
 syllabus of, 236–38
syphilis, 25

Taimur, 116
testimonials, 90, 156, 167, 172–75
Text Book Committee, 86
thermometer, 5, 222
tonics, 149, 183, 224
tribal, 43, 110, 129, 132
tridosha,
 concept of, 147n122
Tripathi, Vaid Guru Prasad, xxiii–xxiv, xxvii n 2–5, 225n9, 240
Tripitakas, 11, 13
tropics, 25, 236–37
 tropical disease 24

'Ugra', Pandey Bechan Sharma, 125
Umballa, 30
 Station Hospital, 30
Unao, 50
United Provinces Indian Medicine Act, 39–40, 73, 199
United Provinces Vaidya Sammelan, 16, 39, 84–85, 88–89, 94, 96, 131
untouchable, 44, 129, 135–36, 140n13, 175
Uttarakhand, 65

vaccination, 2, 62, 81n61
Vagbhata Samhita, 113, 136–37, 143n57, 216n52
vaid-cum-editor, 84–85, 87–88
Vaidya, Vallabhram, 63, 65
Vaishya, 109–10
Varier, P.S., 42, 166, 187n41

Varshaneya, Govind Prasad, 121
vegetarianism/non-vegetarianism,
    129, 136–37
Vibhishana, 113
Victoria, Queen, 130, 134
Vikramaditya, 89
virile, 122, 127, 181
Vishnu, Lord, 9
vitaliser, 149, 183, 224

vivisection, 62, 79n10

washerman, 93, 107
White Man's Burden, 175, 221
widow, 44, 93, 124, 127, 130, 133

zamindar, 2, 94, 100n9, 132, 135,
    150–51, 159, 174
Zandu, 165–66, 183